Pediatric Emergency Medicine

Editors

LE N. LU
DALE WOOLRIDGE
ANN M. DIETRICH

EMERGENCY MEDICINE CLINICS OF NORTH AMERICA

www.emed.theclinics.com

Consulting Editor
AMAL MATTU

August 2013 • Volume 31 • Number 3

ELSEVIER

1600 John F. Kennedy Boulevard • Suite 1800 • Philadelphia, Pennsylvania, 19103-2899

http://www.theclinics.com

EMERGENCY MEDICINE CLINICS OF NORTH AMERICA Volume 31, Number 3
August 2013 ISSN 0733-8627, ISBN-13: 978-0-323-18602-5

Editor: Patrick Manley

Emergency Medicine Clinics of North America (ISSN 0733-8627) is published quarterly by Elsevier Inc., 360 Park Avenue South, New York, NY, 10010-1710. Months of issue are February, May, August, and November. Business and Editorial Offices: 1600 John F. Kennedy Boulevard, Suite 1800, Philadelphia, PA 19103-2899. Customer Service Office: 6277 Sea Harbor Drive, Orlando, FL 32887-4800. Periodicals postage paid at New York, NY, and additional mailing offices. Subscription prices are $149.00 per year (US students), $298.00 per year (US individuals), $507.00 per year (US institutions), $211.00 per year (international students), $428.00 per year (international individuals), $609.00 per year (international institutions), $211.00 per year (Canadian students), $368.00 per year (Canadian individuals), and $609.00 per year (Canadian institutions). International air speed delivery is included in all *Clinics'* subscription prices. All prices are subject to change without notice. **POSTMASTER:** Send address changes to *Emergency Medicine Clinics of North America*, Elsevier Periodicals Customer Service, 11830 Westline Industrial Drive, St. Louis, MO 63146. Customer Service (orders, claims, online, change of address): Elsevier Periodicals Customer Service, 11830 Westline Industrial Drive, St. Louis, MO 63146. Tel: 1-800-654-2452 (U.S. and Canada); 314-453-7041 (outside U.S. and Canada). Fax: 314-453-5170. E-mail: journalscustomerservice-usa@elsevier.com (for print support); journalsonline support-usa@elsevier.com (for online support).

Reprints. For copies of 100 or more of articles in this publication, please contact the Commercial Reprints Department, Elsevier Inc., 360 Park Avenue South, New York, NY 10010-1710. Tel.: 212-633-3812; Fax: 212-462-1935; E-mail: reprints@elsevier.com.

Emergency Medicine Clinics of North America is covered in *MEDLINE/PubMed (Index Medicus)*, *Current Contents/Clinical Medicine*, *EMBASE/Excerpta Medica*, *BIOSIS*, *SciSearch*, *CINAHL*, *ISI/BIOMED*, and *Research Alert*.

Printed and bound by CPI Group (UK) Ltd, Croydon, CR0 4YY

Transferred to digital print 2013

Contributors

CONSULTING EDITOR

AMAL MATTU, MD
Professor and Vice Chair, Department of Emergency Medicine, University of Maryland
School of Medicine, Baltimore, Maryland

EDITORS

LE N. LU, MD
Clinical Assistant Professor, Assistant Program Director, Director, Department of
Emergency Medicine, University of Maryland School of Medicine, Baltimore, Maryland

DALE WOOLRIDGE, MD, PhD
Associate Professor, Departments of Emergency Medicine and Pediatrics, University of
Arizona, Tucson, Arizona

ANN M. DIETRICH, MD
Nationwide Children's Hospital, Columbus, Ohio

AUTHORS

MANEESHA AGARWAL, MD
Fellow in Pediatric Emergency Medicine, Department of Emergency Medicine, Carolinas
Medical Center, Charlotte, North Carolina

ISABEL ARAUJO BARATA, MS, MD
Associate Professor of Pediatrics and Emergency Medicine, Hofstra North Shore-LIJ
School of Medicine; Director of Pediatric Emergency Medicine, North Shore University
Hospital, Manhasset, New York; Attending Physician, Steven and Alexandra Cohen
Children's Medical Center of NY, New Hyde Park, New York

ROSE CHASM, MD
Co-Director, Combined Emergency Medicine and Pediatrics Residency, Assistant Pro-
fessor, Department of Emergency Medicine, University of Maryland School of Medicine;
Director, Pediatric Quality Assurance and Risk Management, University of Maryland
Emergency Medicine Network, Baltimore, Maryland

MARLIE DULAURIER, MD, FAAP
Section of Emergency Medicine, Nationwide Children's Hospital; Assistant Professor of
Pediatrics, OSU College of Medicine, Columbus, Ohio

ANGELIQUE FERAYORNI, DO
Assistant Professor of Emergency Medicine, Department of Pediatrics and Emergency
Medicine, University of Arizona, Tucson, Arizona

SEAN M. FOX, MD
Associate Professor in Emergency Medicine, Department of Emergency Medicine, Carolinas Medical Center, Charlotte, North Carolina

PAUL ISHIMINE, MD
Associate Clinical Professor, Emergency Medicine, University of California, San Diego, UC San Diego health System; Associate Clinical Professor, Pediatrics, Fellowship Director, Pediatric Emergency Medicine, Rady Children's Hospital, University of California, San Diego, San Diego, California

CATHERINE JAMES, MD
Attending Physician, Pediatric Emergency Medicine, UMass Memorial Medical Center, Assistant Professor of Pediatrics, University of Massachusetts Medical School, Worcester, Massachusetts

MARY ELLA KENEFAKE, MD
Resident Physician, PGY5, Departments of Emergency Medicine and Pediatrics, Indiana University School of Medicine, Indianapolis, Indiana

SARAH KLINE-KRAMMES, MD
Attending Physician, Department of Emergency Medicine, Akron Children's Hospital, Akron, Ohio

MATTHEW B. LAURENS, MD, MPH
Assistant Professor of Pediatrics and Medicine, Pediatric Infectious Diseases and Tropical Pediatrics, Howard Hughes Medical Institute/Center for Vaccine Development, University of Maryland School of Medicine, Baltimore, Maryland

BEN LEESON, MD, RDMS, FACEP
Assistant Professor, Christus Spohn Emergency Medicine Residency, Texas A&M Health Science Center, Corpus Christi, Texas

KIMBERLY LEESON, MD, RDMS, FACEP
Assistant Professor, Christus Spohn Emergency Medicine Residency, Texas A&M Health Science Center, Corpus Christi, Texas

AARON N. LEETCH, MD
Assistant Professor, Departments of Emergency Medicine and Pediatrics, University of Arizona, Tucson, Arizona

PATRICK J. MALONEY, MD
Assistant Professor, Department of Emergency Medicine, University of Colorado School of Medicine, Denver Health Medical Center, Denver, Colorado

LAURA OLIVIERI, MD
Department of Emergency Medicine, University of Maryland Medical Center, Baltimore, Maryland

GARRETT S. PACHECO, MD
Department of Pediatrics and Emergency Medicine, University of Arizona, Tucson, Arizona

NIRALI H. PATEL, MD
Attending Physician, Department of Emergency Medicine, Akron Children's Hospital, Akron, Ohio

SHAWN ROBINSON, MD
Pediatric Emergency Medicine Fellow, Department of Emergency Medicine, Akron
Children's Hospital, Akron, Ohio

SEEMA SHAH, MD
Division of Emergency Medicine, Rady Children's Hospital, Associate Clinical Professor,
University of California San Diego, San Diego, California

MICHAEL J. STONER, MD, FAAP, FACEP
Section of Emergency Medicine, Nationwide Children's Hospital; Assistant Professor of
Pediatrics, OSU College of Medicine, Columbus, Ohio

MATTHEW SWARM, MD
Resident Physician, PGY2, Departments of Emergency Medicine and Pediatrics, Indiana
University School of Medicine, Indianapolis, Indiana

JENNIFER WALTHALL, MD
Associate Professor of Clinical Emergency Medicine and Pediatrics, Departments of
Emergency Medicine and Pediatrics, Indiana University School of Medicine, Indianapolis,
Indiana

ROBYN WING, MD
Chief Resident, Department of Pediatrics, Clinical Instructor of Pediatrics, University of
Massachusetts Medical School, Worcester, Massachusetts

DALE WOOLRIDGE, MD, PhD
Associate Professor, Departments of Emergency Medicine and Pediatrics, University of
Arizona, Tucson, Arizona

Contents

diagnose those who have life-threatening intracranial injuries or are victims of abusive head trauma. The goal of the emergency physician is to diagnose and treat the consequences of the primary injury and to limit or prevent secondary injury.

The diagnosis and management of pediatric cardiac emergencies can be challenging and complicated. Early presentations are usually the result of ductal-dependent lesions and appear with cyanosis and shock. Later presentations are the result of volume overload or pump failure and present with signs of congestive heart failure. Acquired diseases also present as congestive heart failure or arrhythmias.

Pediatric asthma is a disease that is managed across outpatient physicians, hospitalists, critical care physicians, and emergency department (ED) physicians. Scoring systems may facilitate a rapid assessment of the child with asthma in the ED. Short-acting beta agonists are still the mainstay of therapy for acute exacerbations along with corticosteroids and ipratropium bromide. ED providers must also know the indications for noninvasive ventilation and intubation. Most patients can be treated and discharged from the ED after acute exacerbation, and should be given a plan for going home that provides educational material and emergency scenarios to help prevent future acute incidents.

Seizures are a commonly encountered condition within the emergency department and, because of this, can engender complacency on the part of the physicians and staff. Unfortunately, there is significant associated morbidity and mortality with seizures, and they should never be regarded as routine. This point is particularly important with respect to seizures in pediatric patients. The aim of this review is to provide a current view of the various issues that make pediatric seizures unique and to help elucidate emergent evaluation and management strategies.

Despite many advances, the incidence of pediatric-onset diabetes and diabetic ketoacidosis (DKA) is increasing. Diabetes mellitus is 1 of the most common chronic pediatric illnesses and, along with DKA, is associated with significant cost and morbidity. DKA is a complicated metabolic state hallmarked by dehydration and electrolyte disturbances. Treatment involves fluid resuscitation with insulin and electrolyte replacement under constant monitoring for cerebral edema. When DKA is recognized and treated immediately, the prognosis is excellent. However, when a patient has prolonged or multiple courses of DKA or if DKA is complicated by cerebral edema, the results can be devastating.

The evaluation of the child with acute abdominal pain often poses as a diagnostic challenge due to the wide range of diagnoses. Surgical emergencies need to be rapidly identified and managed appropriately to minimize morbidity and mortality. Presenting symptoms, clinical examination, and laboratory findings can guide selection of diagnostic imaging. This article reviews common surgical causes of abdominal pain in children.

Otolaryngology (ear, nose, and throat) emergencies are a common complaint in the emergency department. These can present as a result of infection, trauma, foreign bodies, or postprocedure complications. The emergency department physician is called on to offer initial if not definitive management of these patients. This article discusses common ear, nose, and throat emergencies presenting to the emergency department.

Bedside ultrasound (US) was introduced to the emergency department more than 20 years ago. Since this time, many new applications have evolved to aid the emergency physician in diagnostic, procedural, and therapeutic interventions and the scope of bedside ultrasound continues to grow. Many US scanning techniques easily translate from adult applications to the pediatric population. Consequently, US has been adopted by many pediatric emergency providers. This article reviews the use of bedside ultrasound in pediatric emergency medicine.

Sedation and analgesia are vital components of pediatric emergency care. When children present to the emergency department injured, it may be difficult to administer care secondary to the child's anxiety, pain, lack of cooperation, and pressure by the parents to alleviate the child's discomfort. There is much in the emergency physician armamentarium to address these circumstances and provide excellent care, safely.

Child abuse presents commonly to emergency departments. Emergency providers are confronted with medical, social, and legal dilemmas with each case. A solid understanding of the definitions and risk factors of victims and perpetrators aids in identifying abuse cases. Forensic examination should be performed only after the child is medically stable. Emergency providers are mandatory reporters of a reasonable suspicion of abuse. The role of the emergency provider is to identify abuse, facilitate a thorough investigation, treat medical needs, protect the patient, provide an unbiased medical consultation to law enforcement, and to provide an ethical testimony if called to court.

Matthew B. Laurens

Antimicrobial prophylaxis prevents infection and/or complications of infection, and is a routine practice for defined procedures in the hospital. Emergency rooms and pediatric acute care facilities do not have automated procedures for antimicrobial prophylaxis in place. The responsibility thus falls on the physician caring for the child to appropriately prescribe antibiotics to prevent infection and complications of infection. Common indications for antimicrobial prophylaxis in the pediatric acute care setting include traumatic wounds, meningococcal exposures, pertussis exposures, and influenza exposures. For each of these indications, the assessment, management and disposition of pediatric patients are reviewed.

EMERGENCY MEDICINE
CLINICS OF NORTH AMERICA

PROGRAM OBJECTIVE

The goal of *Emergency Medicine Clinics of North America* is to keep practicing emergency medicine physicians and emergency medicine residents up to date with current clinical practice in emergency medicine by providing timely articles reviewing the state of the art in patient care.

TARGET AUDIENCE

All practicing physicians and healthcare professionals who provide patient care utilizing findings from *Emergency Medicine Clinics of North America*.

LEARNING OBJECTIVES

Upon completion of this activity, participants will be able to:

1. Review pediatric ENT emergencies; cardiac emergencies; and gastrointestinal emergencies.
2. Discuss pediatric procedural sedation and analgesia.
3. Recognize child abuse utilizing emergency department evaluation.

ACCREDITATION

The Elsevier Office of Continuing Medical Education (EOCME) is accredited by the Accreditation Council for Continuing Medical Education (ACCME) to provide continuing medical education for physicians.

The EOCME designates this enduringmaterial for a maximum of 15 *AMA PRA Category 1 Credit*(s) ™. Physicians should claim only the credit commensurate with the extent of their participation in the activity.

All other health care professionals requesting continuing education credit for this enduring material will be issued a certificate of participation.

DISCLOSURE OF CONFLICTS OF INTEREST

The EOCME assesses conflict of interest with its instructors, faculty, planners, and other individuals who are in a position to control the content of CME activities. All relevant conflicts of interest that are identified are thoroughly vetted by EOCME for fair balance, scientific objectivity, and patient care recommendations. EOCME is committed to providing its learners with CME activities that promote improvements or quality in healthcare and not a specific proprietary business or a commercial interest.

The planning committee, staff, authors and editors listed below have identified no financial relationships or relationships to products or devices they or their spouse/life partner have with commercial interest related to the content of this CME activity:

Maneesha Agarwal, MD; Isabelle Baratta, MD; Rose Chasm, MD; Marlie Dulaurier, MD; Angelique Ferayorni, MD; Sean Fox, MD; Paul Ishimine, MD; Catherine James, MD; Mary Ella Kenefake, MD; Sarah Kline-Krammes, MD; Indu Kumari; Matthew B. Laurens, MD, MPH; Sandy Lavery; Ben Leeson, MD; Kimberly Leeson, MD; Aaron Leetch, MD; Le N. Lu, MD; Patrick Maloney, MD; Patrick Manley; Amal Mattu, MD; Kristen McFarlane; Jill McNair; Laura Olivieri, MD; Garrett Pacheco, MD; Nirali Patel, MD; Shawn Robinson, MD; Seema Shah, MD; Mike Stoner, MD; Matt Swarm, MD; Jen Walthall, MD; Robyn Wing, MD; Dale Woolridge, MD, PhD.

The planning committee, staff, authors and editors listed below have identified financial relationships or relationships to products or devices they or their spouse/life partner have with commercial interest related to the content of this CME activity:

Ann Dietrich, MD is a consultant/advisor for AHC Inc.

UNAPPROVED/OFF-LABEL USE DISCLOSURE

The EOCME requires CME faculty to disclose to the participants:

1. When products or procedures being discussed are off-label, unlabelled, experimental, and/or investigational (not US Food and Drug Administration (FDA) approved); and
2. Any limitations on the information presented, such as data that are preliminary or that represent ongoing research, interim analyses, and/or unsupported opinions. Faculty may discuss information about pharmaceutical agents that is outside of FDA-approved labelling. This information is intended solely for CME and is not intended to promote off-label use of these medications. If you have any questions, contact the medical affairs department of the manufacturer for the most recent prescribing information.

TO ENROLL

To enroll in the *Emergency Medicine Clinics*Continuing Medical Education program, call customer service at 1-800-654-2452 or sign up online at http://www.theclinics.com/home/cme. The CME program is available to subscribers for an additional annual fee of $212 USD.

METHOD OF PARTICIPATION

In order to claim credit, participants must complete the following:

1. Complete enrolment as indicated above.
2. Read the activity.
3. Complete the CME Test and Evaluation. Participants must achieve a score of 70% on the test. All CME Tests and Evaluations must be completed online.

CME INQUIRIES/SPECIAL NEEDS

For all CME inquiries or special needs, please contact elsevierCME@elsevier.com.

Foreword

Pediatric Emergencies

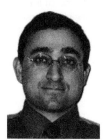

Amal Mattu, MD
Consulting Editor

"Children are not just little adults." This simple phrase could be considered the mantra of pediatric medical care providers around the world, and it is especially common to hear this phrase uttered by pediatricians and specialist pediatric emergency care providers. The belief in this phrase has some benefits. It reminds us that the typical care that we have learned to deliver to adults cannot always be extrapolated to caring for the injured or ill pediatric patient. Children have many different illnesses than adults, and they often suffer their illnesses and injuries through different causes and mechanisms, respectively. The medications with which children are treated, the dosages of those medications, and the side effects and iatrogenic concerns are all frequently different than in adults. Some specialists would have you believe that the ill or injured child can almost be considered a different species! *Almost*.

The mantra has its drawbacks as well. It almost implies that optimal care of children requires a pediatric or pediatric emergency medicine specialist. *Almost*. The fact is that children are *not* a different species. Many of the critically important principles of emergency medicine that apply to adults do successfully extrapolate to children, perhaps with some occasional tweaking of those principles. We know that well-trained general emergency physicians provide outstanding care to pediatric patients. General emergency physicians need not be intimidated by the mantra!

In this issue of *Emergency Medicine Clinics of North America*, three nationally recognized guest editors with expertise in caring for critically ill or injured children have come together to show us all exactly how we can use the general principles of emergency medicine and tweak them to provide optimal care to our pediatric emergency patients. They have assembled an outstanding group of authors, many of whom are general emergency physicians, to teach us how to care for the sickest of these patients. Articles are focused on approaches to general chief complaints and presentations, such as fever, trauma, seizures, and abuse, as well as specific diagnoses such as sepsis, asthma, diabetic ketoacidosis, and concussion. Additional systems are addressed, including cardiac, ear/nose/throat, and gastrointestinal

Emerg Med Clin N Am 31 (2013) xv–xvi
http://dx.doi.org/10.1016/j.emc.2013.06.001
0733-8627/13/$ – see front matter © 2013 Published by Elsevier Inc.

emergencies. Finally, articles are provided to address two more hot topics—procedural sedation and emergency ultrasound.

For those practitioners that are new to emergency medicine, after you read through this issue of *Emergency Medicine Clinics of North America*, I'm certain that you'll see that although "children are not just little adults," they should not be a source of intimidation in the emergency department. And for those practitioners that are well-versed in pediatric emergency medicine already, I know that you, too, will gain some critically useful pearls that will enhance your practice. My thanks to the guest editors and authors for their hard work, which is sure to improve the care of children in the emergency department and to improve the confidence of all emergency practitioners who care for those children.

Amal Mattu, MD
Department of Emergency Medicine
University of Maryland School of Medicine
Baltimore, MD 21201, USA

E-mail address:
amattu@smail.umaryland.edu

Preface

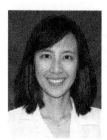 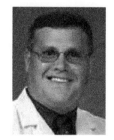 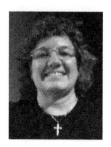

Le N. Lu, MD   Dale Woolridge, MD, PhD   Ann M. Dietrich, MD

Editors

Pediatric emergencies can be overwhelming, and knowledge of current standards, diagnostic evaluations, and effective treatment strategies can have a significant effect on outcome. Clinicians must be able to manage common, benign conditions, such as nasal foreign bodies, requiring relatively simple interventions, as well as recognize the early subtle signs of potentially life-threatening conditions, such as systemic inflammatory response syndrome, sepsis, and septic shock, requiring aggressive goal-directed therapy to give a child the best chance for survival.

Pediatric emergencies encompass a diversity of complaints and disease processes: infections, seizures, concussions, diabetic ketoacidosis, and cardiac arrhythmias. This issue of *Emergency Medicine Clinics of North America* updates the emergency medicine physician on recent advances in the diagnosis and management of specific conditions seen in our pediatric patients.

The authors are experts in the topics selected for this issue and provide clear overviews of each topic area, highlighting critical aspects of diagnosis, illuminating challenges with diagnosis, and presenting the essential elements of treatment. Areas where errors can occur are emphasized, and "tips and tricks" that will help you in your clinical practice are presented. We appreciate the time and effort that each author devoted to the preparation of his or her contribution. We are confident that the information we have compiled will enhance your practice when dealing with your smallest patients.

We thank Amal Mattu for the opportunity to compile this *Emergency Medicine Clinics of North America* issue and Patrick Manley for his support throughout the project. We are grateful for the support of our families and the guidance of our colleagues. We especially acknowledge the inspiration we receive from residents,

Emerg Med Clin N Am 31 (2013) xvii–xviii
http://dx.doi.org/10.1016/j.emc.2013.06.002
0733-8627/13/$ – see front matter © 2013 Published by Elsevier Inc.

fellows, and students—the real reason we choose to undertake projects such as this publication.

Le N. Lu, MD
Department of Emergency Medicine
University of Maryland School of Medicine
110 South Paca Street
Sixth Floor, Suite 200
Baltimore, MD 21201, USA

Dale Woolridge, MD, PhD
Departments of Emergency Medicine and Pediatrics, University of Arizona
1501 North Campbell Avenue
Tucson, AZ 85724, USA

Ann M. Dietrich, MD
Nationwide Children's Hospital
700 Children's Drive
Columbus, OH 43205, USA

E-mail addresses:
mlu@umaryland.edu (L.N. Lu)
dale@aemrc.arizona.edu (D. Woolridge)
Ann.Dietrich@nationwidechildrens.org (A.M. Dietrich)

Sepsis and Septic Shock

Patrick J. Maloney, MD

KEYWORDS

- Systemic inflammatory response syndrome (SIRS) • Sepsis • Septic shock
- Early goal-directed therapy • Vasopressors • Children

KEY POINTS

- Every physician who cares for children is challenged by the difficult tasks of recognizing and managing sepsis and septic shock.
- Early recognition and therapy are the cornerstones of acute care of the septic child. The rapidity and appropriateness of therapy administered in the initial hours significantly affects outcome.
- Septic shock in children is less frequently associated with hypotension than it is in adults. Children are more likely to present with a clinical syndrome referred to as cold shock, in which systemic vascular resistance is high and cardiac output is low. Clinically, these children have tachycardia (although neonates may present with bradycardia), pale, cyanotic, or mottled extremities, and prolonged capillary refill time (>3 seconds). Blood pressures may be normal, low, or high.
- Management of sepsis and septic shock includes respiratory support, aggressive fluid resuscitation, vasopressor therapy, and early antibiotic therapy. The goal is reversal of tissue hypoperfusion.
- The ideal choice of vasopressor agents in children with septic shock depends on the clinical appearance and hemodynamic status of the child.
- Mortality from sepsis in children is significantly lower than in adults.

INTRODUCTION

Infectious diseases have been a leading cause of death throughout the history of the human race, but only recently have we begun to understand their effects on the body. Ancient Greek and Roman philosophers viewed sepsis as a sort of biological decay.[1] It was not until the seventeenth and eighteenth centuries that the germ theory of disease ushered in eras of infection control and modern microbiology. The discovery of antibiotics during the first half of the twentieth century finally armed physicians with a specific weapon to fight infection. As we continue to unravel the mysteries of sepsis and septic shock, more recent research and innovation have focused on the molecular mechanisms and hemodynamics of sepsis and septic shock.[1]

Disclaimer: The author has no financial disclosures or conflicts of interest to acknowledge.
Department of Emergency Medicine, University of Colorado School of Medicine, Denver Health Medical Center, 660 Bannock Street, MC 0108, Denver, CO 80204, USA
E-mail address: patrick.maloney@dhha.org

Emerg Med Clin N Am 31 (2013) 583–600
http://dx.doi.org/10.1016/j.emc.2013.04.006
0733-8627/13/$ – see front matter © 2013 Elsevier Inc. All rights reserved.

Even now, every physician who cares for children is challenged by the difficult tasks of recognizing and managing sepsis and septic shock. In its most fundamental definition, sepsis is a clinical syndrome characterized by systemic inflammation and tissue injury. It represents a clinical continuum of severity, usually triggered by infection, resulting in a cascade of biochemical and pathophysiologic events. If left unabated, microbial toxins together with a dysfunctional host immune response can quickly wreak havoc, resulting in tissue damage, shock, organ failure, and death.

Early recognition and appropriate therapy are the cornerstones of acute care of the septic child. Similar to the severely injured patient, the rapidity and appropriateness of therapy administered in the initial hours affects the outcome. Early goal-directed sepsis management has led to one of the greatest reductions in sepsis-related morbidity and mortality over the past 50 years.[2]

DEFINITIONS

The 1992 joint statement from the American College of Chest Physicians (ACCP) and the Society of Critical Care Medicine (SCCM) introduced the term systemic inflammatory response syndrome (SIRS) to describe the nonspecific inflammatory process in adults that develops in response to significant physiologic insults, such as infection, trauma, burns, and other disease processes.[3] SIRS has since become part of the common medical vernacular.

The original criteria for SIRS contain several clinical signs and laboratory values that are specific to adults and, therefore, are not entirely useful in pediatric populations. In 2005, the International Pediatric Sepsis Consensus Conference (IPSCC) made several modifications and published pediatric-specific definitions based on expert opinion.[4] These definitions are listed in **Box 1**.

Three major differences are noted in the pediatric definitions. Because children are more likely to present with tachycardia or tachypnea unrelated to SIRS, temperature or leukocyte abnormalities must be present. Second, age-appropriate numeric values for normal vital signs, based on consensus expert opinion, were agreed on (**Table 1**). Bradycardia was added as a criterion for SIRS in the newborn age group.

Sepsis, as defined by the 1992 ACCP/SCCM Consensus Conference and accepted unaltered for children by the 2005 IPSCC, is SIRS with an infectious source.[3,4] Infection may be of bacterial, viral, fungal, or rickettsial origin. The diagnosis of infection may be supported by positive culture, tissue stain, or PCR testing, clinical examination, radiologic imaging, or other laboratory test findings (see **Box 1**). Severe sepsis is defined as sepsis plus the presence of cardiovascular dysfunction, ARDS, or 2 or more organ dysfunctions. The definitions of organ dysfunctions are modified for children and listed in **Box 2**.

The clinical definition of septic shock in children is more nebulous than in adults. Contrary to adults, children commonly do not develop hypotension until late in the clinical course of septic shock.[5] Therefore, the 2005 IPSCC agreed on a definition of pediatric septic shock that includes the presence of severe sepsis with signs of cardiovascular dysfunction, defined as, despite 40 or more mL/kg fluid resuscitation, any of 1 of the following criteria: hypotension, a need for vasoactive agents, or 2 or more other signs of organ hypoperfusion (see **Box 2**).[4]

These definitions are useful for standardization of the diagnoses but may be less relevant in the clinical arena. Clinical suspicion for sepsis is more sensitive and should always supersede reliance on the presence of all components of the consensus criteria.[6]

Box 1
Definitions of SIRS, infection, sepsis, severe sepsis, and septic shock in pediatric patients (modifications from the adult criteria are listed in bold)

SIRS

The presence of at least 2 of the following 4 criteria, **1 of which must be abnormal temperature or leukocyte count:**

- Core temperature of more than 38.5°C or less than 36°C (must be measured by rectal, bladder, oral, or central catheter probe).

- Tachycardia, defined as a mean heart rate greater than 2 standard deviations above normal for age in the absence of external stimulus, chronic drugs, or painful stimulus; or otherwise unexplained persistent increase over a 0.5-hour to 4-hour period or for children younger than 1 year: **bradycardia, defined as a mean heart rate less than the 10th percentile for age in the absence of external stimulus, β-blocker drugs, or congenital heart disease; or otherwise unexplained persistent depression over a 0.5-hour period.**

- Mean respiratory rate more than 2 standard deviations higher than normal for age or mechanical ventilation for an acute process not related to underlying neuromuscular disease or the receipt of general anesthesia.

- Leukocyte count increased or depressed for age (not secondary to chemotherapy-induced leukopenia) or greater than 10% immature neutrophils.

Infection

A suspected or proven (by positive culture, tissue stain, or polymerase chain reaction [PCR] test) infection caused by any pathogen or a clinical syndrome associated with a high probability of infection. Evidence of infection includes positive findings on clinical examination, imaging, or laboratory test (eg, white blood cells in a normally sterile body fluid, perforated viscus, chest radiograph consistent with pneumonia, petechial or purpuric rash, or purpura fulminans)

Sepsis

SIRS in the presence of or a result of suspected or proven infection

Severe Sepsis

Sepsis plus 1 of the following: cardiovascular organ dysfunction or acute respiratory distress syndrome (ARDS) or 2 or more organ dysfunctions. Organ dysfunctions are defined in **Box 2**

Septic Shock

Sepsis with cardiovascular organ dysfunction (as defined in **Box 2**)

From Goldstein B, Giroir B, Randolph A. International Pediatric Sepsis Consensus Conference: definitions for sepsis and organ dysfunction in pediatrics. Pediatr Crit Care Med 2005;6(1):4; with permission.

EPIDEMIOLOGY

According to the World Health Organization, more than two-thirds (68%) of the estimated 8.8 million deaths in children younger than 5 years worldwide in 2008 were caused by infectious diseases.[7] The big 4 killers are pneumonia, diarrhea, malaria, and measles.[8] Most of these deaths occur in the developing countries of Asia and sub-Saharan Africa. This situation makes infection, often culminating in severe sepsis and septic shock, the most common cause of death in infants and children in the world.

Among resource-rich countries, large-scale epidemiologic data in children with severe sepsis and septic shock are limited. Furthermore, because childhood immunization programs are constantly altering the microbiological landscape, the data that do

Box 2
Organ dysfunction criteria

Cardiovascular

Despite administration of isotonic intravenous fluid bolus 40 or more mL/kg in 1 hour

- Decrease in blood pressure (BP) (hypotension) less than the fifth percentile for age or systolic BP less than 2 standard deviations less than normal for age or
- Need for vasoactive drug to maintain BP in the normal range (dopamine >5 μg/kg/min or dobutamine, epinephrine, or norepinephrine at any dose) or
- Two of the following:
  - Unexplained metabolic acidosis: base deficit greater than 5.0 mEq/L
  - Increased arterial lactate greater than 2 times upper limit of normal
  - Oliguria: urine output less than 0.5 mL/kg/h
  - Prolonged capillary refill: greater than 5 seconds
  - Core to peripheral temperature gap greater than 3°C

Respiratory

- Pao_2 (partial pressure of oxygen, arterial)/Fio_2 (fraction of inspired oxygen) less than 300 in absence of cyanotic heart disease or preexisting lung disease or
- $Paco_2$ (partial pressure of carbon dioxide, arterial) greater than 65 torr or 20 mm Hg over baseline $Paco_2$ or
- Proven need for more than 50% Fio_2 to maintain saturation $\geq$92% or
- Need for nonelective invasive or noninvasive mechanical ventilation

Neurologic

- Glasgow Coma Scale 11 or greater or
- Acute change in mental status with a decrease in Glasgow Coma Scale 3 points or more from abnormal baseline

Hematologic

- Platelet count greater than 80,000/mm³ or a decline of 50% in platelet count from highest value recorded over the past 3 days (for chronic hematology/oncology patients) or
- International normalized ratio greater than 2

Renal

- Serum creatinine level 2 times or greater than the upper limit of normal for age or 2-fold increase in baseline creatinine

Hepatic

- Total bilirubin level 4 mg/dL or greater (not applicable for newborn) or
- Alanine aminotransferase level 2 times upper limit of normal for age

From Goldstein B, Giroir B, Randolph A. International Pediatric Sepsis Consensus Conference: definitions for sepsis and organ dysfunction in pediatrics. Pediatr Crit Care Med 2005;6(1):5; with permission.

exist may not be applicable to current pediatric populations in most of the developed world. With this caveat, it has been estimated that more than 42,000 children develop severe sepsis each year in the United States.[9] Infants are at highest risk, with rates 10 times that of older children. Low-birth-weight and very-low-birth-weight children make up nearly one-fourth of the pediatric severe sepsis population. Similarly, a recent

Table 1
Age-specific vital signs and laboratory variables (lower values for heart rate, leukocyte count, and systolic BP are for the fifth and upper values for heart rate, respiratory rate, or leukocyte count for the 95th percentiles)

Age Group	Heart Rate (Beats/Min)		Respiratory Rate (Breaths/Min)	Leukocyte Count (Leukocytes × 10^3/mm)	Systolic BP (mm Hg)
	Tachycardia	Bradycardia			
0 d to 1 wk	>180	<100	>50	>34	<65
1 wk to 1 mo	>180	<100	>40	>19.5 or <5	<75
1 mo to 1 y	>180	<90	>34	>17.5 or <5	<100
2–5 y	>140	NA	>22	>15.5 or <6	<94
6–12 y	>130	NA	>18	>13.5 or <4.5	<105
13 to <18 y	>110	NA	>14	>11 or <4.5	<117

From Goldstein B, Giroir B, Randolph A. International Pediatric Sepsis Consensus Conference: definitions for sepsis and organ dysfunction in pediatrics. Pediatr Crit Care Med 2005;6(1):4; with permission.

multicenter study in Columbian pediatric intensive care units estimated that more than half of all admissions for sepsis were children younger than 2 years.[10] Beyond infancy, children with underlying chronic diseases account for about one-half of all cases.[9,10]

In the United States, respiratory infections and primary bacteremia are the most common infections leading to sepsis. Bacteremia predominates in neonates, and respiratory illnesses are more common among older children.[9,11] No specific cause is found in most children presenting to US-based emergency departments with undifferentiated sepsis.[11]

MICROBIOLOGY

Overall, *Staphylococcus aureus* is the most common infecting organism in children with severe sepsis in the developed world (17.5%).[9] Among blood culture isolates, *Staphylococcus aureus*, *Streptococcus pneumoniae*, and group B *Streptococcus* predominate among previously healthy children. In children with chronic medical problems, coagulase-negative *Staphylococcus* species is most common.[9]

Urinary tract infections leading to severe sepsis are most commonly caused by gram-negative bacilli, including *Escherichia coli*, *Klebsiella pneumoniae*, *Enterococcus faecalis*, and *Proteus mirabilis*.[11] Meningococcal infections are rare and even less common among children with comorbidities. Fungal infections, on the contrary, are significantly more common among children with underlying chronic illnesses, especially human immunodeficiency virus (HIV).[9] Herpes simplex virus in neonates may cause either disseminated or central nervous system disease and may be clinically indistinguishable from bacterial infections.

Before widespread immunization, *Haemophilus influenza* serotype b (Hib) was a leading cause of invasive infection and sepsis in children younger than 5 years. Since routine Hib vaccination during infancy in the United States, the rates of Hib-invasive infection has declined to approximately 1 per 100,000 population.[12] With the subsequent widespread implementation of pneumococcal vaccination programs within the last 2 decades, the incidence of invasive pneumococcal infections has similarly decreased significantly.[13] Both of these pathogens continue to exert a huge burden on pediatric populations worldwide.

A more thorough discussion on specific pediatric infections, including urinary tract infections, community-acquired pneumonia, and so forth, is presented in the article on infectious disease emergencies elsewhere in this issue.

RISK FACTORS

Not every infection leads to SIRS, severe sepsis, septic shock, and death. In most cases, the child's immune system and appropriate antimicrobial therapy are able to safely eliminate the offending pathogen and return the child to normal health. The tendency to develop severe sepsis and septic shock is likely more determined by the host response to infection rather than a function of the offending pathogen.[14]

There are several risk factors that may contribute to an increased risk of severe sepsis and septic shock. Age is the single most important factor; neonates are at particularly high risk.[9,10] Beyond infancy, children who have chronic medical problems such as chronic lung disease, congenital heart disease, neuromuscular diseases, and hematologic or oncologic diseases account for nearly half of all cases of pediatric sepsis. In addition, these children have increased mortality.[9,10]

Other unique pediatric populations have an increased risk of sepsis. Sickle cell disease causes splenic dysfunction and impaired ability to combat encapsulated organisms. Host immunosuppression, caused by HIV/AIDS, malignancy, congenital immunodeficiencies, immunomodulating medications, asplenia, malnutrition, among other conditions, also increases the risk. Indwelling medical devices, such as catheters, and anatomic conditions such as congenital heart disease and urinary tract abnormalities predispose children to bacterial seeding and infection.

DIFFERENCES BETWEEN PEDIATRIC AND ADULT SEPSIS PATHOPHYSIOLOGY

The cardiovascular response to severe sepsis in children is complex and more variable than in adults. Systemic vascular resistance (SVR), cardiac contractility, and heart rate may each be affected to different degrees among patients with septic shock. In adults, SVR is almost universally decreased, whereas cardiac output (CO) is usually increased. The result is a distributive shock with hypotension, termed warm shock. Clinically, these patients have warm, well-perfused skin, bounding pulses, and brisk or flash capillary refill time. A few children (approximately 20%) present with signs of warm shock.

The more common cardiovascular response to severe sepsis in children, present in approximately 60% of cases, is an increase in SVR as a result of peripheral vasoconstriction. Consequently, blood flow is redistributed from the nonessential peripheral vascular beds such as the skin to more vital organs, including the brain, heart, kidneys, and lungs. It is also accompanied by a decrease in CO, either as a direct result of impaired cardiac contractility or as a secondary effect of high afterload. This clinical syndrome is referred to as cold shock. Peripheral pulses may be weak or absent; the extremities may appear cool, pale, or cyanotic; and capillary refill time is delayed. An important distinction is that BP is usually maintained and may be supranormal in children with cold shock.

Occasionally, both CO and SVR may be decreased in a child with septic shock. This situation may result in a clinical syndrome that is difficult to classify as either strictly warm or cold shock.

CLINICAL FINDINGS AND RECOGNITION

Recognizing sepsis early in the course of the disease is vital to curbing its natural progression to shock, organ failure, and death. Differentiating a benign, localized infectious illness from sepsis in children is challenging. The clinical signs and symptoms of early sepsis may be subtle and easily missed. Carcillo and colleagues[15] retrospectively reviewed the charts of more than 4000 children transferred from community emergency departments to a large, tertiary pediatric medical center, concluding that physicians failed to recognize and diagnose shock in more than three-quarters (76%) of cases.

There is no single diagnostic tool or clinical decision rule that is both highly sensitive and specific in recognizing sepsis in its early stages. The best approach is a high level of clinical suspicion, combined with the clinical history, vital signs, and physical examination. Often, a parent may describe a vague change from baseline behavior, such as increased fussiness, decreased activity, or poor oral intake, which may be the first clues of a serious infection. Unexplained tachycardia or tachypnea and signs of poor skin perfusion also suggest the presence of sepsis or septic shock.

The Pediatric Assessment Triangle (PAT) is a useful, rapid tool to guide a clinician's initial examination.[16,17] First published in 2000 by the American Academy of Pediatrics as a tool for emergency medical services personnel, it is now included as a standard tool in the pediatric advanced life support (PALS) and advanced pediatric life support (APLS) courses.[18,19] The PAT uses visual and auditory clues to quickly assess a child's general appearance, work of breathing, and circulation (**Fig. 1**). A child's overall appearance is useful as a screening tool of neurologic status. A child with septic shock may appear lethargic or inconsolable, have a weak or absent cry, make poor eye contact or be poorly interactive, or otherwise appear to have an abnormal level of consciousness. Increased work of breathing and tachypnea may be signs of a primary

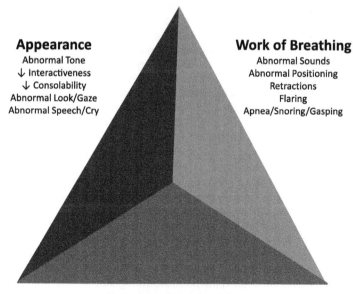

Appearance
Abnormal Tone
↓ Interactiveness
↓ Consolability
Abnormal Look/Gaze
Abnormal Speech/Cry

Work of Breathing
Abnormal Sounds
Abnormal Positioning
Retractions
Flaring
Apnea/Snoring/Gasping

Circulation to the Skin
Pallor
Mottling
Cyanosis

Fig. 1. PAT. (*Adapted from* Dieckmann RA, Brownstein D, Gausche-Hill M. The pediatric assessment triangle: a novel approach for the rapid evaluation of children. Pediatr Emerg Care 2010;26(4):313; with permission.)

respiratory illness, a compensatory mechanism for a primary metabolic acidosis, or secondary to fever, anxiety, or pain.

Evaluating a child's circulatory status and rapidly recognizing signs of inadequate tissue perfusion are often difficult at the child's bedside. Unlike in adults, hypotension is usually a late and ominous finding in children. Tachycardia, bradycardia, and tachypnea, although not highly specific, should never be overlooked. Persistent tachycardia not otherwise caused by fever, anxiety, pain, dehydration, or anemia should always be regarded as a potential sign of early sepsis and shock.

A careful examination of a child's skin may provide vital clues to a child's circulatory status independent of BP measurements. Infants and children with severe sepsis and septic shock often are able to maintain a normal or even increased BP as a result of robust compensatory mechanisms including tachycardia and increased SVR. In these patients with cold shock, capillary refill time is prolonged, and pallor, cyanosis, or mottling may be evident. Children with warm shock, on the other hand, have warm, flushed skin and brisk or flash capillary refill time.

LABORATORY TESTS AND BIOMARKERS

Laboratory tests may be used both in the identification of sepsis as well as in guidance of sepsis management, but none is both highly sensitive and specific in children. The American College of Critical Care Medicine (ACCM) recommends diagnosing sepsis and septic shock in neonates and children using clinical examination rather than any specific biomarkers.[20] However, because this diagnosis may be challenging, using laboratory tests as an adjunct is also recommended by some experts.[20,21]

A complete blood count (CBC) with differential should be obtained in any child suspected of having a serious infection. Age-specific leukocytosis or leukopenia is a criterion for pediatric SIRS (see **Box 1**). The most extensive data regarding the usefulness of the white blood cell count in identifying occult serious bacterial infection are found in children younger than 3 years in the prevaccination eras; several studies identified an increased risk of occult pneumococcal bacteremia among unimmunized febrile children with white blood cells 15,000/μL or greater and absolute neutrophil count 10,000/μL or greater.[22,23] Leukocytosis is less predictive for the presence of a serious bacterial infection in the fully immunized child.[13,24,25] This finding has led some experts to question the routine use of CBC alone to guide the empirical administration of antibiotics.[13]

Lactic acid, which is a by-product of anaerobic metabolism, can be used as a marker of tissue hypoperfusion. In adults with severe sepsis, an increased lactate level (>4 mmol/L) is a negative prognostic indicator and should trigger aggressive septic resuscitation according to the Surviving Sepsis Campaign guidelines.[26] In addition, early lactate clearance, defined as a decrease in serum lactate level by 10% or more after initial fluid resuscitation, is associated with improved outcomes in severe sepsis and septic shock in adults.[27,28]

Lactate levels have not traditionally been used in pediatric sepsis management and data are limited in this population. Nevertheless, an increased lactate level is predictive of serious bacterial infection in the pediatric emergency department as well as an increased risk of death in the pediatric intensive care setting.[29,30] In addition, a recent small, prospective study suggests that an increased lactate level in the emergency department may predict which children have early sepsis and will progress to severe sepsis and septic shock.[31] Further studies are likely needed before routine use of lactate levels is recommended in pediatric sepsis diagnosis and management.

Biomarkers have the potential to diagnose, monitor, and predict outcome in clinical systemic inflammation syndromes such as sepsis. No single biomarker currently available is both highly sensitive and specific to be trusted in isolation. C-reactive protein (CRP) is the most universally available.[32] Although it has limited sensitivity in differentiating bacterial from viral infections, it does aid in identifying children with serious bacterial infections.[24,33] Procalcitonin has more recently been studied in children. Its use as a diagnostic tool is similar to that of CRP.[24] However, its lack of availability and higher cost limits its clinical usefulness. Although there may be some limited added value in combinations of tests to screen for serious infection, any diagnostic test must be interpreted in the context of the child's clinical presentation.[24]

Other routine laboratory tests are less likely to identify the presence of sepsis but may help guide management. A rapid bedside glucose level identifies life-threatening hypoglycemia, which commonly accompanies sepsis in young children and infants. A basic metabolic panel may help identify metabolic acidosis, renal insufficiency, and electrolyte abnormalities. Coagulation studies, fibrinogen, and D-dimer are indicated when there is a clinical suspicion for meningococcal infection or other concerns for disseminated intravascular coagulopathy. Increased total bilirubin and transaminase levels may support the diagnosis of organ dysfunction. Arterial or venous blood gas should be obtained if there is suspicion of acidosis or respiratory insufficiency. Appropriate cultures of all suspected sources of infection should be obtained but should not delay the administration of antibiotics.

MANAGEMENT OF SEPSIS AND SEPTIC SHOCK

The cornerstone of emergency department management of sepsis and septic shock is early recognition and rapid, aggressive resuscitation.[2] The ACCM has developed an algorithm to help guide clinicians (**Fig. 2**).[20] In a prospective study of 91 neonates and children who presented to a community hospital in shock, the children in whom shock was reversed within the first 2 hours had a 96% survival rate and a greater than 9-fold increase in the odds of survival compared with the children in whom shock was not quickly reversed.[34] Moreover, for each hour in which shock was not reversed, there was a significant increase in mortality. Carrillo and colleagues[15] similarly found that early use of PALS/APLS-recommended interventions was associated with reduced mortality and morbidity.

The goal of sepsis management in the emergency department is reversal of tissue hypoperfusion. Physiologic end points include normal BP, capillary refill time 2 seconds or less, normal range heart rate, normal pulses with no differentiation between central and peripheral pulses, urine output 1 mL/kg/h or greater, and restoration of normal mental status.[20,35] Lactate levels and lactate clearance, which are shown in adults to be clinically relevant, are not part of the 2007 ACCM guidelines or 2012 Surviving Sepsis Campaign update but may be clinically useful.[20,35]

Sepsis Protocols

Emergency department-based sepsis protocols are commonly used in adults to aid rapid recognition of sepsis and initiation of resuscitative interventions. These protocols rely on vital signs to initiate prioritized physician evaluation, a standard set of laboratory tests, rapid vascular access and fluid resuscitation, and early antibiotic administration.

There is a limited but growing subset of literature supporting a similar standard approach in pediatric patients. Larsen and colleagues[21] implemented an emergency department sepsis protocol to rapidly identify children with early sepsis and initiate management quickly. Triage nurses relied on a simple reference tool that defined age-appropriate abnormal vital signs and physical findings for patients with possible septic shock. Positive triage screening triggered implementation of a septic shock

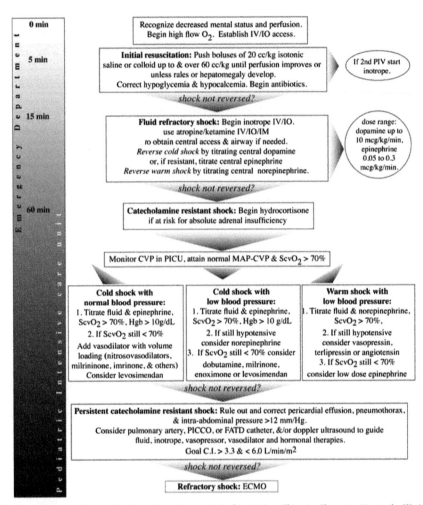

Fig. 2. ACCM septic shock algorithm. (*From* Brierley J, Carcillo JA, Choong K, et al. Clinical practice parameters for hemodynamic support of pediatric and neonatal septic shock: 2007 update from the American College of Critical Care Medicine. Crit Care Med 2009;37(2):677; with permission.)

care guideline based on the 2007 ACCM Consensus recommendations.[20] This triage-based screening tool successfully decreased length of stay in the emergency department and increased compliance with many elements of the recommended guidelines, most important of which were 3 key interventions known to decrease morbidity and mortality (ie, initial fluid resuscitation of ≥20 mL/kg in the first hour, an assessment of serum lactate, and antibiotics within 3 hours of emergency department admission).

Cruz and colleagues[36] similarly studied a triage-based screening tool to recognize vital sign abnormalities and implement a septic shock protocol. Their results showed a significant reduction from the time of triage to the first fluid bolus and antibiotic administration. Overall, emergency department sepsis protocols may improve recognition of early sepsis and compliance with current sepsis guidelines.

ABCs

As in all emergent resuscitation, the initial ABCs (airway, breathing, circulation) should be addressed according to PALS guidelines.[5] Positioning the child's head and neck in the sniffing position to optimize breathing is a basic yet potentially significant intervention. This positioning involves aligning the tragus of the ear with the patient's sternum. In very young children, the sniffing position is usually achieved by placing a towel roll under the shoulders, whereas in older children elevating their head slightly may be necessary. Suctioning excess upper airway secretions, especially within the nasopharyngeal airways, may also be helpful in children younger than 6 months, because they are typically obligate nasal breathers.

Supplemental oxygen should routinely be administered by face mask. In the presence of respiratory distress or hypoxemia, high-flow nasal cannula or nasopharyngeal continuous positive airway pressure (CPAP) may be appropriate.[35] Children are more likely to require mechanical ventilation because they have decreased respiratory reserve and increased oxygen requirements. A definitive airway should be secured by endotracheal intubation if indicated. The decision to intubate is difficult but should be made based on clinical signs of increased work of breathing, inadequate respiratory effort, refractory hypoxemia, or a combination of these signs, rather than any specific laboratory test result.[20] Although endotracheal tube intubation and mechanical ventilation should not be unnecessarily delayed, there is less risk of cardiovascular collapse during rapid sequence intubation (RSI) if the child has been adequately resuscitated before attempting intubation and initiating positive pressure mechanical ventilation.[35]

Venous access should be established as quickly as possible. Peripheral intravenous catheters are preferred, but may be difficult to place in the dehydrated and septic child. If this procedure is unsuccessful, intraosseous access is recommended.[35] Rarely, central venous access is necessary in the emergency department.

When invasive procedures or mechanical ventilation are necessary, procedural sedation or RSI is appropriate. Etomidate has been the induction agent of choice for many clinicians because of its lack of cardiovascular effects. However, although etomidate continues to be recommended by some experts, the current ACCM guidelines discourage the routine use of etomidate in children with septic shock because of concerns that it suppresses adrenal function and may increase mortality.[20] Ketamine may be a more appropriate choice, because it helps maintain cardiovascular stability.[37] Succinylcholine and rocuronium are both acceptable paralytic agents for RSI. However, the recommended dose of succinylcholine in young children (1.5–2 mg/kg) is larger than that usually given to adult patients (1–1.5 mg/kg).[38]

Intravenous Fluids

The current recommendation from the ACCM for neonates and children in septic shock is the rapid intravenous administration of isotonic crystalloid or colloid solution in 20-mL/kg boluses over 5 minutes each (see **Fig. 2**).[20] To accomplish this rapid fluid infusion through a small peripheral or intraosseous catheter, either a pressure bag or the push-pull system is superior to gravity drainage alone.[39] After each bolus, the child's hemodynamic status should be reevaluated for signs of normal perfusion and shock reversal. Children commonly require 40 to 60 mL/kg, and occasionally up to 200 mL/kg, intravenous fluid in the first hour of resuscitation. In general, children with septic shock who receive more fluid in the first hour have reduced morbidity and mortality than children who receive less.[40]

Differentiating septic from cardiogenic shock is a common concern in the emergency department. Consideration should always be given to depressed cardiac contractility either as the primary cause of shock or as a result of septic shock. Aggressive fluid resuscitation in the first several hours in children with septic shock rarely causes ARDS.[41] However, if a child develops rales or hepatomegaly during fluid resuscitation, the clinician should consider inotropic support and emergent echocardiography.

Vasoactive Agents

Vasoactive agents are recommended in children with fluid-refractory septic shock (ie, children who remain in shock despite 40–60 mL/kg or more intravenous fluid resuscitation) (see **Fig. 2**).[5,19,20] Inotropic medications increase CO by increasing cardiac contractility or heart rate. Vasopressors increase SVR by increasing arterial circulation tone. Vasodilators decrease arterial resistance, resulting in a decreased afterload and increased CO. In many cases, a single drug may have combined effects that cause alterations in SVR and contractility or may have dose-dependent effects.

Central venous access is the optimal route of vasoactive drug administration, because it delivers the drug to the central circulation rapidly and eliminates the risk of peripheral extravasation. However, it is preferred that vasopressor administration not be delayed, and, therefore, it is recommended to start vasopressors via a peripheral intravenous or intraosseous catheter if central access is not rapidly available.[5,20]

The choice of vasoactive agent for children with septic shock is a matter of debate, and the recommendations are consensus expert opinion rather than evidence based (see **Fig. 2**). Similar to volume resuscitation, the goal of vasoactive therapy in septic shock is the restoration of normal tissue perfusion. Because the cardiovascular response to severe sepsis is more variable in children than in adults, there is no single vasoactive agent that is appropriate for all children with septic shock. In addition, the age of the child, perfusion of the kidneys and liver, and presence of systemic inflammation may affect the pharmacokinetics and physiologic effects of vasoactive medications. Therefore, recommended agents and dosages are only approximations and should be titrated to clinical effects.[20]

Dopamine traditionally has been used as a first-line medication for the support of circulation, and the ACCM guidelines continue to recommend its use in children with undifferentiated fluid-refractory septic shock.[20] At midrange doses (5–10 μg/kg/min), it is believed that the vasopressive β-adrenergic effects of dopamine predominate, resulting in an increase in SVR. At higher doses, α-adrenergic receptor stimulation adds some inotropic effect as well. However, the dose-related effects of dopamine are unpredictable, and there is some evidence that suggests that adults who receive dopamine have increased morbidity compared with those who do not receive dopamine.[42] In addition, young infants (<6 months old) may be insensitive to dopamine.[43] As a result, many experts discourage the reflexive use of dopamine in septic shock.

Norepinephrine is the preferred vasoactive agent in adults with septic shock, because adults more predictably have increased CO and decreased SVR. There is some controversy regarding its use in children. In children who clinically have fluid-refractory warm shock, the ACCM guidelines recommend the use of norepinephrine (0.03–0.05 μg/kg/min) as the first-line vasopressor rather than dopamine.[20]

In patients with cold shock, inotropic and possibly vasodilatory support is beneficial, because these children have increased SVR and decreased CO. The most commonly used inotropic agents in the emergency department are dopamine and epinephrine. The ACCM guidelines recommend dopamine as the first-line inotrope in cold septic shock. This recommendation is based on wide availability, practitioner familiarity with the drug, and because, unlike in adult populations, dopamine has not been linked to increased mortality in children.[20] For patients who are hypotensive with cold shock, epinephrine (0.05–0.3 μg/kg/min) is the preferred vasoactive agent. However, at doses exceeding 0.1 μg/kg/min, epinephrine may have more pronounced α-adrenergic effects, causing increased systemic vasoconstriction. There are no studies that have directly compared dopamine and epinephrine in the treatment of septic shock in children.

Dopamine is a reasonable first-line drug for undifferentiated septic shock in children. However, norepinephrine for hypotensive warm shock and epinephrine for hypotensive cold shock may be better options. Most children who fail to respond to dopamine respond to norepinephrine or epinephrine.

Overall, the use of vasoactive agents in children with septic shock is a dynamic process in which vasopressors, inotropes, and even vasodilators are titrated to clinical signs of perfusion and shock reversal in each individual patient rather than being administered at a standard infusion rate. This procedure is best achieved by actively attending at the child's bedside. Once the child is in the intensive care unit, other inotropic agents (dobutamine), vasopressors (vasopressin, angiotensin), vasodilators that reduce pulmonary and SVR (sodium nitroprusside), and phosphodiesterase inhibitors that act as inotropes and vasodilators (milrinone) may be indicated.

Antibiotics

Empirical, broad-spectrum antibiotics should be administered as soon as possible in the emergency department whenever sepsis is suspected. The appropriate antibiotic choice is based on suspected infection site, suspected organism, whether the infection was likely acquired in the community or health care setting, host factors such as immunosuppression, and local resistance patterns.

Few studies have analyzed the causes of sepsis and septic shock in all patients presenting to the emergency department, and, therefore, it is difficult to make broad recommendations. In general, all children with septic shock, if not otherwise contraindicated, should receive a third-generation or fourth-generation cephalosporin plus coverage for methicillin-resistant *Staphylococcus aureus*, usually vancomycin. Children who are immunocompromised or are otherwise at risk for infection with *Pseudomonas* species should receive appropriate additional coverage. When gastrointestinal or genitourinary sources are suspected, adding coverage for enteric organisms with an aminoglycoside, piperacillin/tazobactam, clindamycin, or metronidazole is appropriate. Empirical coverage for *Listeria* with ampicillin and for herpes simplex virus with acyclovir should be considered in neonates. It is prudent and recommended to consult a pediatric infectious disease specialist when considering empirical antibiotics in a child with septic shock.

Ideally, appropriate culture should be obtained before antibiotics. However, antibiotics should never be delayed because cultures have not been obtained. The goal is to administer antibiotics within 1 hour of onset of septic shock, because this has been shown to reduce mortality in adults.[44]

Other: Steroids, Glucose, Site Control, Extracorporeal Membrane Oxygenation

If a child is at risk for absolute adrenal insufficiency or adrenal axis failure, such as congenital adrenal hyperplasia, recent systemic steroid therapy, or preexisting hypothalamic/pituitary abnormalities, or there is a clinical concern for purpura fulminans, hydrocortisone should be administered.[20] There is no ideal laboratory method for detecting absolute or relative adrenal insufficiency, but a blood sample for baseline serum cortisol measurement should be obtained before giving hydrocortisone.

Hydrocortisone may be given either as an intermittent bolus dose or as a continuous infusion. The dose ranges for 1 to 2 mg/kg/d for stress coverage to 50 mg/kg/d for reversal of shock. (See further discussion later regarding steroid use in fluid-refractory and catecholamine-resistant septic shock.)[20]

Because hypoglycemia is common among children with sepsis, consideration should always be given to infusing a dextrose-containing fluid at maintenance rate in addition to resuscitative fluid boluses of non–dextrose-containing crystalloid.[20]

Physical measures undertaken to eliminate a focus of infection, referred to as source control, are an important consideration in any patient with septic shock.[26] Specific sources of infection that may require surgical site control include abscesses, empyemas, necrotizing fasciitis, peritonitis, and cholangitis. Other potentially complicated infections that may benefit from removal of a potentially infected device include artificial valve-associated endocarditis, catheter-related bacteremia, and orthopedic hardware-related septic arthritis and osteomyelitis. Infections associated with extensive necrotic tissue may also benefit from surgical debridement.

Although extracorporeal membrane oxygenation (ECMO) is not an emergency department therapy, it is worth mentioning as a viable option for refractory shock. Neonates and children have high survival rates (80% and 50%, respectively) when placed on ECMO for septic shock. This rate is similar to survival rates for refractory respiratory failure. However, thrombotic complications may be more common when ECMO is used for septic shock.[20]

Fluid-Refractory and Catecholamine-Resistant Shock

Pediatric septic shock is usually associated with severe hypovolemia, and children usually respond well to aggressive volume resuscitation and vasoactive therapy. Fluid-refractory, catecholamine-resistant septic shock is defined as persistent cardiovascular dysfunction despite the administration of at least 60 mL/kg of intravenous fluid resuscitation in the first hour and maximum dopamine or norepinephrine or epinephrine therapy.[20] In these patients, it is important to search for alternative causes of persistent shock, including pericardial tamponade, tension pneumothorax, and intra-abdominal compartment syndrome (intra-abdominal pressure >12 mm Hg).[20,35]

The use of hydrocortisone or other steroid therapy in children with fluid-refractory and catecholamine-resistant septic shock remains controversial. Relative or absolute adrenal insufficiency is more common in children.[45] In addition, there is evidence that children who die from septic shock are more likely to have lower cortisol levels than survivors.[46,47] However, another retrospective study found that the mortality among children with septic shock who received steroids was 30% compared with 18% among those who did not receive steroids.[48] Because this study lacked illness severity data, it is impossible to know if steroids were preferentially given to the more ill children. A subsequent study that did account for disease severity found no mortality benefit from steroid therapy.[49] As a result of the limited and potentially flawed data available, the ACCM continues to maintain clinical equipoise of the topic of adjunctive steroid therapy for pediatric septic shock in the absence of a clinical suspicion for absolute adrenal insufficiency, such as children with purpura fulminans and Waterhouse-Friderichsen syndrome, those who have received steroid therapies for chronic illnesses, and children with known pituitary or adrenal abnormalities.[20]

In patients with suspected absolute adrenal insufficiency and catecholamine-resistant shock, the ideal dose of hydrocortisone also remains unknown. The recommendation from the Surviving Sepsis Campaign is an initial stress dose (50 mg/m^2/24 h), with the caveat that some children may require higher infusion rates

($\leq$50 mg/kg/24 h) to reverse shock in the short-term.[35] The ACCM suggests titrating the dose to resolution of shock using between 2 mg/kg/d and 50 mg/kg/d as a continuous infusion.[20] The treatment should be weaned off as quickly as tolerated to minimize potential side effects.

PROGNOSIS

Since the 1960s, the mortality from sepsis in children in the United States has decreased from 97% to less than 10%, which is dramatically lower than the 30% estimated mortality in adults.[9] Mortality is highest among children with chronic medical diseases.[50] However, the overall incidence seems to be increasing. This increase is most likely because of the increased incidence of very-low-weight neonates.

SUMMARY

Despite major advancements in the prevention, recognition, and management of sepsis and septic shock in children, infectious diseases remain a significant burden on childhood health worldwide. Although use of broad-spectrum antibiotic and early goal-directed therapy have together decreased mortality from sepsis in the developed world from more than 90% to approximately 10%, early recognition and aggressive initial management in the emergency department remain obstacles despite their proven benefit.

Early recognition of sepsis and septic shock in children relies on obtaining an attentive clinical history, accurate vital signs, and a physical examination focused on mental status, work of breathing, and circulatory status. Laboratory tests, including a white blood cell count and lactate level, may support the diagnosis but are not reliable in isolation.

The goal of septic shock management is reversal of tissue hypoperfusion. Resuscitation priorities include airway management, respiratory support, aggressive fluid administration, and vasopressor support, as well as early, broad-spectrum, empirical antibiotic therapy. The therapeutic end point is shock reversal, as shown by improved hemodynamic signs on examination rather than laboratory end points.

Overall, children are able to tolerate the physiologic effects of severe sepsis better than adults. Mortality is significantly better among children when managed appropriately; but the stakes remain high. Every physician who cares for children must strive to have a high level of suspicion and keen clinical acumen for recognizing the rare but potentially seriously ill child.

REFERENCES

1. Funk DJ, Parrillo JE, Kumar A. Sepsis and septic shock: a history. Crit Care Clin 2009;25(1):83–101, viii.
2. Rivers E, Nguyen B, Havstad S, et al. Early goal-directed therapy in the treatment of severe sepsis and septic shock. N Engl J Med 2001;345(19):1368–77.
3. Bone RC, Sprung CL, Sibbald WJ. Definitions for sepsis and organ failure. Crit Care Med 1992;20(6):724–6.
4. Goldstein B, Giroir B, Randolph A. International pediatric sepsis consensus conference: definitions for sepsis and organ dysfunction in pediatrics. Pediatr Crit Care Med 2005;6(1):2–8.
5. American Heart Association. 2005 American Heart Association (AHA) guidelines for cardiopulmonary resuscitation (CPR) and emergency cardiovascular

care (ECC) of pediatric and neonatal patients: pediatric basic life support. Pediatrics 2006;117(5):e989–1004.

6. Weiss SL, Parker B, Bullock ME, et al. Defining pediatric sepsis by different criteria: discrepancies in populations and implications for clinical practice. Pediatr Crit Care Med 2012;13(4):e219–26.

7. Black RE, Cousens S, Johnson HL, et al. Global, regional, and national causes of child mortality in 2008: a systematic analysis. Lancet 2010;375(9730): 1969–87.

8. Anon. WHO. Causes of child mortality for the year 2010. Available at: http://www. who.int/gho/child_health/mortality/mortality_causes_text/en/index.html. Accessed January 5, 2013.

9. Watson RS, Carcillo JA, Linde-Zwirble WT, et al. The epidemiology of severe sepsis in children in the United States. Am J Respir Crit Care Med 2003; 167(5):695–701.

10. Jaramillo-Bustamante JC, Marín-Agudelo A, Fernández-Laverde M, et al. Epidemiology of sepsis in pediatric intensive care units: first Colombian multicenter study. Pediatr Crit Care Med 2012;13(5):501–8.

11. Gaines NN, Patel B, Williams EA, et al. Etiologies of septic shock in a pediatric emergency department population. Pediatr Infect Dis J 2012;31(11):1203–5.

12. Talan DA, Moran GJ, Pinner RW. Progress toward eliminating *Haemophilus influenzae* type b disease among infants and children–United States, 1987-1997. Ann Emerg Med 1999;34(1):109–11.

13. Herz AM, Greenhow TL, Alcantara J, et al. Changing epidemiology of outpatient bacteremia in 3- to 36-month-old children after the introduction of the heptavalent-conjugated pneumococcal vaccine. Pediatr Infect Dis J 2006; 25(4):293–300.

14. Marino PL. The ICU book. 3rd edition. Philadelphia: Lippincott Williams & Wilkins; 2006.

15. Carcillo JA, Kuch BA, Han YY, et al. Mortality and functional morbidity after use of PALS/APLS by community physicians. Pediatrics 2009;124(2):500–8.

16. American Academy of Pediatrics. Pediatric education for prehospital professionals: PEPP resource manual. 2nd edition. Sudbury (MA): Jones & Bartlett; 2005.

17. Dieckmann RA, Brownstein D, Gausche-Hill M. The pediatric assessment triangle: a novel approach for the rapid evaluation of children. Pediatr Emerg Care 2010;26(4):312–5.

18. American Academy of Pediatrics, American College of Emergency Physicians. APLS: advanced pediatric life support. 5th edition. Sudbury (MA): Jones and Bartlett Learning; 2011.

19. Chameides L, Samson RA, Schexnayder SM, et al, editors. Pediatric life support provider manual. Dallas (TX): American Heart Association; 2011.

20. Brierley J, Carcillo JA, Choong K, et al. Clinical practice parameters for hemodynamic support of pediatric and neonatal septic shock: 2007 update from the American College of Critical Care Medicine. Crit Care Med 2009;37(2):666–88.

21. Larsen GY, Mecham N, Greenberg R. An emergency department septic shock protocol and care guideline for children initiated at triage. Pediatrics 2011; 127(6):e1585–92.

22. Lee GM, Harper MB. Risk of bacteremia for febrile young children in the post-*Haemophilus influenzae* type b era. Arch Pediatr Adolesc Med 1998;152(7): 624–8.

23. Kuppermann N, Fleisher GR, Jaffe DM. Predictors of occult pneumococcal bacteremia in young febrile children. Ann Emerg Med 1998;31(6):679–87.
24. Van den Bruel A, Thompson MJ, Haj-Hassan T, et al. Diagnostic value of laboratory tests in identifying serious infections in febrile children: systematic review. BMJ 2011;342:d3082.
25. Peltola V, Mertsola J, Ruuskanen O. Comparison of total white blood cell count and serum C-reactive protein levels in confirmed bacterial and viral infections. J Pediatr 2006;149(5):721–4.
26. Dellinger RP, Levy MM, Carlet JM, et al. Surviving Sepsis Campaign: international guidelines for management of severe sepsis and septic shock: 2008. Crit Care Med 2008;36(1):296–327.
27. Arnold RC, Shapiro NI, Jones AE, et al. Multicenter study of early lactate clearance as a determinant of survival in patients with presumed sepsis. Shock 2009; 32(1):35–9.
28. Nguyen HB, Rivers EP, Knoblich BP, et al. Early lactate clearance is associated with improved outcome in severe sepsis and septic shock. Crit Care Med 2004; 32(8):1637–42.
29. Vorwerk C, Manias K, Davies F, et al. Prediction of severe bacterial infection in children with an emergency department diagnosis of infection. Emerg Med J 2011;28(11):948–51.
30. Duke TD, Butt W, South M. Predictors of mortality and multiple organ failure in children with sepsis. Intensive Care Med 1997;23(6):684–92.
31. Scott HF, Donoghue AJ, Gaieski DF, et al. The utility of early lactate testing in undifferentiated pediatric systemic inflammatory response syndrome. Acad Emerg Med 2012;19(11):1276–80.
32. Jaye DL, Waites KB. Clinical applications of C-reactive protein in pediatrics. Pediatr Infect Dis J 1997;16(8):735–46 [quiz: 746–7].
33. Sanders S, Barnett A, Correa-Velez I, et al. Systematic review of the diagnostic accuracy of C-reactive protein to detect bacterial infection in nonhospitalized infants and children with fever. J Pediatr 2008;153(4):570–4.
34. Han YY, Carcillo JA, Dragotta MA, et al. Early reversal of pediatric-neonatal septic shock by community physicians is associated with improved outcome. Pediatrics 2003;112(4):793–9.
35. Dellinger RP, Levy MM, Rhodes A, et al. Surviving Sepsis Campaign. Crit Care Med 2013;41(2):580–637.
36. Cruz AT, Perry AM, Williams EA, et al. Implementation of goal-directed therapy for children with suspected sepsis in the emergency department. Pediatrics 2011;127(3):e758–66.
37. Yamamoto LG. Emergency airway management–rapid sequence intubation. In: Fleisher GR, Lugwig S, editors. Textbook of pediatric emergency medicine. 6th edition. Philadelphia: Lippincott Williams & Wilkins; 2010. p. 74–84.
38. Walls R, Murphy M. Manual of emergency airway management. Lippincott Williams & Wilkins; 2012. p. 464.
39. Stoner MJ, Goodman DG, Cohen DM, et al. Rapid fluid resuscitation in pediatrics: testing the American College of Critical Care Medicine guideline. Ann Emerg Med 2007;50(5):601–7.
40. Carcillo JA, Davis AL, Zaritsky A. Role of early fluid resuscitation in pediatric septic shock. JAMA 1991;266(9):1242–5.
41. Ceneviva G, Paschall JA, Maffei F, et al. Hemodynamic support in fluid-refractory pediatric septic shock. Pediatrics 1998;102(2):e19.

42. Sakr Y, Reinhart K, Vincent JL, et al. Does dopamine administration in shock influence outcome? Results of the Sepsis Occurrence in Acutely Ill Patients (SOAP) Study. Crit Care Med 2006;34(3):589–97.

43. Padbury JF, Agata Y, Baylen BG, et al. Pharmacokinetics of dopamine in critically ill newborn infants. J Pediatr 1990;117(3):472–6.

44. Kumar A, Roberts D, Wood KE, et al. Duration of hypotension before initiation of effective antimicrobial therapy is the critical determinant of survival in human septic shock. Crit Care Med 2006;34(6):1589–96.

45. Pizarro CF, Troster EJ, Damiani D, et al. Absolute and relative adrenal insufficiency in children with septic shock. Crit Care Med 2005;33(4):855–9.

46. Joosten KF, De Kleijn ED, Westerterp M, et al. Endocrine and metabolic responses in children with meningococcal sepsis: striking differences between survivors and nonsurvivors. J Clin Endocrinol Metab 2000;85(10):3746–53.

47. Riordan FA, Thomson AP, Ratcliffe JM, et al. Admission cortisol and adrenocorticotrophic hormone levels in children with meningococcal disease: evidence of adrenal insufficiency? Crit Care Med 1999;27(10):2257–61.

48. Markovitz BP, Goodman DM, Watson RS, et al. A retrospective cohort study of prognostic factors associated with outcome in pediatric severe sepsis: what is the role of steroids? Pediatr Crit Care Med 2005;6(3):270–4.

49. Zimmerman JJ, Williams MD. Adjunctive corticosteroid therapy in pediatric severe sepsis: observations from the RESOLVE study. Pediatr Crit Care Med 2011;12(1):2–8.

50. Odetola FO, Gebremariam A, Freed GL. Patient and hospital correlates of clinical outcomes and resource utilization in severe pediatric sepsis. Pediatrics 2007;119(3):487–94.

Risk Stratification and Management of the Febrile Young Child

Paul Ishimine, MD[a,b,c],*

KEYWORDS

- Fever • Neonate • Child • Bacteremia • Pneumonia • Urinary tract infection
- Rapid viral testing • Pneumococcal vaccination

KEY POINTS

- Febrile neonates require blood, urine, and cerebrospinal fluid cultures, empiric antibiotic therapy, and hospital admission.
- Febrile young infants can be classified as high or low risk for serious bacterial infections. High-risk patients require antibiotic therapy and hospital admission, but most low-risk infants can be discharged home.
- Some febrile older infants and toddlers require testing to identify clinically occult bacterial infections, but most of these children can be discharged home.

Fever is the most frequent complaint of children presenting to the emergency department.[1,2] Most children have viral infections and recover fully, but some febrile children have serious bacterial infections (SBIs), such as meningitis, pneumonia, urinary tract infection (UTI), bacterial gastroenteritis, osteomyelitis, and bacteremia. These patients are at high risk for adverse outcomes. Although these SBIs are often apparent after clinical assessment, some children have fever without an identifiable focus.

Despite the frequency of this complaint, the evaluation and management of these children varies.[3–8] This is particularly true for febrile young children. This variability results from many different factors: limitations of the history and physical examination in young children, the changing epidemiology of SBI, new diagnostic tests, lack of expert consensus, and differing levels of risk acceptance by parents and physicians.[9–11]

Traditional approaches to the febrile young child have relied on risk stratification based on a child's age.[12–14] These age classifications have divided young children

[a] Emergency Medicine, University of California, San Diego, UC San Diego Health System, 200 West Arbor Drive, #8676, San Diego, CA 92103-8676, USA; [b] Pediatrics, University of California, San Diego, Rady Children's Hospital, 3020 Children's Way, #5075, San Diego, CA 92123, USA; [c] Pediatric Emergency Medicine, Rady Children's Hospital, 3020 Children's Way, #5075 San Diego, CA 92123, USA
* Emergency Medicine, University of California, San Diego, UC San Diego Health System, 200 West Arbor Drive, #8676, San Diego, CA 92103-8676.
E-mail address: pishimine@ucsd.edu

Emerg Med Clin N Am 31 (2013) 601–626
http://dx.doi.org/10.1016/j.emc.2013.05.003
0733-8627/13/$ – see front matter © 2013 Elsevier Inc. All rights reserved.

emed.theclinics.com

into 3 general categories: neonates (birth to 28 days old), young infants (children between 1 month and 2 or 3 months of age), and older infants or toddlers (commonly defined as 2 or 3 months of age and older). This categorization schema oversimplifies the heterogeneous level of risk for patients both within and among age categories (eg, the risk of an SBI in a 28-day-old neonate is unlikely to be different from that of a 29-day-old febrile young infant). However, because previous research has used this classification to identify study populations, this arbitrary categorization continues to serve as the foundation for organizing the approach to the febrile young child.

HISTORY AND PHYSICAL EXAMINATION

Fever may have infectious or noninfectious causes,[15] but most febrile children who present to the emergency department (ED) have fevers arising from infections. Although there are fluctuations in the normal body temperature, fever in young children is generally accepted as a temperature of 38.0°C (100.4°F) or higher. Rectal thermometry is the method thought to most closely represent core temperature in the ambulatory setting and is more accurate than oral, axillary, tympanic membrane, and temporal artery thermometry.[16–22] Subjective determination of fever by caretakers at home is a moderately accurate predictor of fever.[23–25] A patient with a fever measured rectally at home should undergo the same evaluation as if this measurement were obtained in the ED.[4,26]

The characteristics of a patient's fever have minimal usefulness in predicting SBI. Hyperpyrexia (temperature ≥40°C) may be associated with increased rates of SBI, especially in young children.[27–31] However, the relationship between height of fever and bacterial infection in older infants and toddlers is less clear.[32–34] The duration of fever does not predict whether a child has occult bacteremia.[35] Response to antipyretic medications does not distinguish between bacterial and viral causes.[36–40] Although bundling a young child may increase the skin temperature, this does not increase the core temperature,[41] and teething does not cause fever.[42] Additional data include associated signs and symptoms, underlying medical conditions, exposure to ill contacts, recent immunizations,[43] and immunization status.[44–46]

The physical examination is a critical part of the assessment of the febrile young child. Although there is an imperfect correlation between physical examination findings and serious bacterial illness, ill-appearing children are more likely than well-appearing children to have SBI. Patients with septic shock presenting with abnormal mental status, weak peripheral pulses and cool extremities, hypotension, and/or delayed capillary refill require aggressive resuscitation and empiric antibiotic therapy.[47] In contrast, most well-appearing children do not have SBI.[48–51] The physical examination may reveal foci of infection, and the identification of a specific infection may decrease the need for additional testing. Febrile children with clinically recognizable viral conditions (eg, croup, chickenpox, and stomatitis) have lower rates of bacteremia than children with no obvious source of infection.[52]

In general, when a source of fever is identified by the history and examination, the clinician can take a more selective approach to diagnostic testing and antibiotic therapy. Young children who have fever without a localizing source of infection pose more of a management dilemma, and the approach to these children is discussed later.

Assumptions

An important limitation posed by the use of existing research as the basis of these recommendations is that most of these studies have excluded patients with preexisting medical conditions. As a result, the following recommendations presume that these children are previously healthy. In addition, most studies of febrile young infants excluded infants born prematurely. Furthermore, most of these studies also assume that these patients appear nontoxic. Patient who appear toxic (with the understanding that clinical toxicity is a subjective assessment) are more likely to have serious underlying disease and thus warrant more aggressive evaluation, empiric treatment, and hospital admission. These recommendations also require the presumption that fever in these children is caused by infection, and, although this assumption will be correct for most febrile children who present to the ED, the clinician needs to recognize that other noninfectious causes of fever (eg, Kawasaki disease, toxins, malignancy) can lead to serious outcomes and may not be identified with the general approach to febrile children with presumed infections.

FEBRILE CHILDREN LESS THAN 2 MONTHS OF AGE
Neonates: Birth to 28 Days Old

Neonates are at a particularly high risk for SBI. Most febrile neonates presenting to the ED are diagnosed as having nonspecific viral illnesses, but approximately 12% to 28% of all febrile neonates presenting to a pediatric emergency department have SBIs.[53–55] The most common bacterial infections in this are group are UTIs and occult bacteremia,[53,55] and these infections are typically caused by more virulent bacteria such as group B *Streptococcus*, *Escherichia coli*, and *Listeria monocytogenes*. In particular, group B *Streptococcus* is associated with high rates of meningitis, nonmeningeal foci of infection, and sepsis.[56] Furthermore, neonates are more likely to become infected with herpes simplex virus (HSV) infections, which may be indistinguishable from bacterial infections during the initial ED assessment.[57]

Evaluation of the febrile neonate

Historical risk factors for significant neonatal infection include maternal fever, prematurity, lethargy, seizures, and rash. Worrisome physical examination findings include temperature abnormalities (both high and low temperatures), lethargy, respiratory distress, and rash. In neonates, the presence of signs suggesting viral illness does not negate the need for a full diagnostic evaluation. Unlike older children, in whom documented respiratory syncytial virus (RSV) infections decrease the likelihood of serious bacterial illness, RSV-infected neonates have the same rate of SBI as RSV-negative neonates.[58]

The physical examination is limited in its ability to identify serious infections in neonates, and so evaluation of febrile neonates must incorporate the use of diagnostic studies. Blood, urine, and cerebrospinal fluid (CSF) cultures should be obtained in these patients.[59] A peripheral white blood cell (WBC) count is often ordered in the evaluation of febrile neonates, but the discriminatory value of the WBC count is insufficient to differentiate between patients with SBI versus nonbacterial infection.[60,61] Additional blood testing may be useful. Thrombocytopenia and increased liver enzymes are associated with herpes simplex infections.[62] No rapid test (eg, urine dipstick, standard urinalysis [UA], and enhanced UA), detects all cases of UTI, so urine cultures must be ordered in all patients.[63,64] Urine should be collected by bladder catheterization or suprapubic aspiration because bag urine specimens are associated with high rates of contamination.[65,66] Because the peripheral WBC is a poor screening test for meningitis,[67] a lumbar puncture should be performed in all febrile neonates. Chest radiographs are indicated in the presence of respiratory symptoms, and stool cultures are indicated in the presence of diarrhea.

Unlike the risk-stratification rules derived for febrile young infants, no risk assessment criteria have been created and validated specifically for neonates, and attempts to extrapolate risk-stratification rules for infants to this neonatal group have been unsuccessful. Dagan and colleagues[68] published the Rochester criteria, used in young children less than 960 days old.[69] Using these criteria, Jaskiewicz and colleagues[14] found that 2 of 227 children younger than 30 days old who met low-risk criteria had SBI. However, Ferrera and colleagues[70] found that 6% of neonates who were retrospectively classified as low risk by the Rochester criteria had SBI. Baker and colleagues[12] retrospectively classified neonates as high-risk and low-risk patients based on the Philadelphia criteria. The neonates who were placed in the high-risk category had a higher incidence of bacterial disease (18.6%), but 4.6% of neonates who were classified as low-risk patients had SBI. Kadish and colleagues[55] found a similar rate of SBI in neonates whom they categorized as low risk when they retrospectively applied both the Philadelphia criteria and the Boston criteria. Other investigators also showed low but significant rates of SBI in neonates initially classified as low risk.[54,71-73]

Treatment and disposition of the febrile neonate

The baseline rates of SBI in febrile neonates are high, and ED screening tools miss a significant number of bacterial infections. Thus, all febrile neonates should receive antibiotics. These patients are typically treated with a third-generation cephalosporins, such as cefotaxime, 50 mg/kg intravenously (IV) (100 mg/kg if there is a concern for meningitis based on CSF results), or gentamicin, 2.5 mg/kg IV. Ceftriaxone is not recommended for neonates who are jaundiced because of the concern of inducing unconjugated hyperbilirubinemia.[74,75] Ampicillin, 50 mg/kg IV (100 mg/kg IV if there is a concern for meningitis) is recommended in the empiric treatment of these patients, although the incidence of L monocytogenes is low.[76,77]

Neonatal HSV infections occur in approximately 1 per 3200 deliveries in the United States.[78] Neonates with HSV infections usually present within the first 2 weeks of life, and only a minority of infected children have fever.[79] Risk factors include primary maternal HSV infection (especially in those neonates delivered vaginally); prolonged rupture of membranes at delivery; the use of fetal scalp electrodes; skin, eye or mouth lesions; and seizures.[78,80,81] Rates of morbidity and mortality are high with neonatal HSV, and delays to treatment are common.[82,83] Acyclovir is not recommended routinely for empiric treatment in febrile neonates[79] but should be considered in neonates with risk factors for neonatal HSV, especially in neonates less than or equal to 21 days of age[84] and with CSF pleocytosis.[85] Treatment with high-dose acyclovir (20 mg/kg IV) improves outcomes in patients.[86]

Outpatient management of these patients has been suggested and occurs frequently when patients present to pediatricians' offices.[4] However, given the lack of prospective studies addressing this approach, as well as the limitations inherent in the screening evaluation in the ED and difficulties in arranging follow-up, hospitalization is strongly recommended.

Young Infants: 1 to 2 Months Old

Evaluation of the febrile young infant

Febrile young infants, defined for the purposes of this article as children between 1 and 2 months of age, are at high risk for bacterial infections. The most common cause of SBI in this age group is UTI[12,13,69,87]; young infants also develop bacteremia (most commonly from E coli),[88] and, less frequently, bacterial meningitis. Evaluation of these young infants has used various criteria to categorize patients as being at high or low risk for SBI. Because relying solely on the clinical examination results in a substantial number of missed SBI, laboratory testing is required in this age group. Although the

3 most commonly used criteria (the Rochester criteria, Boston criteria, and the Philadelphia criteria) differ in the details, they have several components in common:

- Infants must appear well
- No focal infection on physical examination
- Peripheral WBC count within a specified range
- Rapid urine testing without evidence of UTI

Patients who meet low-risk criteria are typically discharged home, whereas patients in the high-risk category are usually started on antibiotics and admitted to the hospital. These criteria are generally effective in identifying patients who are unlikely to have SBI.[89,90]

The Rochester criteria divide children less than 60 days old into high-risk and low-risk groups. The children who meet the low-risk criteria must appear well, have been previously healthy, and have no evidence of skin, soft tissue, bone, joint, or ear infection. In addition, these children must have normal peripheral WBC counts (5000–15,000/mm^3), normal absolute band counts ($\leq$1500/mm^3), less than or equal to 10 WBC/high-power field (hpf) of centrifuged urine sediment, and patients with diarrhea should have less than or equal to 5 WBC/hpf on stool smear.[68,69] Unlike the Boston and Philadelphia criteria, a lumbar puncture is not a required component of the Rochester criteria. In the original study, the Rochester criteria have a negative predictive value of 98.9%.[14]

The Boston criteria are designed for febrile children between 1 and 3 months of age who present to the ED with temperatures greater than or equal to 38.0°C. Patients meet these criteria if they appear well (not strictly defined) and had no ear, soft tissue, joint, or bone infections on physical examination. Furthermore, these patients must have CSF with less than or equal to 10 WBC/hpf, microscopic UA with less than or equal to 10 WBC/hpf or urine dipstick negative for leukocyte esterase, a peripheral WBC count of less than or equal to 20,000/mm^3, and normal findings in patients in whom a chest radiograph is obtained (all tests except the chest radiograph are performed on all patients). Infants were discharged after an intramuscular (IM) injection of ceftriaxone, 50 mg/kg. Twenty-seven of 503 children (5.4%) in the original study were later found to have SBI (bacterial gastroenteritis, UTI, and occult bacteremia).[13]

The Philadelphia criteria similarly seek to identify low-risk patients between 29 and 56 days old with temperatures of greater than or equal to 38.2°C. Patients who appear well (as defined by an Infant Observation Score of 10 or less), have a peripheral WBC count of less than or equal to 15,000/mm^3, a band/neutrophil ratio of less than or equal to 0.2, a UA with fewer than 10 WBC/hpf, few or no bacteria on a centrifuged urine specimen, CSF with fewer than 8 WBC/mm^3, a gram-negative stain, negative results on chest radiographs (obtained on all patients), and stool negative for blood and few or no WBCs on microscopy (ordered on those patients with watery diarrhea) are considered to have a negative screen and are not treated with antibiotics. In the original study, of the 747 consecutively enrolled patients, 65 (8.7%) had SBI. All 65 patients who had SBI were identified using these screening criteria. In a follow-up study (in which fever was defined as $\geq$38.0°C rectally) of 422 consecutively enrolled febrile young infants, 43 (10%) had SBI, and all 101 patients identified as low risk had no SBI. All 43 patients who had SBI were identified prospectively as high risk using the Philadelphia criteria.[91]

Blood and urine testing should be obtained in all febrile young infants. The need for lumbar puncture is controversial. Although the Boston and Philadelphia criteria require CSF analysis, the Rochester criteria do not mandate lumbar puncture. The rarity of bacterial meningitis contributes to the controversy surrounding the usefulness of the lumbar puncture. The prevalence of bacterial meningitis in febrile infants less than 3 months old is 4.1 per 1000 patients. Neither the clinical examination nor the peripheral WBC count is reliable in diagnosing meningitis in this age group[60,67]; therefore, the lumbar puncture should be strongly considered. Although an abnormally high or low peripheral WBC count may increase the concern for bacteremia or meningitis, the WBC count is an imperfect screening tool for bacteremia and meningitis and the decision to obtain blood cultures and spinal fluid should not depend on the WBC results.[60,61,67]

Chest radiographs should be obtained in young febrile infants with signs of pulmonary disease (tachypnea $\geq$50 breaths/min, rales, rhonchi, retractions, wheezing, coryza, grunting, nasal flaring, or cough).[92,93] Stool studies for WBC counts and stool cultures should be ordered in patients with diarrhea.

The results of these screening criteria help to risk stratify these young infants. The WBC count is considered abnormal if the count is greater than 15,000/mm^3 or less than 5000/mm^3 or if the band/neutrophil ratio is greater than 0.2. There should be fewer than 8 WBC/mm^3 and no organisms on Gram stain of the CSF (although sterile CSF pleocytosis can be seen in a small percentage of febrile young infants with UTIs).[94–96] The urine is considered abnormal if the urine dipstick is positive for nitrite or leukocyte esterase, if there are greater than or equal to 5 WBC/hpf on microscopy, or if bacteria are seen on a Gram stained sample of uncentrifuged urine. The most common bacterial infections in this age group are UTIs; correspondingly, the most common bacterial pathogen identified in this age group is E coli.[12,13,97] If obtained, there should be fewer than 5 WBC/hpf on the stool specimen and no evidence of pneumonia on chest radiograph.[59]

The role of viral testing in the febrile young infant
The increased availability of rapid viral testing has added new tools to the diagnostic armamentarium in the young child with fever. Traditional approaches to the febrile young child without an obvious source of infection have been directed toward the identification of an SBI. The diagnosis of viral infection is usually made if, after an evaluation for bacterial causes, no bacterial source is identified. The use of rapid viral testing has introduced evaluation and treatment options that differ from traditional approaches. Some clinicians curtail the search for a bacterial infection if a specific viral infection is identified. However, this approach assumes that the risk of SBI in patients who have positive rapid viral test results are lower than in patients who do not have positive viral test results.

Most studies of rapid viral testing include testing for RSV or influenza. Febrile young infants age 0 to 90 days (some studies analyzed patients up until 60 days of age) enrolled in studies of RSV testing have a 12.5% to 12.6% prevalence of SBI if they were tested negative for RSV, whereas patients who tested positive for RSV in these studies had lower rates of SBI, ranging from 1.15% to 7.0%.[58,98] Most of these SBIs were UTIs.

Patients who test positive for influenza have similar results. Studies of febrile young infants aged 0 to 90 days (some studies analyzed patients up until 60 days of age) undergoing influenza testing have a 13.3% to 17.5% prevalence of SBI if they tested negative for influenza, whereas patients who tested positive for influenza in these studies had significantly lower risks of SBI, ranging from 2.5% to 2.65%.[99–101] Similar to patients who tested positive for RSV, most of these SBIs were UTIs.

Febrile young infants who had positive test viral panels (RSV, influenza, parainfluenza, adenovirus, rotavirus) were at lower risk for SBI compared with infants with negative viral testing panels (4.2% vs 12.3%, $P = .0001$).[102] Patients who were diagnosed clinically with bronchiolitis in physicians' offices also had lower rates of SBI compared with those febrile infants without bronchiolitis (0% vs 11.0%, P<.001),[103] as did febrile infants hospitalized with a clinical diagnosis of bronchiolitis compared with infants who were hospitalized without clinical bronchiolitis (2.2% vs 9.6%, P = .005).[104]

Used in combination with traditional risk-stratification criteria, febrile young infants classified as low risk for SBI are more likely to have positive viral testing.[68,102] Furthermore, febrile young infants categorized as high risk using the Rochester criteria who test positive for viral infections are at lower risk for SBIs than those infants who test negative (5.5% vs 16.7%, P<.0001), although there was no statistically significant difference in rates of SBI in low-risk infants in this study (1.7% vs 3.1%, P = .4).[102] The peripheral WBC count does not help identify RSV-positive patients at higher risk for bacterial infection.[105]

The preponderance of published data show that the risk of SBI decreases in children who have positive viral tests. However, only limited data exist for febrile neonates with positive viral tests, and, in these studies, the investigators found no difference in SBI rates in neonates who were virus test positive compared with those who were virus test negative.[58,106] Furthermore, most of the SBIs in these studies were UTIs; because of the low baseline risk of bacteremia and meningitis, these studies were unable to detect a difference in risk for these infections.[107] Young infants who are RSV positive are at higher risk of serious complications, such as apnea,[108] and the clinician must evaluate and consider this concern, in addition to the other risks of SBI, when making a disposition decision. Although individual studies suggest that rapid viral testing leads to reduction in further testing for bacterial testing,[109–112] a meta-analysis of these data was insufficient to detect a difference in the rates of ancillary testing, antibiotic use, adverse events, or hospital admission in patients who underwent rapid viral testing in the ED.[113] There are insufficient data to conclude that blood and CSF cultures are unnecessary in patients with positive rapid viral tests.

Treatment and disposition of the febrile young infant

Most febrile young infants with fever without a source who are otherwise healthy and born at full term, who appear well, and who have normal results on screening evaluation can be managed on an outpatient basis. If the patient has reliable follow-up within 24 hours, the caretakers have a way of immediately accessing health care if there is a change in the patient's condition, and the parents and the primary care physician understand and agree with this plan of care, then the patient may be discharged home.

The role of empiric antibiotic therapy before discharge of low-risk patients is controversial. Published recommendations state that parenteral antibiotics should be considered if a lumbar puncture is performed.[59] Ceftriaxone, 50 mg/kg IV or IM, can be given before discharge. Although these risk-stratification algorithms perform well, a small subset of patients with SBI, including meningitis, is missed,[114,115] even with strict adherence to these criteria. In addition, there is some concern that performing a lumbar puncture in a bacteremic patient may lead to meningitis.[116,117] However, most children who meet low-risk criteria do not benefit from empiric antibiotic therapy, and so withholding antibiotics in these low-risk patients is an acceptable option. Patients who do not undergo lumbar puncture in the ED should not receive antibiotics because this confounds the evaluation for meningitis if the patient is still febrile on follow-up examination.

Patients who have abnormal test results or who appear too ill for discharge have traditionally been treated with antibiotics and hospitalized. Ceftriaxone (50 mg/kg IV or 100 mg/kg if meningitis is suspected) is commonly used for these patients.

Additional antibiotics should be considered in select circumstances (eg, ampicillin or vancomycin for suspected infection by *Listeria*, gram-positive cocci, or *Enterococcus*). Recent studies suggest that selected patients in this age group (patients who are not clinically ill, without high-risk medical history, peripheral band count of <1250 cells/μL, and peripheral absolute neutrophil count ≥1500 cells/μL) who have UTIs are at low risk for adverse sequelae[96] and may be treated on an outpatient basis, either with oral or parenteral antibiotics.[118–120]

FEBRILE YOUNG CHILDREN 2 MONTHS OF AGE AND OLDER

A temperature of 38.0°C defines a fever and is the usual threshold at which diagnostic testing is initiated in the young infant. However, in febrile children 2 months of age and older, 39.0°C is commonly used as the temperature for initiating further evaluation (some studies restrict this group to include infants 3 months of age and older), This higher temperature cutoff is used largely because, in the era before universal vaccination with the pneumococcal conjugate vaccine, there was some correlation between a patient's temperature and the risk of bacterial infection. Studies of occult bacteremia and UTIs, widely referenced in the medical literature, use this temperature as the study entry criterion.[121–124]

Evaluation of the Child 2 Months of age and Older

The history is often helpful in this age range. Parents and older children are more likely to be able to describe their complaints, and the physical examination is more informative. Clinical assessment as to whether a child appears to be well, ill, or toxic is important. A well appearance does not exclude bacteremia,[125] but children who appear toxic are more likely to have serious illness than ill-appearing or well-appearing children (92% vs 26% vs 3%, respectively).[126] Most children with fever have viral infections, and many bacterial infections can be identified by history and physical examination alone.

Most children with viral infections are diagnosed solely from clinical assessment, but viral testing can be helpful in this age group. Rapid influenza testing may result in a decreased need for diagnostic testing.[127] Febrile children between 3 and 36 months old who are influenza A positive are less likely to have SBIs than those children who are influenza A negative.[101]

In this group, some bacterial infections may be occult. The most common SBIs in this age group that may not be clinically apparent are bacteremia, UTI, and pneumonia. In the absence of a clear cause for a child's fever, diagnostic testing is frequently directed at identification of clinically inapparent bacterial infections.

Occult bacteremia

Febrile young children are at risk for bacteremia, and patients with occult bacteremia are at risk for focal infections, such as meningitis. Although some children with bacteremia may appear overtly ill, others may have occult bacteremia (ie, these children look well). In the first large series describing bacteremia in children seen in an ambulatory setting, 4.4% of febrile children had bacteremia, most commonly from *Streptococcus (diplodocus) pneumoniae* and *Haemophilus influenzae*, type b (Hib).[128] After the inclusion of the Hib vaccine into standard childhood immunization regimens starting in 1985, this pathogen was essentially eliminated as a cause of bacteremia.[121,123]

Pneumococcus has been more difficult to eradicate, and this pathogen remains the most common cause of bacteremia in this age group.[129] In 2000, a heptavalent pneumococcal conjugate vaccine (PCV7) was introduced. This introduction led to a significant reduction in invasive pneumococcal disease, particularly disease caused by the

7 most common pneumococcal serotypes causing invasive pneumococcal disease, and it conferred some protection against some related nonvaccine serotypes and in unimmunized populations through herd immunity.[130–134] Although the overall rate of invasive pneumococcal disease has decreased, this has been tempered by the emerging role of invasive pneumococcal disease caused by serotypes not included in PCV7.[133,135–138] A new pneumococcal conjugate vaccine covering 13 serotypes (PCV13) was licensed in 2010,[139] which includes coverage for 6 additional serotypes. Although this vaccine's efficacy has been shown in prelicensure studies, no epidemiologic studies in the PCV13 era have been published. The full vaccination regimen is a 4-dose series (given at 2, 4, 6, and 12–15 months of age), but significant protection is conferred with at least 2 doses of this vaccine.[140,141]

The second most common cause of bacteremia is *E coli*.[129] *E coli* bacteremia is more common in children younger than 12 months, and most common in children 3 to 6 months of age. *E coli* bacteremia is usually associated with a concomitant UTI[142,143]; in one study, all 27 patients identified with *E coli* bacteremia had UTIs.[129] *Salmonella* causes 4% to 8% of occult bacteremia, occurring in 0.1% of all children 3 to 36 months old who have temperatures greater than or equal to 39.0°C.[121–123,129] Although most of patients with salmonella bacteremia have diarrhea, 5% have primary bacteremia.

Neisseria meningitidis is an infrequent cause of bacteremia but is associated with high rates of morbidity and mortality, and invasive meningococcal disease disproportionately affects young children.[144] These patients are usually overtly sick; however, 12% to 16% of patients with meningococcal disease have unsuspected infection[145–147]; 0.02% of children who appeared to be nontoxic and had temperatures greater than or equal to 39.0°C had meningococcemia.[121,123] Risk factors for meningococcal bacteremia include contact with patients with meningococcal disease, periods of meningococcal disease outbreaks, and presence of fever and petechiae.[148–150]

This changing epidemiology has added to the confusion regarding the usefulness of blood testing in the identification of occult bacteremia. The gold standard for detection of occult bacteremia, the blood culture, is limited by the inability to get results back immediately and by the high rates of contamination. The incidence of true-positive blood cultures in children who present to the ED is less than 1%,[34,130,151–153] and the rate of contaminated blood cultures exceeds the rate of true-positive cultures.[34,121,123,129,154–156] Furthermore, surrogate tests used as predictors of bacteremia are inaccurate. The peripheral WBC count has been the most commonly used test for this purpose. Although there is an increased risk of bacteremia with an increasing WBC count, the sensitivity and specificity of a WBC count greater than or equal to 15,000/mm^3 are only 42% to 86% and 74% to 77%, respectively.[34,123,129,157,158] In the PCV7 era, the positive predictive value of a WBC count greater than or equal to 15,000/mm^3 for detecting bacteremia is 1.5% to 3.2%.[34,155] Patients with *E coli* bacteremia were more likely to have increased WBC counts compared with control subjects without bacteremia.[129] However, the WBC counts in patients with *Salmonella*, *Staphylococcus aureus*, and *N meningitidis* bacteremia do not differ from control patients without bacteremia. Most patients with salmonella bacteremia have peripheral WBC counts in the normal range.[159–162] Although there is an association between younger age and increased band count with meningococcal disease, the positive predictive values of these variables are low, given the low prevalence of this disease, and routine screening for all young febrile children with complete blood counts for meningococcal bacteremia is not useful.[145]

Other blood tests used in screening patients for SBIs perform only marginally better than the peripheral WBC count. Most studies show that both the C-reactive protein[163–165] and procalcitonin[166–172] performed better than the peripheral WBC count in detecting SBIs, with procalcitonin having a higher sensitivity (83%, 95% confidence interval [CI] 70%–91%) than the C-reactive protein (74%, 95% CI 49%–67%) and peripheral WBC count (58%, 95% CI 49%–67%).[173] Given the observed decline in invasive pneumococcal disease; the inconsistent relationship between height of fever and rates of bacteremia; the strong association between E coli UTIs and E coli bacteremia; the relative infrequency of meningococcemia and salmonella bacteremia; and the limited value of the WBC count, C-reactive protein, and procalcitonin, routine blood testing including cultures, and empiric antibiotics therapy are not warranted in children who have received at least 2 Hib and PCV vaccinations.[129,155,174,175]

UTI

UTIs are common sources of fever in young children and, left untreated, can lead to renal damage. Despite the high disease prevalence, this diagnosis is often missed. In older children, historical and examination features such as dysuria, urinary frequency, and abdominal and flank pain may suggest UTI. However, in young children, symptoms are usually nonspecific and the only suggestion of a UTI may be fever.

Although the overall prevalence of UTIs in young children with fever and no obvious source is 7%,[176] differing population subgroups are at higher and lower risk for UTIs. Circumcised boys aged 12 to 24 months with fever and no source have a UTI prevalence of less than 1%, whereas uncircumcised boys aged 0 to 3 months have a UTI prevalence of 20.1%.[176] UTIs were found in 2.7% to 3.5% of febrile children even when these patients had other potential sources of fever (eg, gastroenteritis, otitis media, upper respiratory tract infection, and nonspecific rash).[177,178]

Risk factors for UTI include young age, uncircumcised status, female sex (girls are at higher risk for UTIs than boys in all age categories except for young uncircumcised boys), and nonblack race. Urine testing is generally indicated in girls younger than 2 years with at least 1 risk factor for UTI (history of UTI, temperature >39°C, fever without other apparent source, ill appearance, suprapubic tenderness, fever >24 hours, or nonblack race).[179] Circumcised boys between 3 months and 2 years of age without suprapubic tenderness or with no more than 1 risk factor for UTI (temperature ≥39°C, fever without other apparent source, fever >24 hours, or nonblack race) have a probability of UTI of less than or equal to 2%.[66,179] There are limited data to determine when the risk of UTI in uncircumcised boys decreases to that of circumcised boys, but the increased risk of UTI persists until at least 12 months of age.[178] Some investigators advocate urine testing in uncircumcised up to 2 years of age.[179]

Several rapid urine tests have good sensitivity for detecting UTIs. Enhanced UA (≥10 WBC/hpf or bacteria on Gram stained, uncentrifuged urine)[63,180] or a combination of greater than or equal to 10 WBC/hpf and bacteriuria (on either centrifuged or uncentrifuged urine)[181] are good screening tests. The more readily available urine dipstick (positive for either leukocyte esterase or nitrites) has a sensitivity of 88%.[63] However, because no rapid screening test detects all UTIs, urine cultures should be ordered on all of these patients.[182]

Pneumonia

Young children commonly develop pneumonia, and the most common pathogens are viruses and S pneumoniae.[183] Other pathogens, such as Mycoplasma pneumoniae and S aureus are uncommon in this age range but are emerging as more frequently recognized causes of pneumonia.[184] Group A *Streptococcus*, *Bordetella pertussis*, mycobacterial infections, and fungal infections are rare in young children.

With routine pneumococcal vaccination, all-cause hospital admissions for pneumonia have declined,[185] but pneumonia still presents a significant diagnostic challenge, because the diagnosis of pneumonia based on clinical examination can be difficult.[186] Physician assessment of pneumonia based on history and physical examination findings is only moderately correlated with the radiographic diagnosis of pneumonia.[187] A history of fever and prolonged cough is weakly associated with the presence of pneumonia.[188] Tachypnea as an isolated physical examination finding poorly predicts pneumonia.[189,190] Wheezing as an isolated physical examination finding is not seen commonly in pneumonia.[191] The presence of any pulmonary findings on examination (eg, tachypnea, crackles, respiratory distress, or decreased breath sounds) increases the likelihood of pneumonia, and, conversely, the absence of these findings decreases the likelihood of pneumonia.[192–194] The role of pulse oximetry in detecting pneumonia is unclear; more specifically, although a low pulse oximetry reading is associated with poor outcome in pneumonia, a normal pulse oximetry reading may not exclude the diagnosis of pneumonia.[195–197]

Evaluation of pneumonia is further complicated by the lack of a diagnostic standard.[198] Once considered the gold standard for diagnosing pneumonia, the interpretation of chest radiographs is subject to significant variation, even by pediatric radiologists.[199] In addition, clinical symptoms do not reliably distinguish between bacterial and nonbacterial causes of pneumonia,[200] nor does laboratory testing[201] or radiologic findings.[202,203] Viral testing can be obtained in the evaluation of children with community-acquired pneumonia, because positive viral testing may reduce the need for further evaluation.[204] However, a positive viral test does not necessarily negate the need for antibiotics, because viral coinfection with bacterial pneumonia is common.[205,206] Although serologic testing for *M pneumoniae* can be performed in patients with this suspected diagnosis, no rapid tests to help identify specific bacterial causes of pneumonia are widely available.

Some cases of pneumonia may be clinically occult. A retrospective study after universal PCV7 vaccination showed a 5% occult (ie, no respiratory distress, no tachypnea or hypoxia, and no lower respiratory tract abnormalities on examination) pneumonia rate in patients selected to get chest radiographs. A chest radiograph should be obtained in febrile children if there are physical examination findings with suspected or documented hypoxemia or significant respiratory distress.[204] In patients with suspected pneumonia who look well enough to be treated on an outpatient basis, a chest radiograph may be unnecessary.[207] Obtaining chest radiographs in well-appearing febrile children without respiratory symptoms is generally not indicated.

Treatment and disposition of febrile older infants and toddlers

Most febrile patients in the age group who do not have focal sources of infection do not require antibiotic therapy and can be discharged home. Those patients with suspected bacteremia, UTI, or pneumonia require antibiotic treatment, although only a small proportion of these patients require hospital admission.

Suspected bacteremia The role of antibiotics in children thought to be at high risk for bacteremia is controversial. Using pre-PCV7 data, ceftriaxone was shown to prevent SBI in patients with proven occult bacteremia, although 284 patients at risk for bacteremia would need to be treated with antibiotics to prevent 1 case of meningitis.[208] The bacteremia resolves spontaneously in most patients with pneumococcal bacteremia, which complicates this analysis.[121] Focal infections develop in 15% of bacteremic children[121] and 2.7% to 5.8% of patients with occult pneumococcal bacteremia develop meningitis.[208,209] With the significant decrease in invasive pneumococcal disease[132,210,211] many more children will be treated unnecessarily with antibiotics to prevent a single serious outcome. Thus, empiric antibiotic therapy is generally not warranted, even for patients in whom blood cultures are obtained, and antibiotics should not be given to patients who do not undergo blood culture testing. Patients who had unsuspected meningococcal disease who were treated empirically with antibiotics had fewer complications than patients who were untreated, but there were no differences in rates of permanent sequelae or death.[212] However, given the significantly high rates of morbidity and mortality, testing and empiric treatment may be warranted for children at high risk for meningococcal disease.

Suspected UTI Any positive results from a rapid test should lead to a presumptive diagnosis of a UTI, and antibiotic treatment should be initiated. Most patients with UTIs who appear well can be treated on an outpatient basis with oral antibiotics.[119,204,213] Empiric antibiotic therapy should be tailored to local bacterial epidemiology, but empiric therapy should be directed toward E coli, the most common cause of UTI. The duration of therapy should be from 7 to 14 days.[66]

Suspected pneumonia Most young children with occult pneumonia have viral pneumonia and do not require antibiotic treatment. However, young children with suspected mild to moderate bacterial pneumonia, high-dose amoxicillin is the first-line agent (90 mg/kg divided into 2 daily doses), because this agent is effective against S pneumoniae.[204,207] Although M pneumoniae infection is uncommon in this age group (and mild cases may resolve without antibiotics),[214] azithromycin or other macrolide antibiotics can be used in suspected or confirmed mycoplasma infection.[204,207] Anti-influenza therapy should be initiated if influenza is thought to be either the primary infectious cause or if there is concern for influenza coinfection in someone with suspected bacterial pneumonia.

No decision rules exist for pediatric pneumonia that help with disposition decisions in children who have pneumonia, but most patients are treated on an outpatient basis. Indications for admission for children with community-acquired pneumonia include those children with moderate to severe pneumonia (eg, respiratory distress, hypoxia), infants less than 3 to 6 months of age with suspected bacterial pneumonia, suspected or documented infection by a pathogen with increased virulence (eg, methicillin-resistant S aureus), poor feeding or an inability to take oral medications, and children in whom follow-up or close home observation cannot be ensured.[204,207] Patients who are discharged may benefit from a first dose of parenteral antibiotics in the ED.[215] Patients who need hospital admission should receive ampicillin or ceftriaxone as empiric initial therapy; vancomycin or clindamycin should be also be given to those patients with suspected methicillin-resistant S aureus.[204]

SUMMARY

Fever is a common presenting complaint in children who seek ED care. Most of these children have benign viral infections that cause their febrile illnesses, and most of these children recover fully with only supportive care. However, a small percentage of these patients have serious underlying (typically bacterial) causes of fever and require antibiotic therapy and hospital admission. The challenge for the emergency physician is to categorize patients into groups that are at high risk and low risk for serious outcomes (**Fig. 1**).

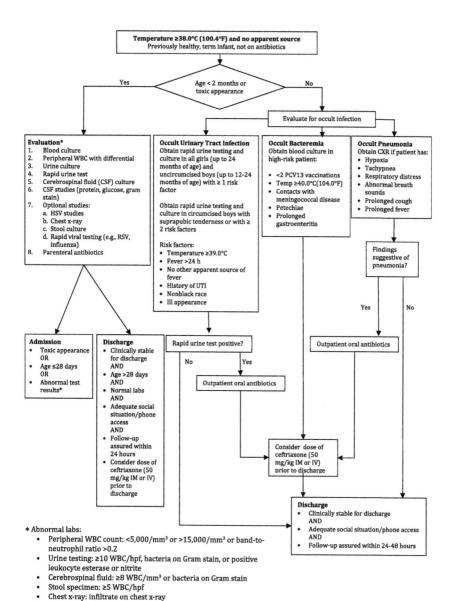

* Abnormal labs:
  * Peripheral WBC count: <5,000/mm³ or >15,000/mm³ or band-to-neutrophil ratio >0.2
  * Urine testing: ≥10 WBC/hpf, bacteria on Gram stain, or positive leukocyte esterase or nitrite
  * Cerebrospinal fluid: ≥8 WBC/mm³ or bacteria on Gram stain
  * Stool specimen: ≥5 WBC/hpf
  * Chest x-ray: infiltrate on chest x-ray

[a]Chest x-rays are indicated in patients with hypoxia, tachypnea, abnormal lung sounds, or respiratory distress. Stool studies are indicated in patients with diarrhea. Herpes simplex virus testing should be considered in the presence of risk factors (e.g., primary maternal infection, prolonged rupture of membranes, use of fetal scalp electrodes, skin, eye, or mouth lesions, seizures, CSF pleocytosis, hemorrhagic CSF). HSV testing is best accomplished by polymerase chain reaction or viral culture. Neonates should receive both ampicillin (50 mg/kg IV; 100 mg/kg IV if concern for meningitis) and cefotaxime (50 mg/kg; 100 mg/kg IV if concern for meningitis). Older children should receive ceftriaxone (50 mg/kg IV; 100 mg/kg IV if concern for meningitis).

Fig. 1. Fever without apparent source in children 0 to 24 months of age. CXR, chest radiograph.

Initial assessment of the febrile young child includes the patient's initial appearance. Children who appear toxic require a comprehensive evaluation, antibiotic treatment, and hospital admission. Furthermore, patients with underlying medical conditions, particularly with medical conditions that cause immunocompromise, are at high risk for serious infectious complications and generally require more comprehensive evaluation than previously healthy children. Children with prolonged fever or children who present to the ED while already taking antibiotics require individualized assessment, because these fevers may be caused by viral illnesses or incompletely treated bacterial infections.

Children can also be categorized as being at high or low risk for serious infection based on age. The febrile neonate is at high risk, even with a normal examination and normal screening laboratory results. These patients need blood, urine, and CSF cultures. Selected patients need HSV testing, as well as chest radiographs and stool cultures. All febrile neonates should receive empiric antibiotic coverage, typically with ampicillin and cefotaxime or gentamicin. Patients thought to be at risk for HSV infection should receive acyclovir as well.

Febrile young infants are a more heterogeneous group. Although these patients are at higher risk for serious infection compared with older children, these patients can be stratified into high-risk and low-risk categories based on results of diagnostic tests. These patients need complete blood counts, blood cultures, urinalyses, and urine cultures. A lumbar puncture with CSF analysis, Gram stain, and culture should be strongly considered because other laboratory tests such as the WBC count are inaccurate in predicting which patients have meningitis. There is insufficient evidence to conclude that blood cultures and lumbar punctures are unnecessary in patients with positive rapid viral testing.

When clinically indicated, chest radiographs and stool studies should be obtained as well. If these test findings are abnormal, these patients should receive ceftriaxone and should be admitted to the hospital. If these initial laboratory results are normal, a patient can be discharged if follow-up within 24 hours can be ensured. A dose of intramuscular ceftriaxone can be considered in patients who have undergone blood, urine, and CSF testing before ED discharge.

The older infant or toddler who has a temperature of greater than or equal to 39.0°C may be evaluated more selectively. For patients who have had at least 2 PCV13 doses, blood testing is generally not indicated in the absence of risk factors for bacteremia (such as high temperatures, petechial rash, or prolonged diarrhea) because the baseline incidence of bacteremia is less than 1%. For those patients who have received fewer than 2 PCV13 doses, blood cultures should be considered, especially for those patients with risk factors for bacteremia. A peripheral WBC count is of limited usefulness, because patients can have bacteremia with normal WBC counts, and, conversely, most patients with increased white blood counts do not have bacteremia. Empiric antibiotics are generally not indicated unless there is a concern for meningococcemia.

Urine testing (typically urethral catheterization and urine culture) is generally indicated in girls younger than 2 years and uncircumcised boys (at least up to age 12 months) with at least 1 risk factor for UTI: history of UTI, temperature greater than 39°C, fever without other apparent source, ill appearance, suprapubic tenderness, fever for longer than 24 hours, or nonblack race. Urine testing can be considered in circumcised boys between 3 months and 2 years of age with suprapubic tenderness or at least 2 of these risk factors for UTI, although the risk of UTI is low. Chest radiographs should be obtained in children with hypoxia or respiratory distress. In addition, a chest radiograph should be considered in a child with prolonged fever and cough.

It is critically important to recognize that these strategies for evaluating and managing febrile young children assist with risk stratification. A systematic plan for the evaluation and treatment of the febrile child may help reduce both unnecessary testing and morbidity associated with serious infection. However, no combination of clinical assessment and diagnostic testing can successfully identify all patients with serious infections at the time of initial presentation. Therefore, the importance of timely reassessment (even for the child with initially normal test results or for the child who has received antibiotic therapy) cannot be overemphasized, and any standardized approach to the febrile young child should serve as an adjunct to, and not a replacement for, the judgment of the treating clinician.

REFERENCES

1. Alpern ER, Stanley RM, Gorelick MH, et al. Epidemiology of a pediatric emergency medicine research network: the PECARN Core Data Project. Pediatr Emerg Care 2006;22(10):689–99.
2. Centers for Disease Control and Prevention/National Center for Health Statistics. NAMCS and NHAMCS web tables: 2010 NHAMCS emergency department summary tables. 2010. Available at: http://www.cdc.gov/nchs/data/ahcd/nhamcs_emergency/2010_ed_web_tables.pdf. Accessed February 15, 2013.
3. Isaacman DJ, Kaminer K, Veligeti H, et al. Comparative practice patterns of emergency medicine physicians and pediatric emergency medicine physicians managing fever in young children. Pediatrics 2001;108(2):354–8.
4. Pantell RH, Newman TB, Bernzweig J, et al. Management and outcomes of care of fever in early infancy. JAMA 2004;291(10):1203–12.
5. Belfer RA, Gittelman MA, Muniz AE. Management of febrile infants and children by pediatric emergency medicine and emergency medicine: comparison with practice guidelines. Pediatr Emerg Care 2001;17(2):83–7.
6. Seow VK, Lin AC, Lin IY, et al. Comparing different patterns for managing febrile children in the ED between emergency and pediatric physicians: impact on patient outcome. Am J Emerg Med 2007;25(9):1004–8.
7. Goldman RD, Scolnik D, Chauvin-Kimoff L, et al. Practice variations in the treatment of febrile infants among pediatric emergency physicians. Pediatrics 2009; 124(2):439–45.
8. Bergman DA, Mayer ML, Pantell RH, et al. Does clinical presentation explain practice variability in the treatment of febrile infants? Pediatrics 2006;117(3): 787–95.
9. Madsen KA, Bennett JE, Downs SM. The role of parental preferences in the management of fever without source among 3- to 36-month-old children: a decision analysis. Pediatrics 2006;117(4):1067–76.
10. Condra CS, Parbhu B, Lorenz D, et al. Charges and complications associated with the medical evaluation of febrile young infants. Pediatr Emerg Care 2010; 26(3):186–91.
11. Bennett JE, Sumner Ii W, Downs SM, et al. Parents' utilities for outcomes of occult bacteremia. Arch Pediatr Adolesc Med 2000;154(1):43–8.
12. Baker MD, Bell LM, Avner JR. Outpatient management without antibiotics of fever in selected infants. N Engl J Med 1993;329(20):1437–41.
13. Baskin MN, O'Rourke EJ, Fleisher GR. Outpatient treatment of febrile infants 28 to 89 days of age with intramuscular administration of ceftriaxone. J Pediatr 1992;120(1):22–7.

14. Jaskiewicz JA, McCarthy CA, Richardson AC, et al. Febrile infants at low risk for serious bacterial infection–an appraisal of the Rochester criteria and implications for management. Pediatrics 1994;94(3):390–6.

15. Alpern E, Henretig F. Fever. In: Fleisher G, et al, editors. Textbook of pediatric emergency medicine. Philadelphia: Lippincott Williams & Wilkins; 2010. p. 266–75.

16. Craig JV, Lancaster GA, Taylor S, et al. Infrared ear thermometry compared with rectal thermometry in children: a systematic review. Lancet 2002;360(9333): 603–9.

17. Craig JV, Lancaster GA, Williamson PR, et al. Temperature measured at the axilla compared with rectum in children and young people: systematic review. BMJ 2000;320(7243):1174–8.

18. Greenes DS, Fleisher GR. When body temperature changes, does rectal temperature lag? J Pediatr 2004;144(6):824.

19. Greenes DS, Fleisher GR. Accuracy of a noninvasive temporal artery thermometer for use in infants. Arch Pediatr Adolesc Med 2001;155(3):376–81.

20. Jean-Mary MB, Dicanzio J, Shaw J, et al. Limited accuracy and reliability of infrared axillary and aural thermometers in a pediatric outpatient population. J Pediatr 2002;141(5):671–6.

21. National Collaborating Centre for Women's and Children's Health. Feverish illness in children: assessment and initial management in children younger than 5 years. London (United Kingdom): RCOG press; 2007.

22. Schuh S, Komar L, Stephens D, et al. Comparison of the temporal artery and rectal thermometry in children in the emergency department. Pediatr Emerg Care 2004;20(11):736–41.

23. Banco L, Veltri D. Ability of mothers to subjectively assess the presence of fever in their children. Am J Dis Child 1984;138(10):976–8.

24. Graneto JW, Soglin DF. Maternal screening of childhood fever by palpation. Pediatr Emerg Care 1996;12(3):183–4.

25. Hooker EA, Smith SW, Miles T, et al. Subjective assessment of fever by parents: comparison with measurement by noncontact tympanic thermometer and calibrated rectal glass mercury thermometer. Ann Emerg Med 1996;28(3):313–7.

26. Yarden-Bilavsky H, Bilavsky E, Amir J, et al. Serious bacterial infections in neonates with fever by history only versus documented fever. Scand J Infect Dis 2010;42(11–12):812–6.

27. Kuppermann N, Fleisher G, Jaffe D. Predictors of occult pneumococcal bacteremia in young febrile children. Ann Emerg Med 1998;31(6):679–87.

28. Bonadio WA, Smith DS, Sabnis S, et al. Relationship of fever magnitude to rate of serious bacterial infections in infants aged 4-8 weeks. Clin Pediatr (Phila) 1991;30(8):478–80.

29. Bonadio WA, Smith DS, Sabnis S. The clinical characteristics and infectious outcomes of febrile infants aged 8 to 12 weeks. Clin Pediatr (Phila) 1994;33(2): 95–9.

30. Stanley R, Pagon Z, Bachur R. Hyperpyrexia among infants younger than 3 months. Pediatr Emerg Care 2005;21(5):291–4.

31. Zorc JJ, Levine DA, Platt SL, et al. Clinical and demographic factors associated with urinary tract infection in young febrile infants. Pediatrics 2005;116(3):644–8.

32. Hsiao AL, Chen L, Baker MD. Incidence and predictors of serious bacterial infections among 57- to 180-day-old infants. Pediatrics 2006;117(5):1695–701.

33. Trautner BW, Caviness AC, Gerlacher GR, et al. Prospective evaluation of the risk of serious bacterial infection in children who present to the emergency

department with hyperpyrexia (temperature of 106 degrees F or higher). Pediatrics 2006;118(1):34–40.

34. Rudinsky SL, Carstairs KL, Reardon JM, et al. Serious bacterial infections in febrile infants in the post-pneumococcal conjugate vaccine era. Acad Emerg Med 2009;16(7):585–90.

35. Teach SJ, Fleisher GR. Duration of fever and its relationship to bacteremia in febrile outpatients three to 36 months old. The Occult Bacteremia Study Group. Pediatr Emerg Care 1997;13(5):317–9.

36. Baker MD, Fosarelli PD, Carpenter RO. Childhood fever: correlation of diagnosis with temperature response to acetaminophen. Pediatrics 1987;80(3):315–8.

37. Baker RC, Tiller T, Bausher JC, et al. Severity of disease correlated with fever reduction in febrile infants. Pediatrics 1989;83(6):1016–9.

38. Huang SY, Greenes DS. Effect of recent antipyretic use on measured fever in the pediatric emergency department. Arch Pediatr Adolesc Med 2004;158(10):972–6.

39. Torrey SB, Henretig F, Fleisher G, et al. Temperature response to antipyretic therapy in children: relationship to occult bacteremia. Am J Emerg Med 1985;3(3):190.

40. Yamamoto LT, Wigder HN, Fligner DJ, et al. Relationship of bacteremia to antipyretic therapy in febrile children. Pediatr Emerg Care 1987;3(4):223–7.

41. Grover G, Berkowitz CD, Thompson M, et al. The effects of bundling on infant temperature. Pediatrics 1994;94(5):669–73.

42. Ramos-Jorge J, Pordeus IA, Ramos-Jorge ML, et al. Prospective longitudinal study of signs and symptoms associated with primary tooth eruption. Pediatrics 2011;128(3):471–6.

43. Wolff M, Bachur R. Serious bacterial infection in recently immunized young febrile infants. Acad Emerg Med 2009;16(12):1284–9.

44. AbdelSalam HH, Sokal MM. Accuracy of parental reporting of immunization. Clin Pediatr (Phila) 2004;43(1):83–5.

45. Williams ER, Meza YE, Salazar S, et al. Immunization histories given by adult caregivers accompanying children 3-36 months to the emergency department: are their histories valid for the *Haemophilus influenzae* B and pneumococcal vaccines? Pediatr Emerg Care 2007;23(5):285–8.

46. Suarez L, Simpson DM, Smith DR. Errors and correlates in parental recall of child immunizations: effects on vaccination coverage estimates. Pediatrics 1997;99(5):E3.

47. Dellinger RP, Levy MM, Rhodes A, et al. Surviving sepsis campaign: international guidelines for management of severe sepsis and septic shock: 2012. Crit Care Med 2013;41(2):580–637.

48. Bonadio WA. The history and physical assessments of the febrile infant. Pediatr Clin North Am 1998;45(1):65–77.

49. Bonadio WA, Hennes H, Smith D, et al. Reliability of observation variables in distinguishing infectious outcome of febrile young infants. Pediatr Infect Dis J 1993;12(2):111–4.

50. McCarthy PL, Lembo RM, Fink HD, et al. Observation, history, and physical examination in diagnosis of serious illnesses in febrile children less than or equal to 24 months. J Pediatr 1987;110(1):26–30.

51. McCarthy PL, Lembo RM, Baron MA, et al. Predictive value of abnormal physical examination findings in ill-appearing and well-appearing febrile children. Pediatrics 1985;76(2):167–71.

52. Greenes DS, Harper MB. Low risk of bacteremia in febrile children with recognizable viral syndromes. Pediatr Infect Dis J 1999;18(3):258–61.

53. Baker MD, Bell LM. Unpredictability of serious bacterial illness in febrile infants from birth to 1 month of age. Arch Pediatr Adolesc Med 1999;153(5):508–11.
54. Chiu CH, Lin TY, Bullard MJ. Identification of febrile neonates unlikely to have bacterial infections. Pediatr Infect Dis J 1997;16(1):59–63.
55. Kadish HA, Loveridge B, Tobey J, et al. Applying outpatient protocols in febrile infants 1-28 days of age: can the threshold be lowered? Clin Pediatr (Phila) 2000;39(2):81–8.
56. Pena BM, Harper MB, Fleisher GR. Occult bacteremia with group B streptococci in an outpatient setting. Pediatrics 1998;102(1 Pt 1):67–72.
57. Caviness AC, Demmler GJ, Almendarez Y, et al. The prevalence of neonatal herpes simplex virus infection compared with serious bacterial illness in hospitalized neonates. J Pediatr 2008;153(2):164–9.
58. Levine DA, Platt SL, Dayan PS, et al. Risk of serious bacterial infection in young febrile infants with respiratory syncytial virus infections. Pediatrics 2004;113(6):1728–34.
59. Baraff L. Management of fever without source in infants and children. Ann Emerg Med 2000;36(6):602–14.
60. Bonsu BK, Harper MB. A low peripheral blood white blood cell count in infants younger than 90 days increases the odds of acute bacterial meningitis relative to bacteremia. Acad Emerg Med 2004;11(12):1297–301.
61. Bonsu BK, Harper MB. Identifying febrile young infants with bacteremia: is the peripheral white blood cell count an accurate screen? Ann Emerg Med 2003;42(2):216–25.
62. Caviness AC, Demmler GJ, Selwyn BJ. Clinical and laboratory features of neonatal herpes simplex virus infection: a case-control study. Pediatr Infect Dis J 2008;27(5):425–30.
63. Gorelick MH, Shaw KN. Screening tests for urinary tract infection in children: a meta-analysis. Pediatrics 1999;104(5):e54.
64. Shaw KN, McGowan KL, Gorelick MH, et al. Screening for urinary tract infection in infants in the emergency department: which test is best? Pediatrics 1998;101(6):E1.
65. Etoubleau C, Reveret M, Brouet D, et al. Moving from bag to catheter for urine collection in non-toilet-trained children suspected of having urinary tract infection: a paired comparison of urine cultures. J Pediatr 2009;154(6):803–6.
66. Roberts KB. Urinary tract infection: clinical practice guideline for the diagnosis and management of the initial UTI in febrile infants and children 2 to 24 months. Pediatrics 2011;128(3):595–610.
67. Bonsu BK, Harper MB. Utility of the peripheral blood white blood cell count for identifying sick young infants who need lumbar puncture. Ann Emerg Med 2003;41(2):206–14.
68. Dagan R, Powell KR, Hall CB, et al. Identification of infants unlikely to have serious bacterial infection although hospitalized for suspected sepsis. J Pediatr 1985;107(6):855–60.
69. Dagan R, Sofer S, Phillip M, et al. Ambulatory care of febrile infants younger than 2 months of age classified as being at low risk for having serious bacterial infections. J Pediatr 1988;112(3):355–60.
70. Ferrera PC, Bartfield JM, Snyder HS. Neonatal fever: utility of the Rochester criteria in determining low risk for serious bacterial infections. Am J Emerg Med 1997;15(3):299–302.
71. Chiu CH, Lin TY, Bullard MJ. Application of criteria identifying febrile outpatient neonates at low risk for bacterial infections. Pediatr Infect Dis J 1994;13(11):946–9.

72. Schwartz S, Raveh D, Toker O, et al. A week-by-week analysis of the low-risk criteria for serious bacterial infection in febrile neonates. Arch Dis Child 2009; 94(4):287–92.
73. Marom R, Sakran W, Antonelli J, et al. Quick identification of febrile neonates with low risk for serious bacterial infection: an observational study. Arch Dis Child Fetal Neonatal Ed 2007;92(1):F15–8.
74. Martin E, Fanconi S, Kalin P, et al. Ceftriaxone–bilirubin-albumin interactions in the neonate: an in vivo study. Eur J Pediatr 1993;152(6):530–4.
75. Robertson A, Fink S, Karp W. Effect of cephalosporins on bilirubin-albumin binding. J Pediatr 1988;112(2):291–4.
76. Sadow KB, Derr R, Teach SJ. Bacterial infections in infants 60 days and younger: epidemiology, resistance, and implications for treatment. Arch Pediatr Adolesc Med 1999;153(6):611–4.
77. Greenhow TL, Hung YY, Herz AM. Changing epidemiology of bacteremia in infants aged 1 week to 3 months. Pediatrics 2012;129(3):e590–6.
78. Brown ZA, Wald A, Morrow RA, et al. Effect of serologic status and cesarean delivery on transmission rates of herpes simplex virus from mother to infant. JAMA 2003;289(2):203–9.
79. Kimberlin DW, Lin CY, Jacobs RF, et al. Natural history of neonatal herpes simplex virus infections in the acyclovir era. Pediatrics 2001;108(2):223–9.
80. Kimberlin D. Herpes simplex virus, meningitis and encephalitis in neonates. Herpes 2004;11(Suppl 2):65A–76A.
81. Kimberlin DW. Neonatal herpes simplex infection. Clin Microbiol Rev 2004;17(1): 1–13.
82. Kimberlin DW, Whitley RJ. Neonatal herpes: what have we learned. Semin Pediatr Infect Dis 2005;16(1):7–16.
83. Benson PC, Swadron SP. Empiric acyclovir is infrequently initiated in the emergency department to patients ultimately diagnosed with encephalitis. Ann Emerg Med 2006;47(1):100–5.
84. Long SS, Pool TE, Vodzak J, et al. Herpes simplex virus infection in young infants during 2 decades of empiric acyclovir therapy. Pediatr Infect Dis J 2011;30(7):556–61.
85. Caviness AC, Demmler GJ, Swint JM, et al. Cost-effectiveness analysis of herpes simplex virus testing and treatment strategies in febrile neonates. Arch Pediatr Adolesc Med 2008;162(7):665–74.
86. Kimberlin DW, Lin CY, Jacobs RF, et al. Safety and efficacy of high-dose intravenous acyclovir in the management of neonatal herpes simplex virus infections. Pediatrics 2001;108(2):230–8.
87. Morley EJ, Lapoint JM, Roy LW, et al. Rates of positive blood, urine, and cerebrospinal fluid cultures in children younger than 60 days during the vaccination era. Pediatr Emerg Care 2012;28(2):125–30.
88. Gomez B, Mintegi S, Benito J, et al. Blood culture and bacteremia predictors in infants less than three months of age with fever without source. Pediatr Infect Dis J 2010;29(1):43–7.
89. Huppler AR, Eickhoff JC, Wald ER. Performance of low-risk criteria in the evaluation of young infants with fever: review of the literature. Pediatrics 2010;125(2):228–33.
90. Garra G, Cunningham SJ, Crain EF. Reappraisal of criteria used to predict serious bacterial illness in febrile infants less than 8 weeks of age. Acad Emerg Med 2005;12(10):921–5.
91. Baker MD, Bell LM, Avner JR. The efficacy of routine outpatient management without antibiotics of fever in selected infants. Pediatrics 1999;103(3):627–31.

92. American College of Emergency Physicians Clinical Policies Committee, American College of Emergency Physicians Clinical Policies Subcommittee on Pediatric Fever. Clinical policy for children younger than three years presenting to the emergency department with fever. Ann Emerg Med 2003;42(4):530–45.

93. Bramson RT, Meyer TL, Silbiger ML, et al. The futility of the chest radiograph in the febrile infant without respiratory symptoms. Pediatrics 1993;92(4):524–6.

94. Shah SS, Zorc JJ, Levine DA, et al. Sterile cerebrospinal fluid pleocytosis in young infants with urinary tract infections. J Pediatr 2008;153(2):290–2.

95. Yam AO, Andresen D, Kesson AM, et al. Incidence of sterile cerebrospinal fluid pleocytosis in infants with urinary tract infection. J Paediatr Child Health 2009; 45(6):364–7.

96. Schnadower D, Kuppermann N, Macias CG, et al. Febrile infants with urinary tract infections at very low risk for adverse events and bacteremia. Pediatrics 2010;126(6):1074–83.

97. Byington CL, Rittichier KK, Bassett KE, et al. Serious bacterial infections in febrile infants younger than 90 days of age: the importance of ampicillin-resistant pathogens. Pediatrics 2003;111(5 Pt 1):964–8.

98. Titus MO, Wright SW. Prevalence of serious bacterial infections in febrile infants with respiratory syncytial virus infection. Pediatrics 2003;112(2):282–4.

99. Krief WI, Levine DA, Platt SL, et al. Influenza virus infection and the risk of serious bacterial infections in young febrile infants. Pediatrics 2009;124(1):30–9.

100. Mintegi S, Garcia-Garcia JJ, Benito J, et al. Rapid influenza test in young febrile infants for the identification of low-risk patients. Pediatr Infect Dis J 2009;28(11): 1026–8.

101. Smitherman HF, Caviness AC, Macias CG. Retrospective review of serious bacterial infections in infants who are 0 to 36 months of age and have influenza A infection. Pediatrics 2005;115(3):710–8.

102. Byington CL, Enriquez FR, Hoff C, et al. Serious bacterial infections in febrile infants 1 to 90 days old with and without viral infections. Pediatrics 2004;113(6): 1662–6.

103. Luginbuhl LM, Newman TB, Pantell RH, et al. Office-based treatment and outcomes for febrile infants with clinically diagnosed bronchiolitis. Pediatrics 2008;122(5):947–54.

104. Bilavsky E, Shouval DS, Yarden-Bilavsky H, et al. A prospective study of the risk for serious bacterial infections in hospitalized febrile infants with or without bronchiolitis. Pediatr Infect Dis J 2008;27(3):269–70.

105. Purcell K, Fergie J. Lack of usefulness of an abnormal white blood cell count for predicting a concurrent serious bacterial infection in infants and young children hospitalized with respiratory syncytial virus lower respiratory tract infection. Pediatr Infect Dis J 2007;26(4):311–5.

106. Yarden-Bilavsky H, Ashkenazi-Hoffnung L, Livni G, et al. Month-by-month age analysis of the risk for serious bacterial infections in febrile infants with bronchiolitis. Clin Pediatr (Phila) 2011;50(11):1052–6.

107. Ralston S, Hill V, Waters A. Occult serious bacterial infection in infants younger than 60 to 90 days with bronchiolitis: a systematic review. Arch Pediatr Adolesc Med 2011;165(10):951–6.

108. American Academy of Pediatrics Subcommittee on the Diagnosis and Management of Bronchiolitis. Diagnosis and management of bronchiolitis. Pediatrics 2006;118(4):1774–93.

109. Doan QH, Kissoon N, Dobson S, et al. A randomized, controlled trial of the impact of early and rapid diagnosis of viral infections in children brought to

an emergency department with febrile respiratory tract illnesses. J Pediatr 2009; 154(1):91–5.

110. Iyer SB, Gerber MA, Pomerantz WJ, et al. Effect of point-of-care influenza testing on management of febrile children. Acad Emerg Med 2006;13(12): 1259–68.

111. Bonner AB, Monroe KW, Talley LI, et al. Impact of the rapid diagnosis of influenza on physician decision-making and patient management in the pediatric emergency department: results of a randomized, prospective, controlled trial. Pediatrics 2003;112(2):363–7.

112. Poehling KA, Zhu Y, Tang YW, et al. Accuracy and impact of a point-of-care rapid influenza test in young children with respiratory illnesses. Arch Pediatr Adolesc Med 2006;160(7):713–8.

113. Doan Q, Enarson P, Kissoon N, et al. Rapid viral diagnosis for acute febrile respiratory illness in children in the Emergency Department. Cochrane Database Syst Rev 2012;(5):
CD006452.

114. Bonsu BK, Harper MB. Accuracy and test characteristics of ancillary tests of cerebrospinal fluid for predicting acute bacterial meningitis in children with low white blood cell counts in cerebrospinal fluid. Acad Emerg Med 2005;12(4): 303–9.

115. Nigrovic LE, Kuppermann N, Macias CG, et al. Clinical prediction rule for identifying children with cerebrospinal fluid pleocytosis at very low risk of bacterial meningitis. JAMA 2007;297(1):52–60.

116. Shapiro ED, Aaron NH, Wald ER, et al. Risk factors for development of bacterial meningitis among children with occult bacteremia. J Pediatr 1986;109(1):15–9.

117. Teele DW, Dashefsky B, Rakusan T, et al. Meningitis after lumbar puncture in children with bacteremia. N Engl J Med 1981;305(18):1079–81.

118. Dayan PS, Hanson E, Bennett JE, et al. Clinical course of urinary tract infections in infants younger than 60 days of age. Pediatr Emerg Care 2004;20(2):85–8.

119. Hoberman A, Wald ER, Hickey RW, et al. Oral versus initial intravenous therapy for urinary tract infections in young febrile children. Pediatrics 1999;104(1 Pt 1): 79–86.

120. Dore-Bergeron MJ, Gauthier M, Chevalier I, et al. Urinary tract infections in 1- to 3-month-old infants: ambulatory treatment with intravenous antibiotics. Pediatrics 2009;124(1):16–22.

121. Alpern ER, Alessandrini EA, Bell LM, et al. Occult bacteremia from a pediatric emergency department: current prevalence, time to detection, and outcome. Pediatrics 2000;106(3):505–11.

122. Fleisher GR, Rosenberg N, Vinci R, et al. Intramuscular versus oral antibiotic therapy for the prevention of meningitis and other bacterial sequelae in young, febrile children at risk for occult bacteremia. J Pediatr 1994;124(4):504–12.

123. Lee GM, Harper MB. Risk of bacteremia for febrile young children in the post-*Haemophilus influenzae* type b era. Arch Pediatr Adolesc Med 1998;152(7): 624–8.

124. Gorelick MH, Shaw KN. Clinical decision rule to identify febrile young girls at risk for urinary tract infection. Arch Pediatr Adolesc Med 2000;154(4):386–90.

125. Teach SJ, Fleisher GR. Efficacy of an observation scale in detecting bacteremia in febrile children three to thirty-six months of age, treated as outpatients. Occult Bacteremia Study Group. J Pediatr 1995;126(6):877–81.

126. McCarthy PL, Sharpe MR, Spiesel SZ, et al. Observation scales to identify serious illness in febrile children. Pediatrics 1982;70(5):802–9.

127. Abanses JC, Dowd MD, Simon SD, et al. Impact of rapid influenza testing at triage on management of febrile infants and young children. Pediatr Emerg Care 2006;22(3):145–9.
128. McGowan JE Jr, Bratton L, Klein JO, et al. Bacteremia in febrile children seen in a "walk-in" pediatric clinic. N Engl J Med 1973;288(25):1309–12.
129. Herz AM, Greenhow TL, Alcantara J, et al. Changing epidemiology of outpatient bacteremia in 3- to 36-month-old children after the introduction of the heptavalent-conjugated pneumococcal vaccine. Pediatr Infect Dis J 2006; 25(4):293–300.
130. Ampofo K, Pavia AT, Chris S, et al. The changing epidemiology of invasive pneumococcal disease at a tertiary children's hospital through the 7-valent pneumococcal conjugate vaccine era: a case for continuous surveillance. Pediatr Infect Dis J 2012;31(3):228–34.
131. Messina AF, Katz-Gaynor K, Barton T, et al. Impact of the pneumococcal conjugate vaccine on serotype distribution and antimicrobial resistance of invasive Streptococcus pneumoniae isolates in Dallas, TX, children from 1999 through 2005. Pediatr Infect Dis J 2007;26(6):461–7.
132. Poehling KA, Talbot TR, Griffin MR, et al. Invasive pneumococcal disease among infants before and after introduction of pneumococcal conjugate vaccine. JAMA 2006;295(14):1668–74.
133. Kyaw MH, Lynfield R, Schaffner W, et al. Effect of introduction of the pneumococcal conjugate vaccine on drug-resistant Streptococcus pneumoniae. N Engl J Med 2006;354(14):1455–63.
134. Lucero MG, Dulalia VE, Nillos LT, et al. Pneumococcal conjugate vaccines for preventing vaccine-type invasive pneumococcal disease and X-ray defined pneumonia in children less than two years of age. Cochrane Database Syst Rev 2009;(4): CD004977.
135. Singleton RJ, Hennessy TW, Bulkow LR, et al. Invasive pneumococcal disease caused by nonvaccine serotypes among Alaska native children with high levels of 7-valent pneumococcal conjugate vaccine coverage. JAMA 2007;297(16): 1784–92.
136. Kaplan SL, Barson WJ, Lin PL, et al. Serotype 19A Is the most common serotype causing invasive pneumococcal infections in children. Pediatrics 2010;125(3): 429–36.
137. Centers for Disease Control and Prevention (CDC). Invasive pneumococcal disease in young children before licensure of 13-valent pneumococcal conjugate vaccine - United States, 2007. MMWR Morb Mortal Wkly Rep 2010;59(9):253–7.
138. Yildirim I, Stevenson A, Hsu KK, et al. Evolving picture of invasive pneumococcal disease in Massachusetts children: a comparison of disease in 2007-2009 with earlier periods. Pediatr Infect Dis J 2012;31(10):1016–21.
139. Centers for Disease Control and Prevention (CDC). Licensure of a 13-valent pneumococcal conjugate vaccine (PCV13) and recommendations for use among children - Advisory Committee on Immunization Practices (ACIP), 2010. MMWR Morb Mortal Wkly Rep 2010;59(9):258–61.
140. Whitney CG, Pilishvili T, Farley MM, et al. Effectiveness of seven-valent pneumococcal conjugate vaccine against invasive pneumococcal disease: a matched case-control study. Lancet 2006;368(9546):1495–502.
141. Mahon BE, Hsu K, Karumuri S, et al. Effectiveness of abbreviated and delayed 7-valent pneumococcal conjugate vaccine dosing regimens. Vaccine 2006; 24(14):2514–20.

142. Bonadio WA, Smith DS, Madagame E, et al. *Escherichia coli* bacteremia in children. A review of 91 cases in 10 years. Am J Dis Child 1991;145(6):671–4.

143. Al-Hasan MN, Huskins WC, Lahr BD, et al. Epidemiology and outcome of Gram-negative bloodstream infection in children: a population-based study. Epidemiol Infect 2011;139(5):791–6.

144. Kaplan SL, Schutze GE, Leake JA, et al. Multicenter surveillance of invasive meningococcal infections in children. Pediatrics 2006;118(4):e979–84.

145. Kuppermann N, Malley R, Inkelis SH, et al. Clinical and hematologic features do not reliably identify children with unsuspected meningococcal disease. Pediatrics 1999;103(2):E20.

146. Wang VJ, Kuppermann N, Malley R, et al. Meningococcal disease among children who live in a large metropolitan area, 1981-1996. Clin Infect Dis 2001;32(7):1004–9.

147. Sullivan TD, LaScolea LJ Jr. *Neisseria meningitidis* bacteremia in children: quantitation of bacteremia and spontaneous clinical recovery without antibiotic therapy. Pediatrics 1987;80(1):63–7.

148. Mandl K, Stack A, Fleisher G. Incidence of bacteremia in infants and children with fever and petechiae. J Pediatr 1997;131(3):398.

149. Nelson DG, Leake J, Bradley J, et al. Evaluation of febrile children with petechial rashes: is there consensus among pediatricians? Pediatr Infect Dis J 1998;17(12):1135–40.

150. Wells LC, Smith JC, Weston VC, et al. The child with a non-blanching rash: how likely is meningococcal disease? Arch Dis Child 2001;85(3):218–22.

151. Benito-Fernandez J, Mintegi S, Pocheville-Gurutzeta I, et al. Pneumococcal bacteremia in febrile infants presenting to the emergency department 8 years after the introduction of pneumococcal conjugate vaccine in the Basque Country of Spain. Pediatr Infect Dis J 2010;29(12):1142–4.

152. Wilkinson M, Bulloch B, Smith M. Prevalence of occult bacteremia in children aged 3 to 36 months presenting to the emergency department with fever in the postpneumococcal conjugate vaccine era. Acad Emerg Med 2009;16(3):220–5.

153. Carstairs KL, Tanen DA, Johnson AS, et al. Pneumococcal bacteremia in febrile infants presenting to the emergency department before and after the introduction of the heptavalent pneumococcal vaccine. Ann Emerg Med 2007;49(6):772–7.

154. Bandyopadhyay S, Bergholte J, Blackwell CD, et al. Risk of serious bacterial infection in children with fever without a source in the post-*Haemophilus influenzae* era when antibiotics are reserved for culture-proven bacteremia. Arch Pediatr Adolesc Med 2002;156(5):512–7.

155. Stoll ML, Rubin LG. Incidence of occult bacteremia among highly febrile young children in the era of the pneumococcal conjugate vaccine: a study from a Children's Hospital Emergency Department and Urgent Care Center. Arch Pediatr Adolesc Med 2004;158(7):671–5.

156. Sard B, Bailey MC, Vinci R. An analysis of pediatric blood cultures in the post-pneumococcal conjugate vaccine era in a community hospital emergency department. Pediatr Emerg Care 2006;22(5):295–300.

157. Bass JW, Steele RW, Wittler RR, et al. Antimicrobial treatment of occult bacteremia: a multicenter cooperative study. Pediatr Infect Dis J 1993;12(6):466–73.

158. Kuppermann N. Occult bacteremia in young febrile children. Pediatr Clin North Am 1999;46(6):1073–109.

159. Zaidi E, Bachur R, Harper M. Non-typhi *Salmonella* bacteremia in children. Pediatr Infect Dis J 1999;18(12):1073–7.

160. Tsai MH, Huang YC, Chiu CH, et al. Nontyphoidal *Salmonella* bacteremia in previously healthy children: analysis of 199 episodes. Pediatr Infect Dis J 2007; 26(10):909–13.

161. Shkalim V, Amir A, Samra Z, et al. Characteristics of non-typhi *Salmonella* gastroenteritis associated with bacteremia in infants and young children. Infection 2012;40(3):285–9.

162. Yang YJ, Huang MC, Wang SM, et al. Analysis of risk factors for bacteremia in children with nontyphoidal *Salmonella* gastroenteritis. Eur J Clin Microbiol Infect Dis 2002;21(4):290–3.

163. Isaacman DJ, Burke BL. Utility of the serum C-reactive protein for detection of occult bacterial infection in children. Arch Pediatr Adolesc Med 2002;156(9): 905–9.

164. Pulliam PN, Attia MW, Cronan KM. C-reactive protein in febrile children 1 to 36 months of age with clinically undetectable serious bacterial infection. Pediatrics 2001;108(6):1275–9.

165. Fernandez Lopez A, Luaces Cubells C, Garcia JJ, et al. Procalcitonin in pediatric emergency departments for the early diagnosis of invasive bacterial infections in febrile infants: results of a multicenter study and utility of a rapid qualitative test for this marker. Pediatr Infect Dis J 2003;22(10):895–903.

166. Thayyil S, Shenoy M, Hamaluba M, et al. Is procalcitonin useful in early diagnosis of serious bacterial infections in children? Acta Paediatr 2005;94(2):155–8.

167. Galetto-Lacour A, Zamora SA, Gervaix A. Bedside procalcitonin and C-reactive protein tests in children with fever without localizing signs of infection seen in a referral center. Pediatrics 2003;112(5):1054–60.

168. Andreola B, Bressan S, Callegaro S, et al. Procalcitonin and C-reactive protein as diagnostic markers of severe bacterial infections in febrile infants and children in the emergency department. Pediatr Infect Dis J 2007;26(8):672–7.

169. Guen CG, Delmas C, Launay E, et al. Contribution of procalcitonin to occult bacteraemia detection in children. Scand J Infect Dis 2007;39(2):157–9.

170. Maniaci V, Dauber A, Weiss S, et al. Procalcitonin in young febrile infants for the detection of serious bacterial infections. Pediatrics 2008;122(4):701–10.

171. Manzano S, Bailey B, Girodias JB, et al. Impact of procalcitonin on the management of children aged 1 to 36 months presenting with fever without source: a randomized controlled trial. Am J Emerg Med 2010;28(6):647–53.

172. Manzano S, Bailey B, Gervaix A, et al. Markers for bacterial infection in children with fever without source. Arch Dis Child 2011;96(5):440–6.

173. Yo CH, Hsieh PS, Lee SH, et al. Comparison of the test characteristics of procalcitonin to C-reactive protein and leukocytosis for the detection of serious bacterial infections in children presenting with fever without source: a systematic review and meta-analysis. Ann Emerg Med 2012;60(5):591–600.

174. Baraff LJ. Editorial: clinical policy for children younger than three years presenting to the emergency department with fever. Ann Emerg Med 2003;42(4):546–9.

175. Kuppermann N. The evaluation of young febrile children for occult bacteremia: time to reevaluate our approach? Arch Pediatr Adolesc Med 2002;156(9):855–7.

176. Shaikh N, Morone NE, Bost JE, et al. Prevalence of urinary tract infection in childhood: a meta-analysis. Pediatr Infect Dis J 2008;27(4):302–8.

177. Hoberman A, Chao HP, Keller DM, et al. Prevalence of urinary tract infection in febrile infants. J Pediatr 1993;123(1):17–23.

178. Shaw KN, Gorelick M, McGowan KL, et al. Prevalence of urinary tract infection in febrile young children in the emergency department. Pediatrics 1998;102(2): e16.

179. Shaikh N, Morone NE, Lopez J, et al. Does this child have a urinary tract infection? JAMA 2007;298(24):2895–904.
180. Zorc JJ, Kiddoo DA, Shaw KN. Diagnosis and management of pediatric urinary tract infections. Clin Microbiol Rev 2005;18(2):417–22.
181. Huicho L, Campos-Sanchez M, Alamo C. Metaanalysis of urine screening tests for determining the risk of urinary tract infection in children. Pediatr Infect Dis J 2002;21(1):1–11, 88.
182. Committee on Quality Improvement and Subcommittee on Urinary Tract Infection. Practice parameter: the diagnosis, treatment, and evaluation of the initial urinary tract infection in febrile infants and young children. Pediatrics 1999; 103(4):843–52.
183. Wubbel L, Muniz L, Ahmed A, et al. Etiology and treatment of community-acquired pneumonia in ambulatory children. Pediatr Infect Dis J 1999;18(2):98–104.
184. Carrillo-Marquez MA, Hulten KG, Hammerman W, et al. *Staphylococcus aureus* pneumonia in children in the era of community-acquired methicillin-resistance at Texas Children's Hospital. Pediatr Infect Dis J 2011;30(7):545–50.
185. Grijalva CG, Nuorti JP, Arbogast PG, et al. Decline in pneumonia admissions after routine childhood immunisation with pneumococcal conjugate vaccine in the USA: a time-series analysis. Lancet 2007;369(9568):1179–86.
186. Margolis P, Gadomski A. Does this infant have pneumonia? JAMA 1998;279(4): 308–13.
187. Neuman MI, Scully KJ, Kim D, et al. Physician assessment of the likelihood of pneumonia in a pediatric emergency department. Pediatr Emerg Care 2010; 26(11):817–22.
188. Murphy CG, van de Pol AC, Harper MB, et al. Clinical predictors of occult pneumonia in the febrile child. Acad Emerg Med 2007;14(3):243–9.
189. Shah S, Bachur R, Kim D, et al. Lack of predictive value of tachypnea in the diagnosis of pneumonia in children. Pediatr Infect Dis J 2010;29(5):406–9.
190. Nijman RG, Thompson M, van Veen M, et al. Derivation and validation of age and temperature specific reference values and centile charts to predict lower respiratory tract infection in children with fever: prospective observational study. BMJ 2012;345:e4224.
191. Mathews B, Shah S, Cleveland RH, et al. Clinical predictors of pneumonia among children with wheezing. Pediatrics 2009;124(1):e29–36.
192. Leventhal JM. Clinical predictors of pneumonia as a guide to ordering chest roentgenograms. Clin Pediatr (Phila) 1982;21(12):730–4.
193. Taylor JA, Del Beccaro M, Done S, et al. Establishing clinically relevant standards for tachypnea in febrile children younger than 2 years. Arch Pediatr Adolesc Med 1995;149(3):283–7.
194. Zukin DD, Hoffman JR, Cleveland RH, et al. Correlation of pulmonary signs and symptoms with chest radiographs in the pediatric age group. Ann Emerg Med 1986;15(7):792–6.
195. Mower WR, Sachs C, Nicklin EL, et al. Pulse oximetry as a fifth pediatric vital sign. Pediatrics 1997;99(5):681–6.
196. Tanen DA, Trocinski DR. The use of pulse oximetry to exclude pneumonia in children. Am J Emerg Med 2002;20(6):521–3.
197. Simon LV, Carstairs KL, Reardon JM, et al. Oxygen saturation is not clinically useful in the exclusion of bacterial pneumonia in febrile infants. Emerg Med J 2010;27(12):904–6.
198. Lynch T, Bialy L, Kellner JD, et al. A systematic review on the diagnosis of pediatric bacterial pneumonia: when gold is bronze. PLoS One 2010;5(8):e11989.

199. Davies HD, Wang EE, Manson D, et al. Reliability of the chest radiograph in the diagnosis of lower respiratory infections in young children. Pediatr Infect Dis J 1996;15(7):600–4.

200. Korppi M, Don M, Valent F, et al. The value of clinical features in differentiating between viral, pneumococcal and atypical bacterial pneumonia in children. Acta Paediatr 2008;97(7):943–7.

201. Flood RG, Badik J, Aronoff SC. The utility of serum C-reactive protein in differentiating bacterial from nonbacterial pneumonia in children: a meta-analysis of 1230 children. Pediatr Infect Dis J 2008;27(2):95–9.

202. Courtoy I, Lande AE, Turner RB. Accuracy of radiographic differentiation of bacterial from nonbacterial pneumonia. Clin Pediatr (Phila) 1989;28(6):261–4.

203. McCarthy PL, Spiesel SZ, Stashwick CA, et al. Radiographic findings and etiologic diagnosis in ambulatory childhood pneumonias. Clin Pediatr (Phila) 1981; 20(11):686–91.

204. Bradley JS, Byington CL, Shah SS, et al. The management of community-acquired pneumonia in infants and children older than 3 months of age: clinical practice guidelines by the Pediatric Infectious Diseases Society and the Infectious Diseases Society of America. Clin Infect Dis 2011;53(7):e25–76.

205. Cilla G, Onate E, Perez-Yarza EG, et al. Viruses in community-acquired pneumonia in children aged less than 3 years old: high rate of viral coinfection. J Med Virol 2008;80(10):1843–9.

206. Techasaensiri B, Techasaensiri C, Mejias A, et al. Viral coinfections in children with invasive pneumococcal disease. Pediatr Infect Dis J 2010;29(6):519–23.

207. Harris M, Clark J, Coote N, et al. British Thoracic Society guidelines for the management of community acquired pneumonia in children: update 2011. Thorax 2011;66(Suppl 2):ii1–23.

208. Bulloch B, Craig WR, Klassen TP. The use of antibiotics to prevent serious sequelae in children at risk for occult bacteremia: a meta-analysis. Acad Emerg Med 1997;4(7):679–83.

209. Baraff LJ, Oslund S, Prather M. Effect of antibiotic therapy and etiologic microorganism on the risk of bacterial meningitis in children with occult bacteremia. Pediatrics 1993;92(1):140–3.

210. Haddy RI, Perry K, Chacko CE, et al. Comparison of incidence of invasive *Streptococcus pneumoniae* disease among children before and after introduction of conjugated pneumococcal vaccine. Pediatr Infect Dis J 2005;24(4):320–3.

211. Black S, Shinefield H, Baxter R, et al. Postlicensure surveillance for pneumococcal invasive disease after use of heptavalent pneumococcal conjugate vaccine in Northern California Kaiser Permanente. Pediatr Infect Dis J 2004;23(6): 485–9.

212. Wang VJ, Malley R, Fleisher GR, et al. Antibiotic treatment of children with unsuspected meningococcal disease. Arch Pediatr Adolesc Med 2000;154(6): 556–60.

213. Hodson EM, Willis NS, Craig JC. Antibiotics for acute pyelonephritis in children. Cochrane Database Syst Rev 2007;(4):CD003772.

214. Bradley JS, Arguedas A, Blumer JL, et al. Comparative study of levofloxacin in the treatment of children with community-acquired pneumonia. Pediatr Infect Dis J 2007;26(10):868–78.

215. Chumpa A, Bachur RG, Harper MB. Bacteremia-associated pneumococcal pneumonia and the benefit of initial parenteral antimicrobial therapy. Pediatr Infect Dis J 1999;18(12):1081–5.

Nuances in Pediatric Trauma

Mary Ella Kenefake, MD[a,b,*], Matthew Swarm, MD[a,b],
Jennifer Walthall, MD[b,c]

KEYWORDS

- Pediatric trauma • Pediatric primary survey • Pediatric secondary survey
- Pediatric airway • Pediatric C-spine • Pediatric head trauma
- Pediatric abdominal trauma

KEY POINTS

- Pediatric trauma is a significant cause of morbidity and mortality in children under the age of 18 years.
- Pediatric patients require special considerations when addressing their assessment and evaluation after trauma.
- Pediatric patients have unique injury patterns compared with their adult counterparts. Consideration and recognition of these variants are of utmost importance.

INTRODUCTION

In the United States, approximately 17,000 children and adolescents die annually of unintentional and intentional injuries.[1] According to the National Center for Injury Prevention and Control, unintentional injury was the number 1 cause of death in children 1 to 18 years of age in 2007, accounting for 41.5% of childhood deaths, followed by homicide (11.2%), malignant neoplasms (9.0%), and suicide (6.1%). In infants under a year of age, unintentional injury accounts for 4.4% of deaths. When further broken down by injury type, injuries sustained in motor vehicle accidents account for more than half of these deaths. The leading causes of traumatic death in children and adolescents from 2007 are listed in **Table 1**.

Childhood injury is a major focus for trauma research, both for prevention and best practices for coordination of care from acute stabilization through rehabilitation. Several advancements in injury prevention have dramatically decreased unintentional

Disclosures: None.
[a] Department of Emergency Medicine, Indiana University School of Medicine, 1701 North Senate Boulevard, AG012, Indianapolis, IN 46202, USA; [b] Department of Pediatrics, Indiana University School of Medicine, Riley Hospital for Children, 705 Riley Hospital Drive, Indianapolis, IN 46202, USA; [c] Department of Emergency Medicine, Indiana University School of Medicine, 1701 North Senate Boulevard, Indianapolis, IN 46202, USA
* Corresponding author. Department of Emergency Medicine, Indiana University School of Medicine, 1701 North Senate Boulevard, AG012, Indianapolis, IN 46202.
E-mail address: mekenefake@gmail.com

Table 1 Leading causes of injury deaths in 2007		
Children <1 y		
Cause of Death	**Number of Deaths**	**Percentage of Deaths**
Unintentional suffocation	959	54.9
Homicide unspecified	174	10.0
Unintentional MVC	122	7.0
Homicide other spec, classifiable	86	4.9
Unintentional drowning	57	3.3
Children 1–18 y		
Cause of Death	**Number of Deaths**	**Percentage of Deaths**
Unintentional MVC	4.910	40.1
Homicide firearm	1553	12.7
Unintentional drowning	918	7.5
Unintentional poisoning	645	5.3
Suicide suffocation	566	4.6

From Centers for Disease Control and Prevention. Injury prevention & control: data & statistics (WISQARSTM). Available at: http://www.cdc.gov/injury/wisqars/fatal.html. Accessed October 15, 2012.

injury mortality, including enhanced child restraints for most states, pool fencing, and bicycle helmet laws, although universal compliance has not yet been achieved. A Centers for Disease Control and Prevention vital signs report renewed prevention efforts in research, education, and outreach programming when surveillance revealed unintentional injury remained the leading cause of childhood morbidity despite a 40% decrease since 2005. Suffocation and poisoning subsets have substantially increased in that time frame as well.[2]

PHYSIOLOGIC CONSIDERATIONS IN THE PEDIATRIC PATIENT

Children have unique anatomy and physiology that must be taken into consideration when managing them as trauma patients. First and foremost, compared with adults, children are much more susceptible to multiple and more severe injuries given the same amount of force in any given trauma. This force is more widely distributed throughout their bodies, often resulting in more significant internal organ damage, sometimes without significant external signs. Additionally, the proportionately larger surface area of children's bodies to their weight exposes them to significant heat loss and subsequent secondary negative effects. These effects include decreased cardiac function, cardiac inotropy, left ventricular contractility, catecholamine responsiveness, platelet function, renal and hepatic drug clearance, and a higher metabolic demand that potentiates metabolic acidemia.[3]

Knowledge of or access to a chart of normal vital signs broken down by age helps facilitate recognition of critically injured children (**Table 2**).[4] Multiple platforms exist online and via electronic tablets or mobile devices to access this information in real time during a trauma resuscitation. Blood pressure is not listed to help reinforce a pediatric patient's capacity to maintain a normal blood pressure despite significant loss of up to 25% to 30% of total blood volume.[3] Changes in heart rate, respiratory rate, and peripheral perfusion can indicate imminent cardiopulmonary collapse and should be closely monitored throughout a patient's stabilization period.

Table 2
Normal vitals signs, ages 0–18 years—50th percentile (1st–99th percentiles)

Age	Heart Rate	Respiratory Rate
0 mo	139 (90–165)	43 (26–68)
1 mo	145 (110–182)	42 (25–67)
2 mo	143 (108–180)	42 (24–66)
3 mo	142 (105–178)	41 (23–65)
6 mo	136 (100–170)	40 (22–62)
9 mo	130 (95–165)	39 (22–60)
12 mo	125 (93–160)	38 (21–67)
2 y	110 (80–150)	30 (18–42)
4 y	105 (70–135)	25 (16–31)
6 y	95 (60–130)	22 (16–28)
8 y	90 (55–120)	20 (15–25)
10 y	85 (55–115)	20 (14–25)
12 y	80 (50–110)	19 (12–24)
14–18 y	75 (45–105)	15 (10–22)

Data from Fleming S, Thompson M, Stevens R, et al. Normal ranges of heart rate and respiratory rate in children from birth to 18 years of age: a systematic review of observational studies. Lancet 2011;377(9770):1011–8.

Lastly, when injured, pediatric patients have a significantly higher energy and caloric requirement than at baseline. Their oxygen extraction and consumption as well as glucose use is much higher per kilogram than their adult counterparts. Therefore, maintaining adequate oxygenation and consideration of early initiation of glucose-containing fluids are important in the management of injured children.

INTRODUCTION TO THE PEDIATRIC PRIMARY SURVEY

The initial assessment and survey of pediatric patients is not vastly different from those of adults. This brief and focused assessment is necessary to rule out the presence of life-threatening injury and set in motion life-saving interventions within 5 minutes of presentation. During the primary survey, vital signs should be continuously monitored, allowing for early notification of impending compromise for patients. The primary survey is composed of A for airway, B for breathing, C for circulation, D for disability, E for exposure, and F for family.[3] If at any time during this initial assessment a patient begins to deteriorate, the provider should start at the top and reassess each step again to stabilize the patient.

Primary Survey: Airway

Effective management of a pediatric airway is challenging because it poses both anatomic and physiologic differences from the adult airway. Children become hypoxemic much more quickly and thus require careful preparation and swift intervention. In pediatrics, effective airway management is a critical component to successful cardiopulmonary resuscitation. Respiratory arrest usually precedes cardiac arrest in children.[3] When assessing the pediatric airway, the first priority is to ensure the airway is clear and patent. Can the child speak? Or is he or she crying if not yet verbal? If the voice seems muffled, the provider may consider an oral foreign body and should sweep the mouth for debris, teeth, and other items. Additionally, evidence of facial fractures or tracheal injury should be noted as potential for a complicated airway. Once the airway has been deemed clear and intubation is eminent, the differences in the pediatric airway (summarized in **Table 3**) should be considered before intubation (**Box 1**).

Rapid sequence intubation with both sedation and a paralytic is the optimal setting for airway control. Prior to intubating a pediatric trauma patient, a contingency plan should be in place. Although rapid sequence intubation is safe and effective, especially in emergent situations, there are times when this method fails and a back-up method must be ready to be executed immediately, which may be in the form of a supraglottic airway adjunct or video laryngoscopy. More recently, there is evidence showing that, although the duration of intubation is slightly longer (36 seconds vs 23.8 seconds), video laryngoscopy provides a better view than direct laryngoscopy in the pediatric airway.[8]

There has been some controversy surrounding the consistent use of continuous cricoid pressure (Sellick maneuver) during intubation. Although this method may be considered during sedation and paralysis to aid in the reduction of gastric aspiration, it should be at the discretion of the intubating practitioner once airway manipulation begins[9] because of the significant risk of obstruction and delayed tube placement if not used skillfully.[10] In the pediatric airway, it takes as little as 0.2 lb of force to obstruct the airway; thus, careful steps must be taken when manipulating the cricoid externally.[3]

Cervical spine considerations with intubation
If intubating a pediatric patient who has been involved in trauma, the patient should have continuous attention to cervical spine (C-spine) immobilization during the procedure. During intubation there should be minimal to no movement of the neck. It is most helpful for another person to hold in-line C-spine immobilization while the front of the

Table 3
Anatomic differences in the pediatric airway

Airway Differences	Interventions
Prominent occiput	Place a rolled towel under the shoulders May not be possible in cervical spine precautions
Larger tongue that falls against the hypopharynx	Use of an oropharyngeal airway, optimize head positioning, jaw-thrust position
Larger adenoid tissues contribute to obstruction[5]	Use of an oropharyngeal airway, optimize head positioning, jaw-thrust position
Floppy, U-shaped epiglottis	Use of a straight blade
Larynx more cephalad and anterior	May need to be closer to the patient at a 45° angle[3]
Cricoid ring is the narrowest portion of the airway	Have a size smaller tube ready because the larger may pass the cords but not the cricoid
Narrow tracheal diameter and distance between the rings	Must do needle cricothyrotomy rather than surgical
Shorter tracheal length resulting in frequent right-mainstem intubations or dislodgement	Use 3 times the tube size to estimate accurate depth of placement, minimize head movement once placed[6]

Box 1
Indications for intubating pediatric trauma patients

- Glasgow Coma Scale (GCS) score <8 or obtunded
- Inadequate oxygenation or ventilation—poor effort or color
- Inability to maintain or protect airway—gag reflex not especially helpful because it does not correlate with GCS[7]
- Inability to ventilate by bag-valve-mask (BVM) or need for prolonged control
- Severe head injury
- Potential for clinical deterioration (thermal inhalation injuries)
- Respiratory failure from flail chest
- Decompensated shock resistant to initial fluid resuscitation

---

cervical collar is released to allow for mandibular manipulation. Often this is a situation where video laryngoscopy is considered first line; however, a small prospective case study in 2012 revealed a decreased view of the glottis entrance when used with C-spine precautions.[11]

Selecting equipment

The endotracheal (ET) tube size should be determined by a length-based resuscitation tape or age-based calculation:

Uncuffed: 4 + (age in years/4)[12]
Cuffed: 3.5 + (age in years/4)[12]

It is important to prepare ET tubes both one-half size larger and one-half size smaller before initiating intubation. When considering a laryngoscope blade, the straight blade is usually preferred for children under 2 years of age due to its ability to manipulate the epiglottis. Additionally, a straight blade may be more useful in situations where there is concern for C-spine injury because it results in less motion of the neck.[13] Depth of placement is most accurately estimated by multiplying the tube size by 3, resulting in correct placement more than 80% of the time.[14] Immediately after placement, typical methods of ET tube placement confirmation should be completed, such as equal chest rise and breath sounds, air fogging in the ET tube, absence of gastric sounds with bagging, and color change on colorimetric capnography. There is no substitute for direct visualization of the ET tube passing through the cords and a decompensating patient should always have airway placement reevaluated. Consideration of end-tidal capnography for the most accurate confirmation of continued correct placement is becoming a part of regular ongoing monitoring practice for intubated patients.[9]

Cuffed or uncuffed?

Beyond the newborn period, a cuffed ET tube is a safe option for airway management.[9] In some instances, placement of a cuffed tube is favorable because it helps reduce the risk of aspiration, allows for management of airway swelling, and helps those who may require higher ventilator settings. This practice is supported by the American Heart Association Pediatric Advanced Life Support guidelines.[9] Traditionally, uncuffed ET tubes were preferred for children under 8 years of age because there was concern for pressure-induced ischemic damage to their tracheal mucosa from the cuff, mostly due in part to the cricoid cartilage being the narrowest part of the airway as opposed to adults where the narrowest part is the vocal cords. Several studies have shown, however, there is no increase in postextubation stridor, need for racemic epinephrine, or long-term complications when cuffed tubes are used in pediatric airway control.[15,16] It is important to keep cuff pressures no greater than 20 mm H_2O to 25 mm H_2O to avoid harm to a patient's airway.[9]

Primary Survey: Breathing and Ventilation

The breathing and ventilation assessment of trauma patients begins with observation of the neck and chest. Specific areas for inspection include tracheal deviation, abnormal chest wall movement, use of accessory muscles, and injury to the chest wall. Identification of these signs trigger recognition of the following life-threatening injuries: tension pneumothorax, flail chest, impending respiratory failure, and cardiothoracic injury, respectively. As the provider moves through this portion of the trauma assessment, action may be required before moving on to the next step to address life-threatening conditions. Considerations when managing breathing and ventilation in pediatric trauma patients are

Physiologic considerations in pediatric breathing

- Respiratory rate: age dependent. A chart with normal ranges should be readily available to the provider (see **Table 2**).
- Increased vagal tone: tendency to result in bradycardia with tongue blade manipulation. It is no longer standard practice, however, to pretreat with atropine for intubation.
- Smaller tidal volumes: for all children, set initial tidal volumes at 6–8 mL/kg. Careful setting of the ventilator helps avoid iatrogenic barotrauma.
- Lower functional residual capacity: children have little intrapulmonary oxygen reserve and become hypoxic more precipitously than adults. Optimal preoxygenation with BVM and passive oxygenation with a nasal cannula help avoid this phenomenon. Additionally, the nasal cannula should remain in place for passive oxygenation while intubating.[17]
- Higher oxygen metabolism: leads to a shorter safe apnea time.[18]
- Respiratory fatigue: children are diaphragmatic breathers at baseline. They do not possess the chest wall musculature to aid in respiration; therefore, fatigue happens more quickly.
- Positioning is of utmost importance. Anatomic alignment for both C-spine precautions and sniffing position is preferred; hyperextension often leads to obstruction.
- Jaw-thrust maneuvers help open the airway in unresponsive children. Consider placement of oral airway to lift the tongue and pharyngeal soft tissues to aid with BVM ventilation.

Bag-valve-mask ventilation

BVM ventilation is a temporizing method of ventilating pediatric patients; it is commonly used in prehospital settings and has been shown to be even more effective than intubation for emergency medical services providers.[19] It is important to ensure the proper size, and methods are used to reduce the risk of barotrauma to patients. All pediatric BVM units should be equipped with a safety pop-off valve along with a manometer that limits peak inspiratory pressures between 35 cm H_2O and 40 cm H_2O per breath. Each breath administered should be just enough to make the chest rise. The mask should only cover the mouth and nose to ensure a proper seal. Additionally, use of an oropharyngeal airway is particularly useful in children with macroglossia or tonsillar hypertrophy. To select the correct size of the oral airway, hold it along the side of a child's face with the flange at the corner of the mouth. The opposite end of the oropharyngeal airway should reach the angle of the mandible. With optimal use of BVM ventilation, children may be ventilated for long periods of time if necessary or until a more definitive airway is established.

Finally, once the airway is established and the child placed on the ventilator, it is important to understand the potential harm that hyperoxemia presents postintubation. In recent adult studies, hyperoxemia has been shown to significantly increase patient risk for in-hospital mortality.[20] When subsequently studied in children, however, one group of researchers did not find a difference in mortality with hyperoxia after cardiac arrest.[21] Hyperoxemia is likely to be studied more extensively in the future and should remain a consideration when managing intubated pediatric patients.

Primary Survey: Circulation

Assessment of pediatric patients' circulation and volume status involves examination of central and peripheral pulses, skin color, and capillary refill. Blood pressure is not an initial measure of circulation because pediatric patients have excellent compensatory measures that allow for blood pressure maintenance even in the face of significant volume loss (**Table 4**). These measures include an increase in heart rate and systemic vascular resistance to aid in central shunting. When these fail, however, children quickly convert from compensated to decompensated shock and risk complete cardiopulmonary failure. Signs of decompensated shock in pediatric patients include cool pale extremities, weak peripheral pulses, mottled/cyanotic skin, altered mental status, and delayed capillary refill. The avoidance of decompensated shock is possible with attention to specific signs and symptoms that are aggressively addressed in this initial evaluation.

When treating shock in pediatric patients, it is helpful to understand the category of shock. Three types of shock exist in traumatized patients: hemorrhagic, cardiogenic, and distributive. Hemorrhagic shock may present externally or internally. Either way, until the source of blood loss is identified, temporarily compressed, and then stopped, other resuscitative efforts minimally improve a patient's clinical status. Cardiogenic shock can occur in the setting of severe thoracic trauma from cardiac contusion or rupture inhibiting the heart from pumping normally. Finally, distributive shock typically occurs in the setting of poor circulation as a result of either obstruction of return or loss of vascular tone in the setting of spinal cord injuries. In each of these types of shock, fluid or blood product resuscitation likely is required in conjunction with specific interventions to address patient injuries.

Because hemorrhagic shock is most common in trauma, initial intervention should begin with a 20-mL/kg bolus of isotonic intravenous/intraosseous fluids for resuscitation. If no significant response has been achieved after 2 20-mL/kg fluid

Table 4 Systolic blood pressures—5th percentile	
Neonates (0–28 d)	60 mm Hg
1–12 mo	70 mm Hg
1–10 y	70 + (2 × age in years)
>10 y	90 mm Hg

Data from Kleinman ME, Chameides L, Schexnayder SM, et al. Part 14: pediatric advanced life support: 2010 American Heart Association Guidelines for Cardiopulmonary Resuscitation and Emergency Cardiovascular Care. Circulation 2010;122:S876.

boluses, reassessment and consideration of packed red blood cell transfusion (10–20 mL/kg) follows. The overall goal is to improve oxygen delivery and reduce consumption to reverse the state of shock.

Primary Survey: Disability

Rapid identification of neurologic deficits takes place during the disability portion of the primary survey. Use of the GCS or another validated neurologic evaluation tool is the quickest way to complete this assessment. The American Heart Association Pediatric Advanced Life Support program recommends the use of the AVPU scale.[9] This mnemonic stands for decreasing levels of consciousness: alert, responds to voice, responds to pain, and unresponsive. It should also be recognized that a child's mental status can be dramatically affected by hypoglycemia in this setting. Rapid bedside evaluation of glucose and correction can help in accurately assessing a child's disability.

Primary Survey: Exposure

In order to adequately examine pediatric trauma patients, they must be fully undressed, log rolled, and thoroughly examined for any hidden injuries. During this assessment, there is a potential for hypothermia and heat loss, so careful attention to maintaining normothermia is paramount, which can be done through use of warm blankets, warm humidified oxygen, warm ambient temperature in the room, and warmed resuscitative fluids.

Primary Survey: Family

In the resuscitation and evaluation of children, families should be given the opportunity to be present in the room with their children.[9] In general, children do not cope well in unknown, loud, and scary environments. Because the emergency department trauma bay is usually all of these things, children's assessments may be altered as a result. By allowing family to be present, emergency physicians allow comfort and guidance from a family directed to the child, providing a more accurate assessment of mental status. Families report that they wish to be present during their child's resuscitation and would recommend it to other families when reflecting on their experience.[22] In fact, their presence has shown to be beneficial to both the patient and the family in their grieving process.[22] It is important, however, that there is a point person in the room who serves as home base for the family. Social work, chaplaincy, and child life specialists can be helpful in this role. These individuals can be instrumental in helping a family know what is going on, where they can stand, when they can touch their child, and any other questions that arise during the resuscitation. Preexisting family presence policies and procedures should be considered for any emergency department that has the potential to evaluate pediatric trauma patients. Medical provider comfort and experience have been shown to be major barriers to implementing this practice.

INTRODUCTION TO THE PEDIATRIC SECONDARY SURVEY

After the primary assessment and stabilization of pediatric trauma patients, the second portion of the evaluation serves to fully examine patients head to toe. Specific injuries are discussed with recommendations regarding clinical testing and treatment.

Secondary Survey: Head Trauma

Pediatric head trauma accounts for approximately 600,000 emergency department visits and 7400 fatalities annually in the United States, making it the leading cause of death in children ages 0 to 18 years.[23] Fortunately, most of these traumatic injuries are not life threatening. The evaluation of pediatric patients with reported head trauma must be thorough and systematic, because patients in this age range may not present with symptoms normally found in their adult counterparts with head injuries. The goal of a systematic approach is to limit the number of unnecessary CT scans performed on young children, without overlooking clinically significant injuries.

As with any emergency evaluation, patient history and physical examination should guide the work-up. It is important for physicians to elicit the mechanism of patient injury, especially in younger children who are preverbal. Most pediatric head traumas are caused by falls, whereas motor vehicle crashes (MVCs) and pedestrian injuries account for slightly less than 20% each of these types of injuries. The height from which a child fell and type of surface on which he or she landed are important prognostic factors. It is also important to ask if a child involved in an MVC was properly restrained in an appropriately sized car seat or booster seat. Lastly, nonaccidental trauma (NAT) in pediatric head injuries must always be considered, especially in newborns and infants.

Pediatric patients are more vulnerable to the forces of head trauma for several reasons. First, the relative size of a pediatric patient's head compared with the trunk makes a patient more vulnerable to increased torque along the C-spine axis. Children under the age of 2 have more pliability to their skull, specifically due to sutures that may not be completely fused yet, accounting for the high number of intraparenchymal injuries without associated skull fractures. Finally, the pediatric brain is more vulnerable to shear injury because it is less myelinated and underdeveloped in size relative to the cranium.[24,25]

The physical examination should be focused around assessment of a patient's neurologic status along with any obvious extracranial injury to the head or neck. Focal neurologic defects, including unreactive pupils, the absence of a gag or corneal reflex, and any motor or sensory deficits, should increase provider suspicion of an intracranial injury. Nonfrontal scalp hematomas are particularly worrisome. Any temporal, parietal, or occipital scalp hematoma may be indicative of an intracranial abnormality, especially in children less than 2 years of age. In a study of head injuries in this age group, 93% of children with brain injuries had associated scalp hematomas.[26] In younger children, physicians should palpate the anterior fontanelle, which generally closes at approximately 1 year of age. Any evidence of anterior fontanelle fullness or bulging should increase provider suspicion of elevated intracranial pressure as a result of hemorrhage.

Even within the pediatric population, age subcategories based on developmental milestones change the approach to trauma. Specifically, children under the age of 2 present a variety of challenges to providers. First, children this age are typically not able to express an accurate history of the traumatic event. Stranger anxiety is at its height between 6 months and 2 years of age, making the physical examination particularly difficult. Also, the anatomic differences (discussed previously) predispose children less than 2 years old to intracranial injuries with subtle to no findings on physical examination. GCS also has limited usefulness in the younger pediatric population because it is based on a patient's ability to comprehend and cooperate with provider instructions.

In an attempt to decrease the amount of unnecessary radiation exposure to children, a prospective cohort study was published in 2009 to establish clinical guidelines for the use of CT in the setting of pediatric head trauma.[23] This set of rules, known as the *Pediatric Emergency Care Applied Research Network* (PECARN) head injury guidelines, was developed between 2004 and 2006 after evaluating 42,412 patients between the ages of 0 and 18, with traumatic head injuries within 24 hours of presentation. **Table 5** outlines the results of this landmark study and provides guidelines for obtaining a CT scan based on symptomatology. These rules should not outweigh physician gestalt and experience. CT scans should also be considered if a child has any preexisting condition that increases risk for an intracranial hemorrhage, including hemophilias, a known arteriovenous malformation, use of anticoagulation, and indwelling hardware, such as a ventriculoperitoneal shunt. **Table 5** lists the indications for obtaining a CT scan to assess for intracranial hemorrhage based on the PECARN head injury guidelines.

Children who do not meet these criteria for immediate CT scan but do have an intermediate risk for an acute intracranial injury should be observed for 4 to 6 hours in an emergency department. If a patient has any worsening clinical symptoms during the observation period, a CT scan should be obtained at that time.

A significant portion of children who have suffered isolated head trauma are sent home from the emergency department after a normal CT or suitable observation period. Prior to discharge, patients should be easily arousable with a normal neurologic examination. The provider should have a patient's parents compare the child's baseline mentation to his or her current state. The child should also be able to tolerate oral liquids without vomiting before discharge. Finally, provide strict and specific return precautions to the parents for any change in the child's mental status or further concern. The provider should also attempt to establish follow-up with the patient's primary pediatrician before a child is discharged. In the setting of a concussion, there is no need to instruct parents to wake their child from sleep after discharge.

Recently, there has been increased focus on concussions and their sequelae. Concussions are defined by the American Academy of Neurology as any traumatically

Table 5	
Indications for CT scan in pediatric trauma patients based on PECARN	
Children Less than 2 y of Age	**Children Older than 2 y of Age**
Age <3 mo	GCS ≤14 or any signs of altered mental status
Palpable skull fracture	Signs of basilar skull fracture
GCS <14 or any signs of altered mental status	Battle sign—ecchymosis of the mastoid process
Agitation/irritability	Raccoon eyes—periorbital ecchymosis
Somnolence	CSF otorrhea or rhinorrhea
Slow response to verbal communication	Loss of consciousness
Occipital, parietal, or temporal scalp hematoma (any nonfrontal hematoma)	Vomiting
Loss of consciousness >5 s	Severe headache
Not acting appropriately per parent	Severe mechanism
Severe mechanism	Falls >3 feet
Falls >3 feet	MVC with passenger ejection, rollover, or death of another passenger
MVC with passenger ejection, rollover, or death of another passenger	Pedestrian or bicycle passenger unhelmeted and hit by a motor vehicle
Pedestrian or bicycle passenger unhelmeted and hit by a motor vehicle	
Struck in head by a high-impact object	

Data from Jaffe D, Wesson D. Emergency management of blunt trauma in children. N Engl J Med 1991;324(21):1477–82.

induced disturbance of neurologic function and mental state, occurring with or without actual loss of consciousness. Concussions may present in a similar fashion as an intracranial lesion secondary to a traumatic event. Typically, patients with a concussion present with a headache and amnesia. Vomiting is not uncommon. These symptoms are generally short-lived and often resolve spontaneously. A CT scan is not indicated for simple concussive symptoms.

In any pediatric head trauma, the provider must consider NAT, which is especially true in children less than 1 year of age because these patients are more vulnerable and physical findings of injury may be more obscure. It is important for providers to elicit a detailed history and complete a thorough physical examination with a child completely undressed. The provider must determine if the reported mechanism is compatible with the child's injury given a child's age and correlating developmental milestones. Classically, the injury pattern associated with nonaccidental head trauma includes subdural hemorrhages, retinal hemorrhages, and diffuse brain injury.[27,28] The provider must be judicious and search for other injuries in a child with suspected NAT, because approximately 20% to 50% of children with abusive head trauma have extracranial skeletal fractures.[29–34] The American Academy of Pediatrics recommends a full skeletal survey in any child less than 2 years of age with suspected NAT. Between the ages of 2 and 5 years old, the use of a skeletal survey diminishes but can still provide useful information if there is a presence of any injury consistent with abuse. There is little value in obtaining a skeletal survey in children greater than 5 years of age because these children are often verbal and can express specific areas of pain or injury.[35] **Box 2** outlines the specific radiographic films to be obtained in a skeletal survey as outlined by the American College of Radiology. In any cases where NAT is suspected, physicians must be proactive in involving the appropriate resources, including Child Protective Services.

Box 2
Plain radiographs to be obtained in a complete skeletal survey

Appendicular skeleton

- Arms (anteroposterior [AP])

- Forearms (AP)

- Hands (AP)

- Thighs (AP)

- Legs (AP)

- Feet (AP or posteroanterior)

Axial skeleton

- Chest/thorax (AP and lateral)

- AP abdomen, lumbosacral spine, and bony pelvis

- Lumbar spine (lateral)

- C-spine (AP and lateral)

- Skull (frontal and lateral)

Data from American College of Radiology. ACR practice guideline for skeletal surveys in children. In: American College of Radiology. ACR Standards. Reston (VA): American College of Radiology; 2006. p. 203–7.

Secondary Survey: Cervical Spine

The stabilization, evaluation, and subsequent clearance of the C-spine are of utmost importance in a pediatric trauma. C-spine injuries are rare in children although they must be considered and properly evaluated in an emergency department.

There are approximately 1100 pediatric spinal injuries annually in the United States.[36] A majority of these injuries are attributed to a small number of mechanisms, which are mostly age dependent. MVCs make up the highest percentage of pediatric C-spine injuries in all age groups, whereas contact sports make up a more significant percentage of C-spine injuries in children older than 8 years of age.[37–40]

Anatomic differences in the pediatric cervical spine

C-spine injuries in children vary from their adult counterparts due to anatomic differences. Specifically, children under the age of 8 are more susceptible to injuries of the upper C-spine. These anatomic differences are illustrated in **Box 3**.[37,41–45]

Certain pediatric populations also have genetic predisposition to C-spine injuries. Up to 15% of children with Down syndrome have atlantoaxial instability along the C1-C2 interface. Less common genetic disorders, including Klippel-Feil syndrome and Morquio syndrome, also have increased risk of C-spine injury.[46–49] The C-spine does not fully mature until approximately 16 years of age in developmentally normal children.[50]

Initial evaluation of the pediatric cervical spine

Any child involved in a trauma with the potential for a C-spine injury should be treated as if the injury exists until proved otherwise, either by physical examination or radiography. The C-spine should be adequately immobilized as soon as possible, ideally in a prehospital setting. Failure to immobilize the C-spine during resuscitation and transport has lead to neurologic deficits in an estimated 3% to 25% of patients with a spinal cord injury.[51–53] If concern exists after the initial evaluation for a C-spine injury, patients ought to remain immobilized until an injury is excluded both clinically and radiographically.[54] **Box 4** illustrates indications for spinal cord immobilization.

Pediatric C-spine collars are available in multiple sizes for ideal immobilization of the neck in a neutral position. The child's head should be place in a supine position relative to their torso and a properly positioned backboard. The Advanced Trauma Life Support (ATLS) guidelines define the neutral position as "supine without rotating or bending the spinal column."[55]

Determining a C-spine injury is difficult in children, especially those who are unable to give a reliable history. ATLS protocol should be followed in all trauma cases, with

---

Box 3
Anatomic differences in pediatric patients predisposing them to cervical spine injury

- Larger head size and weight compared with the neck and trunk
- Weaker C-spine musculature
- Increased laxity of the spinal ligaments
- Immature vertebral joints and ossification centers
- Increased elasticity of the spinal column
- Lack of uncinate processes until approximately age 10

Data from Refs.[37,41–45]

Box 4
Indications for immobilizing the pediatric cervical spine in a trauma

- High-risk mechanism (MVCs, diving, contact sports, acceleration-deceleration injury)
- Altered mental status
- C-spine midline tenderness
- Decreased range of motion
- Neurologic deficits
- Distracting injury
- Multiple system trauma

Data from Hoffman JR, Mower WR, Wolfson AB, et al. Validity of a set of clinical criteria to rule out injury to the cervical spine in patients with blunt trauma. National Emergency X-Radiography Utilization Study Group. N Engl J Med 2000;343:94.

---

evaluation of the C-spine taking place in the secondary survey. Most spinal cord injuries are a result of direct compression on the cord itself or disruption of the cord by a fractured or subluxed vertebrae.[56] Symptoms of a C-spine injury are extremely variable. Neurologic complaints may be vague or transient. In some cases, children with spinal cord injuries are asymptomatic. The evaluation of a C-spine injury on physical examination focuses on vital signs, neck examination, and neurologic examination. A child who presents with apnea or hypoventilation may have damage to the phrenic nerve (C3-C5), which controls the movement of the diaphragm. Spinal shock, also known as distributive shock, may be the presenting sign in some cases of spinal cord injury, with hypotension and bradycardia most commonly found on examination.

Physical examination should center on a thorough neck and neurologic evaluation. The C-spine should be palpated down the midline. This can be safely completed with the removal of the immobilization collar; however, it is recommended that a second provider hold the patient's head in a neutral position during the examination. Any midline deformities or point tenderness are concerning for a C-spine injury. Second, a thorough neurologic examination is an integral part of the assessment for a spinal cord injury. Isolated sensory deficits are far more common than motor deficits. It is also important to assess and document muscle tone, muscle strength, and deep tendon reflexes. In patients with abnormal vital signs and an abnormal neurologic examination, a rectal examination may help rule out spinal shock. The lack of a bulbocavernous reflex is indicative of an injury leading to spinal shock. This particular reflex is elicited and measured by squeezing the glans penis or pulling on an indwelling Foley catheter while monitoring anal sphincter tone.

The assessment of children with a C-spine injury is challenging to providers. Because of the likelihood of a high mechanism causing the injury, children are often scared and uncooperative during a physician's physical examination. It is important for physicians to use the available resources to thoroughly examine patients. Early and aggressive pain management techniques, including the use of intranasal or intravenous opioids, allow practitioners to provide adequate analgesia while assessing a child's injury. Other resources, including child life specialists, are valuable when available, because they can provide distraction and comforting measures to patients. Finally, a patient's family should be allowed to accompany the child during the evaluation as long as they do not impede the examination or necessary resuscitation.

Common cervical spine injuries in pediatric trauma

Given the anatomic differences in pediatric patients, clinical presentations of C-spine injuries can vary widely. Hyperflexion injuries are the most common type of C-spine injury. Such injuries include the clay-shoveler's fracture, which is an avulsion fracture of a single spinous process, usually located within the lower cervical vertebrae. Clay-shoveler's fractures are stable; however, neurosurgical consultation is warranted in any vertebral fracture. The teardrop fracture is another common C-spine fracture that occurs when extreme flexion causes a vertebral body to come in contact with the vertebral body below. This particular mechanism leads to a fracture of the ante-roinferior vertebral body, resembling a teardrop. The teardrop fracture of the C-spine is considered unstable and can present with anterior cord symptoms including paralysis and loss of pain sensation.

Radiology for assessment of a cervical spine injury

Any child with a suspected C-spine injury must undergo radiographic evaluation. Many of the C-spine decision rules for imaging do not apply to the pediatric population. The National Emergency X-Radiography Utilization Study must be applied with caution to children less than 8 years of age, because only 2.5% of the study population was under the age of 8 years old and thus is not validated for this age group. Preverbal children are notoriously difficult to clear clinically because the surroundings, stress, and nature of their emergency department visits make a calm environment difficult to attain. Also, ambulation is not a predictor of C-spine injury in pediatric patients. The Canadian C-spine rule is a second well-known clinical decision rule that has been validated in adult populations; however, this particular study excluded patients under the age of 16 and, therefore, cannot be applied to a majority of the pediatric population.[57]

If indicated after the initial assessment, radiographic evaluation should include AP, cross-table lateral, and open-mouth odontoid views of the patient's C-spine. Cross-table lateral plain films identify approximately 80% of fractures, dislocations, and subluxations.[58] Adding the AP and open-mouth odontoid views increases the sensitivity of the evaluation to approximately 90%.[59] Flexion-extension and oblique views provide minimal information and are not recommended.[60,61]

CT scan has increased sensitivity and specificity of 98% or higher for the detection of C-spine fractures or injuries but is not recommended as the initial radiographic modality.[62,63] Children are at a much higher risk of developing malignancy of soft tissues, including the skin and thyroid, when exposed to the radiation of a helical CT scan. CT scans do have a place in the evaluation of pediatric C-spine injuries in certain instances. CT of the C-spine should be obtained in the following instances: inadequate plain films, suspicious findings on plain films, fracture or displacement seen on plain films, or if the provider has a high clinical suspicion of C-spine injury.[64,65]

MRI is the imaging modality recommended in any patient with persistent neurologic symptoms and normal plain films or CT. MRI is more sensitive for identifying injuries, including soft tissue abnormalities, vertebral disk herniation, ligamentous injury, or acute spinal cord injury.[66–73] MRI does have a limited use in the acute setting because it is not readily available, expensive, and time-intensive.

Spinal cord injuries without radiographic abnormality

Not all C-spine injuries are detected on plain film or CT. Spinal cord injuries without radiographic abnormality (SCIWORA) is the term used to describe spinal cord injuries without radiographic abnormality. SCIWORA is suspected in patients with neurologic deficits, including transient parasthesias, numbness, or paralysis, without any pathology found on plain radiographs, flexion-extension radiographs, and/or CT scan.[74] MRI has greatly decreased the number of such cases, because this particular modality better assesses the soft tissue components of the spinal column and is recommended in any child who displays transient or persistent neurologic deficits despite having no abnormalities with other imaging modalities.[49,75] Transient neurologic complaints are especially worrisome because approximately 25% of children with transient neurologic complaints or deficits can develop permanent symptoms ranging from complete paralysis to distinct neurologic deficits.[76–79] SCIWORA continues to be a controversial entity, with few well-powered or long-term studies to assess the true incidence and outcome of this injury. Current literature suggests it is more likely to occur in children less than 8 years old, with incidence ranging between 4.5% and 35% of children with spinal cord injuries.[49,78]

Secondary Survey: Cardiothoracic Injury

In pediatric trauma, thoracic injury occurs infrequently and is generally the result of forceful mechanisms that tend to cause other concomitant injuries. In an observational study from 1990, only 4.4% of traumatic victims had intrathoracic injuries.[80] The most common injuries include pulmonary contusion (48%); pneumothorax, hemothorax, or pneumohemothorax (39%); and rib fractures (32%).[80] Of those children with thoracic injury, 82% had other involved systems and significantly higher trauma severity scores.[80] Blunt trauma, generally from MVCs, is responsible for most thoracic injuries. Penetrating injury to the chest often results, however, in higher mortality with gunshot wounds, making up 60% of these injuries.[81] Overall, the mortality rate for children with thoracic trauma is between 15% and 26%.[82]

Anatomic and physiologic considerations

Injury patterns as the result of thoracic trauma in children are different from those seen in adults, mostly due to the differences in pediatric anatomy and physiology (**Box 5**). Most importantly, children have a more compliant chest wall that is able to absorb and distribute forces, resulting in fewer rib fractures than seen in their adult counterparts. Conversely, this compliance can often mask serious underlying injury because patients exhibit minimal signs externally.[83] Additionally, the mediastinum is more freely

---

Box 5
Physical evaluation—what to look for in pediatric thoracic trauma

Respiratory

- Abnormal rate
- Nasal flaring or retractions
- Paradoxic chest wall movement
- Chest wall injuries or defects
- Abnormal lung sounds on auscultation

Cardiac

- Distant or muffled heart tones
- Murmur
- Irregular rhythm
- Distended neck veins

mobile often, resulting in greater displacement with intrathoracic injury, leading to decreased venous return to the heart and subsequently decreased cardiac output and hypotension with the risk of complete circulatory collapse.

In a study from 2002, researchers looked for a clinical decision rule for predicting thoracic injury in children after blunt trauma.[84] They found that significant predictors included low systolic blood pressure, elevated respiratory rate, abnormal findings on thoracic examination, abnormal auscultation findings, and a GCS score of less than 15.[84] Of the patients they reviewed, 98% had at least 1 of these predictive factors.[84] These findings should be used to guide laboratory and radiologic investigation in traumatic patients suspected of intrathoracic injury.

Diagnostic evaluation of cardiothoracic injury

After a thorough historical and physical evaluation, diagnostic studies are the next step in identifying a patient's injuries. There is a growing use of CT for evaluating children in the setting of trauma. As a result, there is also a growing concern that CT is unnecessarily overused in traumatic evaluation, especially given the concern for excessive radiation exposure at a young age.[85] When considering thoracic trauma specifically, there is significant evidence that a plain film chest radiograph remains an effective screening tool for significant injury in pediatric patients. It is recommended that a chest CT not be the primary imaging tool but, rather, an adjunct to clinical evaluation and plain film imaging.[86]

Other modalities to consider using to evaluate chest trauma in children include ECG, cardiac troponins, and a cardiac view on bedside ultrasound via the Focused Assessment with Sonography for Trauma (FAST) examination. ECG should be considered in any child with anterior chest trauma, sternal fracture, or any arrhythmia. In the setting of possible cardiac contusion, a 12-lead ECG and cardiac troponin levels are helpful, although not routinely recommended. In a recent study, stable patients with suspected intrathoracic trauma with normal troponin levels and normal ECGs were unlikely to have significant myocardial injury; however, this is not standard practice in most pediatric trauma centers.[87] Additionally, the bedside FAST examination can reveal cardiac tamponade and, in the hands of a skilled ultrasonographer, pneumothorax.

Specific cardiothoracic injuries common in pediatric trauma

Diaphragmatic injury Although a rare event in pediatric patients, a diaphragmatic injury can result in rapid respiratory deterioration and failure if not quickly addressed. Often this injury is a predictor of other serious associated injuries in trauma.[88] These children often present with chest pain and tachypnea but tend to lack external signs of injury unless caused by a penetrating wound that suggests diaphragmatic involvement.[88] In general, this injury is easily identified on plain film chest radiograph where loops of intestine are seen above the diaphragm, the tip of the nasogastric tube lies above the diaphragm, or the hemidiaphragm appears elevated or obscured. Definitive treatment requires surgical intervention. Therefore, the focus in an emergency department should include resuscitation, definitive airway control, gastric decompression, and stabilization of other injuries.

Traumatic asphyxia A unique and rare injury to the pediatric population, traumatic asphyxia occurs as a result of the increased compliance of pediatric the chest wall. Typically, this entity follows a marked increase in intrathoracic pressure due to direct chest compression in conjunction with deep inspiration against a closed glottis experienced during a crush injury. This dramatic increase in pressure is transmitted directly to the superior and inferior vena cava, resulting in significant facial and neck petechial hemorrhages, cyanosis, subconjunctival hemorrhages, and facial swelling.[89] Occasionally, neurologic and ocular involvement is seen in severe cases. Neurologic findings include altered mental status, brachial plexus injuries, and coma, although ocular findings, including hemorrhage into the retina, vitreous body, or optic nerve, can result in vision loss. Generally speaking, this injury does not result in significant morbidity and mortality, but is often associated with other severe injuries. Treatment involves elevating the head of the bed and addressing other associated injuries.

Commotio cordis This disease entity, commotio cordis, described almost solely in pediatric trauma, is a combination of ventricular fibrillation and sudden cardiac death secondary to a sudden impact to the anterior chest wall. Frequently it is described in association with sudden cardiac death that occurs after direct impact to the chest when playing sports, specifically baseball. According to the National Commotio Cordis Registry, victims have a mean age of 15 years, with a 95% male predominance, and are frequently struck in the chest with projectiles rather than blunt bodily contact.[90] Although usually a fatal event, the survival rate has risen to 35% over the past decade due to improved public awareness, increased availability of automatic external defibrillators, and earlier activation of first responders.[90]

There are several factors that contribute to the risk of commotio cordis. These relate to the timing, location, and velocity of impact to the chest wall. Most importantly, there is only a 20-millisecond to 40-millisecond window during the cardiac cycle in which the trauma must occur to result in ventricular fibrillation.[91] Commotio cordis is best diagnosed by the appropriate clinical scenario, ECG data demonstrating ventricular fibrillation, and the absence of structural heart damage on subsequent studies after resuscitation.

One study in 2006 aimed at looking at the effectiveness of commercially available chest wall protectors in the prevention of commotio cordis. Unfortunately, it found these protectors were mostly ineffective in preventing ventricular fibrillation in pig models.[92] A study from 1998, however, found that the likelihood of ventricular fibrillation was proportional to the hardness of the ball, with soft safety baseballs providing the lowest risk of ventricular fibrillation.[91] As a result, it has been recommended that age-appropriate baseballs be used to help reduce the incidence of this potentially fatal event.

Secondary Survey: Blunt Abdominal Trauma

Blunt abdominal trauma in pediatric patients is the third leading cause of traumatic death behind head and chest injuries. The mechanism of blunt abdominal trauma is especially important in the pediatric population, because certain mechanisms often correlate with specific injuries. Motor vehicle collisions are the most common cause of lethal blunt abdominal trauma in this age group. The mortality of these traumatic events is directly proportional to the number of intra-abdominal organs injured.[81] Children are inherently more susceptible to serious intra-abdominal injuries because of their anatomic structure. Children have larger solid organs, less-protective subcutaneous fat and abdominal musculature, more-flexible rib cages, and a smaller torso, allowing for wide transmission of significant force.

The extent of injury in a child with blunt abdominal trauma is often difficult to determine. Generally, patients with severe abdominal trauma also present with other traumatic injuries, which can make obtaining a detailed history difficult. Children who present with obvious traumatic injuries should be considered as having an intra-abdominal injury until proved otherwise; this is especially true in patients who are hemodynamically unstable. It is important to remember that the assessment of the abdomen is part of the secondary survey, and serial examinations of the abdomen aid in ongoing evaluation.

The physical examination is an important part of the evaluation of abdominal trauma and can provide clues to clinicians regarding specific injuries that may be potentially life threatening. On initial evaluation, a patient's vital signs should be obtained. A child found tachycardic, hypotensive, or tachypneic may have significant intra-abdominal injuries.

In children who are hemodynamically stable, the physical examination can yield clues to potential injuries. It is important to completely undress children to do a thorough examination, specifically looking for bruising, tire tracks, or any missed injuries. Patients with presumed abdominal trauma and subsequent abdominal distension should have an orogastric or nasogastric tube placed for abdominal decompression. Doing so improves ventilatory abilities of the child and decreases the risk for aspiration. Any ecchymosis of the abdominal wall should greatly increase provider suspicion of severe intra-abdominal injury. The seat belt sign is a transverse bruise over the inferior portion of the abdomen. This particular bruising pattern may be associated with small bowel injuries, Chance fractures of the lumbar spine, and, rarely, injuries of the abdominal aorta. A seat belt sign may be present in up to 10% of motor vehicle collisions.[93–95] Bruising of the flank may be indicative of injuries to retroperitoneal structures, including the kidney. Point tenderness of the abdomen may also increase the probability of injury to the underlying structure but is unreliable in younger children. Potentially dangerous splenic injuries may be manifested only by pain in the left shoulder, known as Kehr sign.

Solid organs, including the liver and spleen, are the most commonly injured structures in the setting of blunt trauma in children. These particular organs are highly vascularized, and injury can cause significant blood loss with rapid decompensation. Pancreatic injuries are far less common than hepatic or splenic insults but may be present, especially in patients with epigastric pain. Hollow viscous organ injury is less common than solid organ injuries but potentially life threatening. In descending order, the jejunum, duodenum, colon, and stomach are the most commonly injured hollow viscus organs damaged in pediatric abdominal trauma. Duodenal injuries are often associated with bicycle accidents, specifically by handlebars contacting the epigastric and right upper quadrant regions of the abdomen. Hematomas of the duodenum occur when the structure is compressed against the vertebral column, momentarily interrupting the blood flow. Duodenal hematomas can expand causing partial or complete small bowel obstructions. These particular obstructions may be manifested as bilious vomiting and often occur 24 to 48 hours after the injury. Duodenal hematomas and their subsequent obstructions generally resolve with conservative management including nothing by mouth status, bowel rest, gastric decompression, and parenteral nutrition.

Beyond the physical examination, there are a few laboratory and radiographic tests that may aid providers in determining the extent of underlying abdominal injury. During the initial assessment, intravenous access should ideally be established. Laboratory tests, including a complete blood cell count (CBC), lipase, and comprehensive metabolic panel (including electrolytes and liver function tests), are particularly useful. Other laboratory tests, including coagulation studies, and a urinalysis may also aid physicians but are not as sensitive nor specific for intra-abdominal injuries. The CBC provides physicians with patients' intravascular blood volume. Abnormally low hemoglobin may indicate internal hemorrhage requiring emergent intervention by pediatric surgeons or interventional radiologists. A blood type and crossmatch should also be obtained quickly as to not delay any potential surgical care. Elevated transaminases have been shown sensitive and specific for the presence of intra-abdominal injury in the setting of blunt trauma.[96,97] Specifically, patients with an aspartate aminotransferase (AST) greater than 200 IU/L or alanine aminotransferase (ALT) greater than 125 IU/L should raise clinician suspicion of injury and warrant further investigation of his abdomen with imaging. Pancreatic enzymes, such as amylase and lipase, are not sensitive for acute pancreatic or other intra-abdominal organ injury. They are useful as a baseline when monitoring the development of a pancreatic complication or unexplained abdominal pain in trauma patients. An elevated lipase is fairly specific for pancreatic injury, but an elevated level is not a clear indication for imaging, especially without epigastric pain. A urinalysis is another routinely obtained laboratory test in trauma patients, and the presence of gross blood may indicate injury to the genitourinary system. No single laboratory test has acceptable sensitivity or negative predictive value to safely and effectively screen patients after undergoing blunt abdominal trauma when used alone (**Box 6**).[98]

The gold standard radiographic method for identifying intra-abdominal injury after a traumatic event is the abdominal CT with intravenous contrast in hemodynamically stable patients. **Box 7** lists indications for obtaining an abdominal CT. Patients who are hemodynamically unstable with suspected abdominal injury should be evaluated by a surgeon immediately. The FAST examination is another modality often used in the emergency department to assess for free fluid in the peritoneum or pericardium secondary to trauma. The FAST examines 4 specific locations: Morison pouch (hepatorenal interface in the right upper quadrant), subxyphoid cardiac view, splenorenal interface, and bladder. A positive FAST that indicates free fluid in a patient's abdomen or pericardium should prompt a physician to obtain an abdominal CT with intravenous contrast if the patient is hemodynamically stable. Patients with a positive FAST examination and hemodynamic instability should undergo prompt surgical evaluation. A negative FAST does not rule out serious intra-abdominal injury. Patients with a high suspicion of solid organ injury should undergo an abdominal CT (**Box 7**).

In hemodynamically unstable children with suspected intra-abdominal injury who are unable to go to CT scan, a diagnostic peritoneal lavage (DPL) may be useful. The discussion of performing a DPL versus an emergent laparotomy should be held with a pediatric surgeon. The DPL is much less invasive than laparotomy. The DPL, however, is less specific, cannot detect retroperitoneal injury, has potentially harmful side effects, and may lead to unnecessary exploratory laparotomy because many children with intra-abdominal blood are safely observed without surgical intervention.[99] Because of the aforementioned risks and the availability of high-resolution

Box 6
Laboratory testing indicated in pediatric abdominal trauma
CBC
Comprehensive metabolic panel, including transaminases
Blood type and crossmatch
Urinalysis
Serum amylase and lipase
Urine pregnancy test

Box 7
Indications for obtaining an abdominal CT in pediatric trauma in hemodynamically stable patients trauma

History suggestive of severe intra-abdominal injury

Physical examination concerning for intra-abdominal injury (ie, abdominal tenderness, guarding, or rebound tenderness)

Presence of the seat belt sign or other abdominal bruising

AST >200 or ALT >125

Decline in hemoglobin or hematocrit <30% from baseline

Gross or microscopic blood on urinalysis (≥50 red blood cells)

Positive FAST examination

CT scanners, the DPL has mostly fallen out of favor with most pediatric surgeons when assessing the need for operative management. **Box 8** outlines the indications for emergency laparotomy in pediatric patients who present after blunt abdominal trauma.

A substantial portion of children with acute abdominal trauma are managed without surgical intervention. Children who have any indication of hemodynamic instability or required volume resuscitation should be admitted to an intensive care unit for continuous monitoring. Patients with stable vital signs and physical examination or laboratory findings suggestive of acute intra-abdominal injury can be safely monitored on a pediatric ward. In both settings, patients should undergo serial abdominal examinations to assess for clinical worsening and the need for subsequent intervention. Specifically, the American Pediatric Surgical Association has developed guidelines for the management of clinically stable patients who have isolated liver or spleen injuries. The guidelines recommend that all pediatric patients who are hemodynamically stable with grades I to IV liver or splenic lacerations secondary to blunt abdominal trauma should receive nonoperative management.[97,103] In addition, immunization against encapsulated organisms is standard practice and should be given during the hospital stay for children with severe splenic injuries. Pediatric studies that indicate the optimal timing of immunization as it relates to the grade of liver injury are limited, but two randomized trials suggest that two weeks post-splenectomy generates the best immune response.[104,105]

Box 8
Indications for emergency laparotomy after blunt abdominal trauma

Intra-abdominal bleeding with persistent hemodynamic instability despite aggressive crystalloid and blood transfusion (transfusion >20 mL/kg packed red blood cells),

Perforation of a hollow viscous injury leading to pneumoperitoneum

Increasing abdominal tenderness or the development of peritoneal signs on examination

Solid organ injury with persistent bleeding

Pancreatic injury with ductal disruption

Data from Refs.[24,100–102]

SUMMARY

The evaluation of pediatric trauma patients involves several various nuances, differentiating it from that of an adult counterpart. It is important to develop a structured yet focused approach when dealing with children with traumatic injuries. With the completion of a thorough physical examination, appropriate laboratory and radiographic adjuncts, and adherence to ATLS protocol, the evaluation of pediatric patients involved in a trauma can be managed in a safe and efficient manner.

REFERENCES

1. Centers for Disease Control and Prevention. National Center for Injury Prevention and Control. Injury and violence prevention and control: data and statistics. 1 Dec. 2011. Web. 31 Oct. 2012. Available at: http://www.cdc.gov/injury/wisqars/index.html.
2. Centers for Disease Control and Prevention (CDC). Vital signs: unintentional injury deaths among persons aged 0-19 years—United States, 2000-2009. MMWR Morb Mortal Wkly Rep 2012;61:270-6.
3. Marx JA, Hockberger RS, Walls RM, et al, editors. Rosen's emergency medicine concepts and clinical practice. Philadelphia: Mosby/Elsevier; 2010.
4. Fleming S, Thompson M, Stevens R, et al. Normal ranges of heart rate and respiratory rate in children from birth to 18 years of age: a systematic review of observational studies. Lancet 2011;377(9770):1011-8.
5. Arens R, McDonough JM, Costarino AT, et al. Magnetic resonance imaging of the upper airway structure of children with obstructive sleep apnea syndrome. Am J Respir Crit Care Med 2001;164:698.
6. Weiss M, Knirsch W, Kretschmar O, et al. Tracheal tube-tip displacement in children during head-neck movement—a radiological assessment. Br J Anaesth 2006;96:486.
7. Moulton C, Pennycook AG. Relation between Glasgow coma score and cough reflex. Lancet 1994;343(8908):1261-2.
8. Kim JT, Na HS, Bae JY, et al. GlideScope video laryngoscope: a randomized clinical trial in 203 paediatric patients. Br J Anaesth 2008;101(4):531-4.
9. Kleinman ME, Chameides L, Schexnayder SM, et al. Part 14: Pediatric Advanced Life Support: 2010 American Heart Association guidelines for cardiopulmonary resuscitation and emergency cardiovascular care. Circulation 2010; 122:S876.
10. Harris T, Ellis DY, Foster L, et al. Cricoid pressure and laryngeal manipulation in 402 pre-hospital emergency anaesthetics: essential safety measure or a hindrance to rapid safe intubation? Resuscitation 2010;81(7):810-6.
11. Vlatten A, Litz S, Macmanus B, et al. A comparison of the glidescope video laryngoscope and standard direct laryngoscopy in children with immobilized cervical spine. Pediatr Emerg Care 2012;28(12):1317-20.
12. King BR, Baker MD, Braitman LE, et al. Endotracheal tube selection in children: a comparison of four methods. Ann Emerg Med 1993;22:530.
13. Gerling MC, David DP, Hamilton RS, et al. Effects of cervical spine immobilization technique and laryngoscope blade selection on an unstable cervical spine in a cadaver model of intubation. Ann Emerg Med 2000;36:293.
14. Phipps LM, Thomas NJ, Gilmore RK, et al. Prospective assessment of guidelines for determining appropriate depth of endotracheal tube placement in children. Pediatr Crit Care Med 2005;6:519.

15. Weiss M, Dullenkopf A, Fischer JE, et al. Prospective randomized controlled multi-centre trial of cuffed or uncuffed endotracheal tubes in small children. Br J Anaesth 2009;103(6):867.

16. Newth CJ, Rachman B, Patel N, et al. The use of cuffed versus uncuffed endotracheal tubes in pediatric intensive care. J Pediatr 2004;144(3):333–7.

17. Taha SK, Siddik-Sayyid SM, El-Khatib MF, et al. Nasopharyngeal oxygen insufflation following pre-oxygenation using the four deep breath technique. Anaesthesia 2006;61(5):427–30.

18. Patel R, Lenczyk M, Hannallah RS, et al. Age and the onset of desaturation in apnoeic children. Can J Anaesth 1994;41(9):771.

19. Gausche M, Lewis RJ, Stratton SJ, et al. Effect of out-of-hospital pediatric endotracheal intubation on survival and neurological outcome: a controlled clinical trial. JAMA 2000;283(6):783–90.

20. Kilgannon JH, Jones AE, Parrillo JE, et al. Relationship between supranormal oxygen tension and outcome after resuscitation from cardiac arrest. Circulation 2011;123(23):2717–22.

21. Del Castillo J, Lopez-Herce J, Matamoros M, et al. Hyperoxia, hypocapnia and hypercapnia as outcome factors after cardiac arrest in children. Resuscitation 2012;83(12):1456–61.

22. Tinsley C, Hill JB, Shah J, et al. Experience of families during cardiopulmonary resuscitation in a pediatric intensive care unit. Pediatrics 2008;122(4):e799–804.

23. Kuppermann N, Holmes JF, Dayan PS, et al. Identification of children at very low risk of clinically-important brain injuries after head trauma: a prospective cohort study. Lancet 2009;374(9696):1160–70.

24. Jaffe D, Wesson D. Emergency management of blunt trauma in children. N Engl J Med 1991;324(21):1477–82.

25. Ghajar J. Management of pediatric head injury. Pediatr Clin North Am 1992;39:1093.

26. Palchak MJ, Holmes JF, Vance CW, et al. A decision rule for identifying children at low risk for brain injuries after blunt head trauma. Ann Emerg Med 2003;42:492.

27. Caffey J. The whiplash shaken infant syndrome: manual shaking by the extremities with whiplash-induced intracranial and intraocular bleedings, linked with residual permanent brain damage and mental retardation. Pediatrics 1974;54:396.

28. Duhaime AC, Christian CW, Rorke LB, et al. Nonaccidental head injury in infants—the "shaken-baby syndrome". N Engl J Med 1998;338:1822.

29. Keenan HT, Runyan DK, Marshall SW, et al. A population-based study of inflicted traumatic brain injury in young children. JAMA 2003;290:621.

30. King WJ, MacKay M, Sirnick A, Canadian Shaken Baby Study Group. Shaken baby syndrome in Canada: clinical characteristics and outcomes of hospital cases. CMAJ 2003;168:155.

31. Alexander R, Sato Y, Smith W, et al. Incidence of impact trauma with cranial injuries ascribed to shaking. Am J Dis Child 1990;44:724.

32. Atwal GS, Rutty GN, Carter N, et al. Bruising in non-accidental head injured children; a retrospective study of the prevalence, distribution and pathological associations in 24 cases. Forensic Sci Int 1998;96:215.

33. Merten DF, Osborne DR, Radkowski MA, et al. Craniocerebral trauma in the child abuse syndrome: radiological observations. Pediatr Radiol 1984;14:272.

34. Lazoritz S, Baldwin S, Kini N. The Whiplash Shaken Infant Syndrome: has Caffey's syndrome changed or have we changed his syndrome? Child Abuse Negl 1997;21:1009.

35. Di Pietro MA, Brody AS, Cassady CI, et al. American Academy of Pediatrics Section on Radiology Policy Statement. Diagnostic imaging of child abuse. Pediatrics 2009;123(5):1430–5.

36. Apple J. Cervical spine fractures and dislocations in children. Pediatr Radiol 1987;17:45.

37. Baker C, Kadish H, Schunk JE. Evaluation of pediatric cervical spine injuries. Am J Emerg Med 1999;17:230.

38. Orenstein JB, Klein BL, Gotschall CS, et al. Age and outcome in pediatric cervical spine injury: 11-year experience. Pediatr Emerg Care 1994;10:132.

39. Brown RL, Brunn MA, Garcia VF. Cervical spine injuries in children: a review of 103 patients treated consecutively at a level 1 pediatric trauma center. J Pediatr Surg 2001;36:1107.

40. Peclet MH, Newman KD, Eichelberger MR, et al. Patterns of injury in children. J Pediatr Surg 1990;25:85.

41. Patel JC, Tepas JJ, Mollitt DL, et al. Pediatric cervical spine injuries: defining the disease. J Pediatr Surg 2001;36:373.

42. Chen LS, Blaw ME. Acute central cervical cord syndrome caused by minor trauma. J Pediatr 1986;108:96.

43. Hill SA, Miller CA, Kosnik EJ, et al. Pediatric neck injuries. A clinical study. J Neurosurg 1984;60:700.

44. Fesmire FM, Luten RC. The pediatric cervical spine: developmental anatomy and clinical aspects. J Emerg Med 1989;7:133.

45. Mohseni S, Talving P, Branco BC, et al. Effect of age on cervical spine injury in pediatric population: a National Trauma Data Bank review. J Pediatr Surg 2011; 46:1771.

46. Hall DE, Boydston W. Pediatric neck injuries. Pediatr Rev 1999;20:13.

47. Atlantoaxial instability in Down syndrome: subject review. American Academy of Pediatrics Committee on Sports Medicine and Fitness. Pediatrics 1995;96:151.

48. Herman MJ, Pizzutillo PD. Cervical spine disorders in children. Orthop Clin North Am 1999;30:457.

49. Ruge JR, Sinson GP, McLone DG, et al. Pediatric spinal injury: the very young. J Neurosurg 1988;68:25.

50. Pang D. Spinal cord injury without radiographic abnormality in children, 2 decades later. Neurosurgery 2004;55:1325.

51. Riggins RS, Kraus JF. The risk of neurologic damage with fractures of the vertebrae. J Trauma 1977;17:126.

52. Podolsky S, Baraff LJ, Simon RR, et al. Efficacy of cervical spine immobilization methods. J Trauma 1983;23:461.

53. Bonadio WA. Cervical spine trauma in children: Part I. General concepts, normal anatomy, radiographic evaluation. Am J Emerg Med 1993;11:158.

54. Skellett S, Tibby SM, Durward A, et al. Lesson of the week: Immobilisation of the cervical spine in children. BMJ 2002;324:591.

55. Committee on Trauma. Spine and spinal cord trauma. In: Advanced Trauma Life Support for Doctors. Chicago: American College of Surgeons; 1998. p. 265.

56. Jaffe DM, Binns H, Radkowski MA, et al. Developing a clinical algorithm for early management of cervical spine injury in child trauma victims. Ann Emerg Med 1987;16:270.

57. Jacobs LM, Schwartz R. Prospective analysis of acute cervical spine injury: a methodology to predict injury. Ann Emerg Med 1986;15:44.

58. Stiell IG, Wells GA, Vandemheen KL, et al. The Canadian C-spine rule for radiography in alert and stable trauma patients. JAMA 2001;286(15):1841–8.

59. Mower WR, Hoffman JR, Pollack CV Jr, et al. Use of plain radiography to screen for cervical spine injuries. Ann Emerg Med 2001;38:1.

60. Pollack CV Jr, Hendey GW, Martin DR, et al. Use of flexion-extension radiographs of the cervical spine in blunt trauma. Ann Emerg Med 2001;38:8.

61. Freemyer B, Knopp R, Piche J, et al. Comparison of five-view and three-view cervical spine series in the evaluation of patients with cervical trauma. Ann Emerg Med 1989;18:818.

62. McCulloch PT, France J, Jones DL, et al. Helical computed tomography alone compared with plain radiographs with adjunct computed tomography to evaluate the cervical spine after high-energy trauma. J Bone Joint Surg Am 2005; 87:2388.

63. Sanchez B, Waxman K, Jones T, et al. Cervical spine clearance in blunt trauma: evaluation of a computed tomography-based protocol. J Trauma 2005;59:179.

64. Borock EC, Gabram SG, Jacobs LM, et al. A prospective analysis of a two-year experience using computed tomography as an adjunct for cervical spine clearance. J Trauma 1991;31:1001.

65. Hockberger RS, Kirshenbaum KJ, Doris PE. Spinal injuries. In: Rosen P, editor. Emergency medicine: concepts and clinical practice. 4th edition. St Louis (MO): Mosby-Year Book; 1998. p. 462.

66. Levitt MA, Flanders AE. Diagnostic capabilities of magnetic resonance imaging and computed tomography in acute cervical spinal column injury. Am J Emerg Med 1991;9:131.

67. Selden NR, Quint DJ, Patel N, et al. Emergency magnetic resonance imaging of cervical spinal cord injuries: clinical correlation and prognosis. Neurosurgery 1999;44:785.

68. Grabb PA, Pang D. Magnetic resonance imaging in the evaluation of spinal cord injury without radiographic abnormality in children. Neurosurgery 1994;35:406.

69. Felsberg GJ, Tien RD, Osumi AK, et al. Utility of MR imaging in pediatric spinal cord injury. Pediatr Radiol 1995;25:131.

70. Matsumura A, Meguro K, Tsurushima H, et al. Magnetic resonance imaging of spinal cord injury without radiologic abnormality. Surg Neurol 1990;33:281.

71. Flynn JM, Closkey RF, Mahboubi S, et al. Role of magnetic resonance imaging in the assessment of pediatric cervical spine injuries. J Pediatr Orthop 2002;22: 573.

72. Hyman RA, Gorey MT. Imaging strategies for MR of the spine. Radiol Clin North Am 1988;26:505.

73. Fehlings MG, Rao SC, Tator CH, et al. The optimal radiologic method for assessing spinal canal compromise and cord compression in patients with cervical spinal cord injury. Part II: Results of a multicenter study. Spine 1999;24:605.

74. Pang D, Wilberger JE. Spinal cord injury without radiographic abnormalities in children. J Neurosurg 1982;57:114.

75. Yucesoy K, Yuksel KZ. SCIWORA in MRI era. Clin Neurol Neurosurg 2008;110: 429.

76. Pang D, Pollack IF. Spinal cord injury without radiographic abnormality in children—the SCIWORA syndrome. J Trauma 1989;29:654.

77. Hamilton MG, Myles ST. Pediatric spinal injury: review of 174 hospital admissions. J Neurosurg 1992;77:700.

78. Osenbach RK, Menezes AH. Spinal cord injury without radiographic abnormality in children. Pediatr Neurosci 1989;15:168.

79. Martin BW, Dykes E, Lecky FE. Patterns and risks in spinal trauma. Arch Dis Child 2004;89:860.

80. Peclet MH, Newman KD, Eichelberger MR, et al. Thoracic trauma in children: an indicator of increased mortality. J Pediatr Surg 1990;25(9):961–5.
81. Cooper A, Barlow B, DiScala C, et al. Mortality and truncal injury: the pediatric perspective. J Pediatr Surg 1994;29(1):33.
82. Reyes Mendez D. Initial evaluation and stabilization of children with thoracic trauma. In: Bachur RG, editor. UpToDate. Waltham (MA): UpToDate; 2012.
83. Avarello JT, Cantor RM. Pediatric major trauma: an approach to evaluation and management. Emerg Med Clin North Am 2007;25(3):803–36.
84. Holmes JF, Sokolove PO, Brant WE, et al. A clinical decision rule for identifying children with thoracic injuries after blunt torso trauma. Ann Emerg Med 2002; 39(5):492–9.
85. Markel TA, Kumar R, Koontz NA, et al. The utility of computed tomography as a screening tool for the evaluation of pediatric blunt chest trauma. J Trauma 2009; 67(1):23–8.
86. Renton J, Kincaid S, Ehrlich PF. Should helical CT scanning of the thoracic cavity replace the conventional chest x-ray as a primary assessment tool in pediatric trauma? An efficacy and cost analysis. J Pediatr Surg 2003;38(5):793–7.
87. Velmahos GC, Karaiskakis M, Salim A, et al. Normal electrocardiography and serum troponin I levels preclude the presence of clinically significant blunt cardiac injury. J Trauma 2003;54(1):45–50.
88. Ramos CT, Koplewitz BZ, Babyn PS, et al. What have we learned about traumatic diaphragmatic hernias in children? J Pediatr Surg 2000;35(4):601.
89. Hurtado TR, Della-Giustina DA. Traumatic asphyxia in a 6-year-old boy. Pediatr Emerg Care 2003;19(3):167–8.
90. Maron BJ, Estes NA. Commotio cordis. N Engl J Med 2010;362(10):917–27.
91. Link MS, Wang PJ, Pandian NG, et al. An experimental model of sudden death due to low-energy chest-wall impact (commotio cordis). N Engl J Med 1998; 333(25):1805.
92. Weinstock J, Maron BJ, Song C, et al. Failure of commercially available chest wall protectors to prevent sudden cardiac death induced by chest wall blows in an experimental model of commotio cordis. Pediatrics 2006;117(4):e656–62.
93. Sivit C. Safety-belt injuries in children with lap-belt ecchymosis: CT findings in 61 patients. Am J Radiol 1991;157:111–4.
94. Sturm P. Lumbar compression fractures secondary to lap belt use in children. J Pediatr Orthop 1995;15:521.
95. Saladino R. The spectrum of liver and spleen injuries in children: failure of the PTS and clinical signs to predict isolated injuries. Ann Emerg Med 1991;20: 636.
96. Holmes JF, Sokolove PE, Brant WE, et al. Identification of children with intra-abdominal injuries after blunt trauma. Ann Emerg Med 2002;39:500.
97. Hennes HM, Smith DS, Schneider K, et al. Elevated liver transaminase levels in children with blunt abdominal trauma: a predictor of liver injury. Pediatrics 1990; 86:87.
98. Capraro AJ, Mooney D, Waltzman ML. The use of routine laboratory studies as screening tools in pediatric abdominal trauma. Pediatr Emerg Care 2006;22:480.
99. Pediatric trauma. In: American College of Surgeons Committee on Trauma, editor. Advanced trauma life support for doctors: student course manual. 8th edition. Chicago: American College of Surgeons; 2008. p. 225.
100. Saladino RA, Lund DP. Abdominal trauma. In: Fleisher GR, Ludwig S, editors. Textbook of pediatric emergency medicine. 6th edition. Philadelphia: Lippincott Williams and Wilkins; 2010. p. 1271.

101. DuBose J, Inaba K, Barmparas G, et al. Bilateral internal iliac artery ligation as a damage control approach in massive retroperitoneal bleeding after pelvic fracture. J Trauma 2010;69:1507.

102. Schafermeyer R. Pediatric trauma. Emerg Med Clin North Am 1993;11:187.

103. Moretz JA, Campbell DP, Parker DE, et al. Significance of serum amylase level in evaluating pancreatic trauma. Am J Surg 1975;130:739.

104. Shatz DV, Romero-Steiner S, Elie CM, et al. Antibody responses in postsplenectomy trauma patients receiving the 23-valent pneumococcal polysaccharide vaccine at 14 versus 28 days postoperatively. J Trauma 2002;53(6):1037–42.

105. Shatz DV, Schinsky MF, Pais LB, et al. Immune responses of splenectomized trauma patients to the 23-valent pneumococcal polysaccharide vaccine at 1 versus 7 versus 14 days after splenectomy. J Trauma 1998;44(5):760–6.

Pediatric Head Injury and Concussion

Robyn Wing, MD[a], Catherine James, MD[a,b],*

KEYWORDS

- Head injury • Concussion • Mild traumatic brain injury • Return to play
- Postconcussive syndrome • Abusive head trauma • Pediatric

KEY POINTS

- The Pediatric Glasgow Coma Scale can be used for serial evaluation of mental status in head-injured infants and young children.
- Decision rules can be used to decide which head-injured pediatric patients need to undergo further imaging studies.
- The diagnosis of concussion, a subclassification of the mild traumatic brain injury group, involves the assessment of a range of domains, including somatic and cognitive symptoms, physical signs, emotional and behavioral changes, and sleep disturbances.
- After a suspected concussion, patients should be withdrawn from physical activities immediately. Treatment for patients with concussion is centered on physical and cognitive rest, symptom management, and education of the patient, family, and other significant contacts. A graduated return-to-play protocol should be used for gradual reintroduction of physical activity in patients with concussion.
- The clinician must remain alert for the possibility of abusive head trauma when evaluating the head-injured pediatric patient.

Children with head injuries frequently present to emergency departments (EDs). Emergency medicine providers are often the first medical professionals to evaluate these children. The challenge for the provider is to determine which children have significant intracranial injuries that require intervention. Medical providers must rapidly stabilize injured patients and diagnose the primary injury while limiting secondary brain injury. There has been increased awareness of the damaging effects of even mild traumatic brain injuries, or concussions, leading to campaigns for prompt evaluation and education of health care providers, families, and athletic staff.

The authors have nothing to disclose.
[a] Department of Pediatrics, University of Massachusetts Medical School, 55 Lake Avenue North, Worcester, MA 01655, USA; [b] Pediatric Emergency Medicine, UMass Memorial Medical Center, 55 Lake Avenue North, Worcester, MA 01655, USA
* Corresponding author. Pediatric Emergency Medicine, UMass Memorial Medical Center, 55 Lake Avenue North, Worcester, MA 01655.
E-mail address: Catherine.james@umassmemorial.org

Emerg Med Clin N Am 31 (2013) 653–675
http://dx.doi.org/10.1016/j.emc.2013.05.007
0733-8627/13/$ – see front matter © 2013 Elsevier Inc. All rights reserved.

It is also imperative to identify the children who are victims of abusive head trauma to protect them from future injury.

INTRODUCTION/EPIDEMIOLOGY

Head injuries are a common reason for ED visits for children in the United States. Although most children suffer only minor injury, there are almost 600,000 ED visits, 60,000 hospitalizations, and more than 6000 deaths per year for children ages 19 years and younger.[1] Head injuries are the most common cause of injury-related pediatric hospitalizations and deaths, with a total cost of more than $1 billion in 2000.[2] The causes of trauma vary based on the child's age and developmental level. In patients 19 years and younger, the most common cause of head injuries is falls, followed by being struck by or against an object, other or unknown causes, motor vehicle accidents (occupant or pedestrian), and assaults. Falls are the most common cause of head injury for patients 0 to 4 years of age, whereas motor vehicle–related injuries are the most common cause of head injury in the 15 to 19-year age group. The rate of ED visits is higher for younger patients, but the hospitalization and death rates are higher for older children. Boys outnumber girls for both ED visits and deaths in all age groups. Motor vehicle accidents are the most common cause of head injury deaths for all age groups.[1–3]

Head injury in children differs from adults in several aspects. Clinical evaluation can be challenging in the young patient because they are unable to provide a history of the event and do not always cooperate with the physical examination. The developing anatomy and age-specific biomechanical properties of the head and neck result in different injuries in different age groups. Children's heads are proportionally larger and heavier in relation to their bodies than adults, the occiput and forehead are more prominent, and the facial bones are proportionally smaller. The pediatric skull is more compliant than the adult, thus it can absorb more force without a fracture, but this also increases the shearing forces between the skull, dura, subdural vessels, and brain. Children also have relatively weaker necks than adults, which allows more movement of the head when forces are applied to the torso. The pediatric brain has higher water content and lesser degree of myelination, so it is less dense and may sustain more acceleration-deceleration injury than adults.

INJURY TYPES

The *primary injury* is the mechanical damage to the scalp, skull, and brain that occurs at the time of trauma. Many children evaluated for head injury have only superficial injuries, such as a scalp laceration or hematoma, or a nondepressed skull fracture without intracranial injury. Concussion is a type of primary brain injury that does not involve structural derangements and will be discussed in more detail in a later section. Depressed, open, and basilar skull fractures may be associated with intracranial injuries. Brain injuries can be extra-axial (epidural hematoma, subdural hematoma, subarachnoid hematoma, intraventricular hemorrhage) or intra-axial (cerebral contusion, intracerebral hematoma, diffuse axonal injury). More than one type of injury may occur simultaneously.

- *Epidural hematomas* develop from bleeding into the space between the skull and dura mater. Although classically resulting from shearing of the middle meningeal artery, they may also be caused by venous bleeding. They are less common in infants and young children than adults because the dura is more firmly adherent to the skull. They usually result from a fall or direct blow to the head and can occur without skull fracture. Computed tomography (CT) scans demonstrate lens-shaped convexities that do not usually cross suture lines.

- *Subdural hematomas* are caused by injury to the bridging cortical veins between the dura and arachnoid membranes. The mechanism usually involves sudden acceleration/deceleration of the head. They are more common in younger children. They can also occur without skull fracture and may be bilateral. They are crescent-shaped on CT scans and can cross suture lines. Abusive head trauma is a common cause in infants and toddlers.
- *Subarachnoid hematomas* result from tearing of small pial vessels due to blunt trauma or shearing forces. They are often widely distributed and do not usually cause mass effect.
- *Intraventricular hemorrhages* may result from bleeding from an intracerebral hematoma, extension of a subarachnoid hematoma, or tearing of subependymal veins or periventricular structures. They are often associated with other injuries. Premature infants often suffer from spontaneous intraventricular bleeding.
- *Cerebral contusions* are localized areas of neuronal injury with associated bleeding. They are caused by blunt trauma to the head, which causes movement of the brain against the skull.
- *Intracerebral hematomas* result from tearing of intraparenchymal vessels. They may cause mass effect.
- *Diffuse axonal injury* is widespread damage to axons in multiple parts of the brain and usually results from acceleration/deceleration or rotational forces. It is often caused by motor vehicle collisions or abusive head trauma.

Secondary injury is further damage to neuronal cells that occurs as a consequence of hypoxia, hypoperfusion, metabolic derangements, and increased intracranial pressure (ICP). This process begins immediately after the injury and may progress over days to months, leading to impaired oxygen and glucose delivery to neurons, and eventual cell death. Types of secondary injury include brain herniation, cerebral edema, infarction, and hydrocephalus. Since the primary injury occurs before the patient presents for care, a major goal of the emergency provider is to prevent secondary injury.

INITIAL EVALUATION OF THE HEAD-INJURED CHILD

The initial evaluation and management of the head-injured child focuses on diagnosing the primary brain injury and stabilizing the patient to prevent or limit secondary brain injury. As for any injured patient, the airway must be stabilized, and breathing and circulation must be ensured while taking precautions to protect the cervical spine. Once these concerns have been addressed, full assessment of the child may be performed and the provider must determine whether imaging studies are needed.

History

The history should focus on the mechanism and timing of the injury as well as previous and current symptoms. If the child is conscious and mature enough, much of the history can be obtained directly from the patient. The parent and any witnesses to the event may also provide additional information. Details about the mechanism of injury should include the height and surface for falls; a description of the object that struck the head; and whether protective devices like seatbelts, car seats, and helmets were used. If the injury involved a motor vehicle, questions should include the approximate speed of the vehicle, amount of damage to the vehicle, and any injuries other occupants sustained. The provider should inquire about the presence and duration of loss of consciousness, seizures (time of onset, length, and focality), nausea/vomiting, headache, visual disturbances, amnesia, and confusion. In addition, the provider should obtain information about the progression of symptoms and concomitant injuries.

Physical Examination

The physical examination begins with a rapid assessment of airway, breathing, circulation, neurologic status and an evaluation for other life-threatening injuries. Abnormal vital signs, such as bradycardia, tachycardia, hypotension, or hypoxia should be noted and addressed. Examination of the head should be performed to look for scalp swelling, hematomas, abrasions, and lacerations; obvious fracture or deformity; fullness of the fontanel in infants; hemotympanum; Battle sign (bruising over the mastoid) or raccoon eyes (periorbital bruising); and bleeding or drainage from the ears or nose concerning for cerebrospinal fluid leak. The clinician should assess pupillary symmetry, size, and responsiveness, and perform a fundoscopic examination to look for retinal hemorrhages and papilledema. The cervical spine should be inspected and palpated. The remainder of the body should be assessed for associated injuries.

The neurologic examination includes evaluation of mental status, cranial nerves, and motor, sensory, and cerebellar functions. The mental status examination is one of the most important parts of the physical examination and should be serially monitored. The provider should ask the parent if the patient is acting at his or her baseline, especially if the child is preverbal. The Glasgow Coma Scale (GCS) is an important part of this assessment and has been modified for use in infants and young children. The remainder of the neurologic examination must be tailored to the child's age and developmental stage.

Pediatric GCS

The GCS has long been used as a scoring system for serial evaluation of patients with head trauma[4]; however, verbal and motor responses must be evaluated with respect to a child's age. For example, the normal babbling of infants could be termed "incomprehensible sounds" and they are not able to understand commands. Even a fully conscious but frightened (or stubborn) toddler may not follow instructions. A modified GCS for infants and young children was therefore developed to allow assignment of a score to preverbal children.[5] Eye opening is evaluated similarly to adults, but verbal and motor scores are modified (**Table 1**). The verbal component of the modified GCS score may be affected by the injured child's fear or discomfort. Therefore, the GCS should be reassessed once the child has been calmed and has received pain medications.

Table 1
Pediatric Glasgow Coma Scale (GCS)

Eye Opening		Best Verbal Response		Best Motor Response	
Spontaneous	4	Smiles, coos, babbles, interacts, oriented to sounds	5	Normal spontaneous movement	6
To speech	3	Cries but consolable	4	Withdraws to touch	5
To pain	2	Cries to pain	3	Withdraws to pain	4
None	1	Moans to pain	2	Abnormal flexion	3
		None	1	Abnormal extension	2
				None	1

In pediatric trauma patients of all ages, the initial GCS has been found to correlate well with overall mortality, death on arrival to the ED, and major injury.[6] When applied to children 2 years and younger, the pediatric GCS has been found to perform similarly to the standard GCS for children older than 2 years, especially regarding the need for acute intervention for children with blunt head trauma.[7] The GCS is also an important component of the published pediatric head injury decision rules, as described in the next section.

IMAGING STUDIES

CT of the head provides rapid identification of most life-threatening injuries, including intracranial blood collections that require emergency evacuation. However, these injuries are uncommon and the risks of radiation to a developing brain, sedation of a pediatric patient, and the cost of the study are not negligible. The lifetime risk of fatal cancer from a single head CT has been estimated to be 1 in 1500 for a 1-year-old and 1 in 5000 for a 10-year-old.[8] Other reports have also shown increased risks of both brain tumors and leukemia associated with CT scans in childhood and encourage physicians to weigh the risks and benefits before ordering these studies.[9–12] In addition, children often require procedural sedation to obtain a CT scan because of fear, agitation, or young age and procedural sedation carries the risk of airway and hemodynamic compromise.

Decision Rules for Head CT

Young children are more difficult to assess than adults, and signs and symptoms of intracranial injury vary in different age groups. Therefore, many decision rules have been developed to help the emergency provider identify which head-injured pediatric patients require imaging studies. A systematic review of clinical decision rules for pediatric head injury was published in 2012.[13] The 3 studies found to have the highest quality and accuracy were the CHALICE (Children's Head Injury Algorithm for the Prediction of Important Clinical Events),[14] CATCH (Canadian Assessment of Tomography for Childhood Head Injury),[15] and the PECARN (Pediatric Emergency Care Applied Research Network)[16] studies. They are all large multicenter studies and all perform with high sensitivity and negative predictive value.

There are several differences among the 3 studies. Slightly different age groups were included in each study. CHALICE included patients with any severity of injury without specified time after the injury, whereas both CATCH and PECARN include only children with minor head injuries evaluated within the first 24 hours of injury. CATCH and PECARN both include observation as a strategy to determine which children require imaging. The CATCH and CHALICE rules were derived to identify which head-injured children needed a head CT, whereas the PECARN rule was derived to identify which children did not. For these reasons, the 3 studies cannot be directly compared. The review's investigators suggest that the 3 decision rules should be compared and validated in a single population.[13] This comparison has not been published at the time of this writing; however, the PECARN study is the largest of the 3 and includes a separate algorithm for children younger than 2 years. At this time, the PECARN rule is the only one of the three that has been validated.

CHALICE

The CHALICE decision rule was derived by the UK Emergency Medicine Research Group and was published in 2006. The study enrolled 22,722 children younger than 16 years. The goal of the CHALICE study was to identify which head-injured children are at high risk of clinically significant intracranial injury, defined as death as a result of head injury, need for neurosurgical intervention, or marked abnormality on CT scan.[14] This rule had a sensitivity of 98% and specificity of 87% for clinically significant intracranial injury. The CHALICE rule recommends a head CT scan for a head-injured child with the following (CT scan rate of 14%):

- Witnessed loss of consciousness (LOC) greater than 5 minutes
- Amnesia of more than 5 minutes
- Abnormal drowsiness
- 3 or more episodes of emesis
- Suspicion of nonaccidental trauma
- Seizure in a patient without epilepsy
- An injury mechanism of high-speed motor vehicle collision (MVC), fall of more than 3 m, or head struck by a high-velocity object
- GCS less than 14 (or <15 if younger than 1 year)
- Penetrating or depressed skull injury
- Bulging fontanel
- Signs of basilar skull fracture
- Abnormal neurologic examination
- Scalp swelling, bruising, or laceration larger than than 5 cm if younger than 1 year

CATCH

The CATCH decision rule was derived by the Pediatric Emergency Research Canada (PERC) Head Injury Study Group and published in 2010. The study enrolled 3866 children age 16 years and younger. The goal of the CATCH study was to determine which children with minor head injury within the past 24 hours needed neurologic intervention.[15] Minor head injury was defined as blunt trauma to the head with GCS of 13 to 15 with witnessed loss of consciousness, amnesia, disorientation, persistent vomiting, or irritability. The rule was 100% sensitive and 70% specific in determining the need for surgical intervention in the "high-risk" group. It was 98% sensitive and 50% specific for identifying visible brain injury on CT in the medium-risk group.

Head-injured children were considered "high risk" if they had any of the following (CT scan rate of 30%):

- GCS less than 15 at 2 hours after injury
- Suspected open or depressed skull fracture
- Worsening headache
- Irritability

They were considered "medium risk" if they had any of the following (CT scan rate of 52%):

- Signs of basilar skull fracture
- A large, boggy scalp hematoma
- A dangerous mechanism of injury (fall >3 feet or 5 stairs, MVC, fall from a bicycle without helmet)

PECARN

The PECARN decision rule was developed by the Pediatric Emergency Care Applied Research Network in the United States and was published in 2009. The goal of the PECARN study was to identify which head-injured children were at very low risk of clinically important traumatic brain injuries and therefore did not require head CT scans.[16] They defined a clinically important traumatic brain injury (ciTBI) as an injury that resulted in death, neurosurgical intervention, intubation for more than 24 hours for brain injury, or hospital admission of 2 nights or more associated with TBI on CT scan. Skull fractures were not considered a ciTBI unless the fracture was depressed by more than the width of the skull.

The PECARN investigators performed a prospective cohort study of head-injured patients younger than 18 years with GCS of 14 to 15 who presented within 24 hours of injury. They analyzed more than 42,000 patients with blunt head trauma in the derivation and validation phases of the study. Preverbal children (younger than 2 years) were analyzed separately from children older than 2 years. The Pediatric GCS was used for preverbal children. Overall, ciTBI occurred in 376 children and 60 children required neurosurgery. In the validation group of children younger than 2 years, the prediction rule (**Table 2**) had a sensitivity of 100% for ciTBI and a negative predictive value of 100% if none of the predictors were present. In the validation group of children 2 years and older, the prediction rule had a sensitivity of 96.8% for ciTBI and a negative predictive value of 99.95% if none of the predictors were present.

In the PECARN study, altered mental status was defined as agitation, somnolence, repetitive questioning, or slow response to verbal communication. Severe mechanisms of injury included MVC with ejection, death of another passenger or rollover, unhelmeted bicyclist or pedestrian struck by a motorized vehicle, a fall of more than 3 feet in a child younger than 2 years or more than 5 feet in a child 2 years or older, or head struck by a high-velocity object.

A secondary analysis of the PECARN data found that children with only a severe mechanism of injury and no other predictors had a lower risk of ciTBI than children with more than one predictor (relative risk 0.07 for children <2 years and 0.11 for children ≥2 years).[17] The risk was even lower if they did not have other signs of trauma, seizures, abnormal neurologic examination, scalp hematoma, loss of consciousness, headache, or amnesia. Another analysis of the PECARN data found that children with ventricular shunts did not have higher risk of ciTBI than children without shunts, although they were scanned more often.[18] Because these children will likely have many head CT scans in their lifetime, it would be beneficial to avoid unnecessary scans. Children with bleeding disorders have traditionally been thought to be at high risk for

Table 2	
PECARN head injury decision rule	
Children Under 2 years of Age	**Children 2 years and Older**
Head CT scan recommended if the following features are present (CT scan rate 14%):	
Pediatric GCS = 14	GCS = 14
Other signs of altered mental status	Other signs of altered mental status
Palpable skull fracture	Signs of basilar skull fracture
If none of the above are present, head CT vs a period of observation recommended if any of the following features are present (about 30% of patients):	
Nonfrontal scalp hematoma	History of loss of consciousness
History of loss of consciousness of 5 sec or more	History of vomiting
Severe mechanism of injury	Severe mechanism of injury
Are not acting normally per parents	Severe headache
If none of the above are present, head CT is not recommended	

Adapted from Kuppermann N, Holmes JF, Dayan PS, et al. Identification of children at very low risk of clinically-important brain injuries after head trauma: a prospective cohort study. Lancet 2009;374(9696):1160–70.

intracranial hemorrhage after minor head injuries. An analysis of the PECARN data found that only 1% of head-injured children with bleeding disorders in their study population had intracranial hemorrhage and that these children had symptoms that would recommend a CT scan based on the PECARN decision rule.[19]

Observation The PECARN investigators recommend observation as a possible alternative to CT scan depending on other clinical factors, including age younger than 3 months, the presence of single versus multiple findings, worsening signs or symptoms, clinician experience, and parental preference.[16] Observing a head-injured child in the ED instead of obtaining an immediate CT scan allows time to see whether their symptoms improve or worsen. Children who clinically deteriorate (which may be due to an intracranial hemorrhage or cerebral edema) during that time should undergo a CT scan. The provider must keep a high index of suspicion for ciTBI in infants younger than 3 months because clinical signs are more difficult to evaluate in this age group. A subanalysis of the PECARN data investigated the effect of observation on head CT use and outcomes.[20] The investigators found that the rate of head CT scan use was lower among children who were observed without a higher rate of ciTBI, especially if their symptoms improved during the observation period. The length of the observation period is not specified.

A recent study found that parents of children with minor head injuries (as determined by triage evaluation) were slightly more likely to prefer observation to immediate CT (57% vs 40%) when they were given information about the risks and benefits of CT scan for head-injured children.[21] Most parents in this study preferred to be allowed to choose from all management options (89%) rather than have the physician decide the management plan (9%).

A recent retrospective study of the incidence of delayed diagnosis of intracranial hemorrhage in children with uncomplicated minor head injuries found this to be a rare event.[22] Investigators reviewed approximately 18,000 cases of head-injured children younger than 14 years who had a GCS of 15, normal neurologic examination, no loss of consciousness of more than 1 minute, and no amnesia. Ten children had diagnosis of intracranial hemorrhage not apparent until at least 6 hours after the time of injury. Three of these children presented more than 6 hours after the injury and the others had been discharged after an evaluation performed less than 6 hours after the injury. These data suggest that an observation period of 6 hours is sufficient for most children with minor head injuries.

Other Imaging Studies

Magnetic resonance imaging (MRI) is usually impractical from the ED as the initial study in the acutely injured patient due to lack of availability, time required to perform the study, need for sedation, and difficulty monitoring an unstable patient in the MRI scanner. Although they expose the child to less radiation than a CT scan, skull x-rays have fallen out of favor (except as part of the skeletal survey for suspected child abuse) because they do not provide information about intracranial injury, as infants may have intracranial hemorrhage without fracture. Bedside ED ultrasound may prove to be useful to diagnose skull fractures.[23,24] It is rapid, noninvasive, and does not require sedation or movement of the patient out of the ED; however, it cannot be used to diagnose intracranial injury in patients without open fontanels.

MANAGEMENT

Management of a head-injured child focuses on limiting or preventing secondary injury. If imaging studies reveal an intracranial lesion that requires neurosurgical evacuation, the emergency provider must continue to stabilize the patient until the patient can be taken to the operating room or transferred to a higher level of care. Other patients with severe injuries that do not require surgical management may still require admission for further monitoring and treatment. The provider should perform serial examinations to evaluate for signs of deterioration. Important aspects of management are discussed as follows.

Airway and Breathing

Hypoxia is a leading cause of secondary brain injury and must be promptly recognized and treated. Cervical spine precautions must be maintained while the airway is opened and during endotracheal intubation. If a head-injured pediatric patient requires intubation, medication selection should balance prevention of intracranial hypertension with preservation of systemic blood pressure. Rapid-sequence intubation with sedation and paralysis should be performed. Atropine has been used to blunt the vagal response to laryngoscopy, but recent data suggest that it may not be useful.[25,26] The use of lidocaine to blunt ICP response to laryngoscopy is also controversial.[27–29] Etomidate may be considered as a sedative because it has been shown to reduce ICP without significantly reducing systemic blood pressure, which improves cerebral perfusion pressure.[30,31] It has a rapid onset and short duration of action, which allows for serial neurologic assessments. Ketamine has been found to reduce ICP in mechanically ventilated head-injured children in an ICU setting, and may also be useful in the ED setting.[31,32] It has a short duration of action and maintains systemic blood pressure. Thiopental may also be considered to decrease ICP,[31] but should not be used in hypotensive patients. Rocuronium or succinylcholine may be used as paralytic agents.

Circulation

Once the airway has been secured and ventilation established, adequate circulating volume must be ensured. Systemic hypotension contributes to secondary brain injury because cerebral perfusion pressure (CPP) is the difference between mean arterial pressure (MAP) and ICP (ie, CPP = MAP – ICP). Initial resuscitation usually begins with isotonic fluids. Hypotonic fluids should be avoided; normal saline has a higher sodium content than lactated Ringer solution. Hypertonic saline may prove to be useful for fluid resuscitation in the head-injured patient.[31,33] Blood products may be needed if there are associated injuries.

Hyperosmolar Therapy

Increased ICP decreases cerebral perfusion pressure and contributes to secondary brain injury. Hyperosmolar therapy has long been used to reduce ICP in head-injured patients. The 2 most commonly used agents are mannitol and hypertonic saline. Current pediatric guidelines recommend the use of hypertonic saline rather than mannitol for head-injured pediatric patients with intracranial hypertension.[31] Hypertonic saline increases serum osmolarity directly and has been found to be more effective in reducing ICP than mannitol.[34] Concentrations of 3.0%, 7.5% and 23.4% are available; though a central line is preferred, 3% saline can be given safely through a peripheral intravenous line at a dose of 6 ml/kg over 15 minutes or as a continuous infusion of 0.1–1 ml/kg/hour to maintain ICP <20 mmg/hg.[34–36] In contrast, mannitol increases serum osmolarity by acting as an osmotic diuretic, and risks of its use include dehydration, electrolyte abnormalities, and renal failure if euvolemia is not maintained.[36] It may be used if hypertonic saline is not available. Mannitol is given at a dose of 0.5 to 1.0 mg/kg. These therapies should be avoided until the patient is adequately volume-resuscitated unless there are clear signs of herniation.

Antiseizure Prophylaxis

Posttraumatic seizures increase metabolic demand on the brain and may contribute to secondary brain injury. They occur in about 10% of children with TBI and are usually focal.[31] Early posttraumatic seizures occur within 7 days of injury and late seizures occur more than 7 days after the injury. Risk factors for early posttraumatic seizures include age younger than 2 years, GCS less than 8, and nonaccidental trauma.[37] Adult consensus guidelines recommend phenytoin prophylaxis for the first 7 days after severe brain injuries to lower the rate of early posttraumatic seizures, though it has not been found to affect the occurrence of late seizures.[38] Although there are no consensus guidelines for children, antiseizure prophylaxis with phenytoin or fosphenytoin may be considered for children with severe brain injuries.[31]

Antiemetics

Many head-injured patients present to the ED with vomiting; it is one of the predictors in the CHALICE and PECARN rules and one of the inclusion criteria for CATCH. Patients with known intracranial injuries often receive antiemetics, but providers may be concerned about masking serious injuries if antiemetics are given to patients who have not undergone a head CT or to patients with planned discharge home. A recent retrospective study showed a reduction in repeat ED visits within 72 hours for head-injured patients with negative head CT scans who received ondansetron for nausea or vomiting while in the ED.[39] The likelihood of hospital admission was not affected. A small number of patients in this study received ondansetron but did not have a head CT performed. None of the patients who returned to the ED within 72 hours had a missed diagnosis of ciTBI. However, because the number of patients in this study was small, this practice cannot be definitively recommended at this time.

Other Therapies

For a severely head-injured child, the head of the bed should be elevated to 30° and the head kept midline to promote venous drainage. There are limited data on the use of *therapeutic hypothermia* to prevent secondary brain injury in severely head-injured children. The rationale for use of therapeutic hypothermia is to reduce cerebral metabolic demands, but so far, it has not been shown to improve neurologic outcomes or mortality rates.[31,40] Although *corticosteroids* are beneficial for reducing cerebral edema in children with brain tumors, they have not been found to reduce ICP or improve outcomes for children with brain injuries and are therefore not recommended.[31] *Hyperventilation* to $Paco_2$ lower than 30 reduces ICP by causing reduction of cerebral blood flow, but it may induce brain ischemia and decrease cerebral oxygenation; therefore, it is not recommended.[31]

DISPOSITION AND FOLLOW-UP OF HEAD-INJURED CHILDREN

Children with severe head injuries that require neurosurgical intervention or have respiratory and/or hemodynamic compromise require hospital admission. Additional indications for admission include other traumatic injuries requiring intervention, evaluation for child abuse, or intractable vomiting. Children with isolated minor head injuries (GCS 14 and 15) and normal head CT results may be safely discharged because the risk for neurologic deterioration is very low.[41] Children who did not undergo a head CT but remained asymptomatic after a period of observation may also be discharged.[22]

   All children who sustain head injuries should be discharged with written instructions and with a responsible adult who will remain with the child for the next 24 hours.

Indications to return to the ED include persistent vomiting, worsening headache, or worsening neurologic symptoms. In the absence of neurologic decline, repeat CT imaging is not indicated for patients with an initial negative scan.[42–46] Children should be instructed not to return to gym class or sports until all of their symptoms have resolved and they have been reevaluated by a physician. They should be given instructions to follow-up with their primary care provider or in a specialized head injury clinic within the next few days for reevaluation.

CONCUSSION

Concussion, a common complaint in the pediatric ED, represents a subclassification of the mild TBI group.[47,48] Traditionally, concussion has been defined in various ways and grading scales that relied mainly on loss of consciousness and amnesia to dictate physician management of concussions.[49,50] In 2008, a consensus group of international experts met in Zurich to update concussion guidelines based on the most current evidence. Concussion was defined as a "complex pathophysiological process affecting the brain, induced by traumatic biomechanical forces."[51] Several common features used to further define a concussive head injury include a "rapid onset of short-lived impairment of neurologic function that resolves spontaneously" and the requirement that "no abnormality on standard structural neuroimaging studies is seen."[51] The American Academy of Neurology's (AAN) 2013 concussion guidelines define concussion as a "clinical syndrome of biomechanically induced alteration of brain function, typically affecting memory and orientation, which may involve loss of consciousness."[52]

Up to 3.8 million recreation-related and sport-related concussions occur annually in the United States.[53] This number could certainly be an underestimation because of underreporting and the lack of injury surveillance systems in youth sports.[54,55] Overall, the incidence of concussion is greater for males than females because of the greater number of male participants in sports. However, concussion risk is higher for female athletes participating in soccer and basketball than for male athletes participating in these sports. Sports that present the highest risk of concussion are American football and ice hockey (AAN guidelines).[52]

Pathophysiology

The biomechanics and pathophysiology of the brain tissue damage in concussion have been investigated in animal models in the laboratory setting; however, it is still unclear whether these results can be applied to clinical concussions. It is hypothesized that concussion results from acceleration-deceleration and rotational forces on the brain, causing deformation of the brain through compressive, tensile, or shearing forces.[56] This transient deformation may alter the function in astrocytes and neurons through various proposed mechanisms, including abrupt neuronal depolarization, changes in glucose metabolism, and alterations in cerebral blood flow, which allow for initiation of biochemical pathways leading to cell death within hours to days.[57,58] In addition, it has been proposed that a hypometabolic state may persist for up to 4 weeks after the injury, which may account for prolonged symptoms in some patients.[59,60]

Signs and Symptoms of Concussion

The diagnosis of concussion involves the assessment of a range of domains, including somatic and cognitive symptoms, physical signs, emotional and behavioral changes, and sleep disturbances (**Table 3**).[51,53,61] Headache is the most common presenting symptom.[62] Brief loss of consciousness occurs in fewer than 10% of concussions.[53]

Table 3
Signs and symptoms of concussion

Somatic	Cognitive	Physical	Emotional/ Behavioral	Sleep
Headache	Mental "fogginess"	Loss of consciousness	Irritability	Drowsiness
Nausea/vomiting	Difficulty answering questions	Amnesia (anterograde or retrograde)	Nervousness	Difficulty wakening
Visual changes	Difficulty concentrating		Sadness	Insomnia
Balance difficulties	Difficulty remembering			
Fatigue	Confusion about recent events			
Photophobia	Repetition of questions			
Phonophobia	Disorientation			
Dizziness				

Patients may initially be asymptomatic and then develop symptoms several hours after the time of concussion.[51] An important part of the evaluation of a patient with a possible concussion is discussion with eyewitnesses to the injury and parents or coaches to determine whether the patient has improved or deteriorated since the time of injury. Worsening symptoms or failure to improve are indications for imaging.[63]

Several versions of standardized symptom tools and sideline assessment tools exist to aid physicians and trainers in objectively evaluating postconcussive cognitive deficits. The Standardized Assessment of Concussion (SAC), Sports Concussion Assessment Tool 2 (SCAT2), and the Sports Concussion Office Assessment Tool (SCOAT) which can easily be found online, can be used for baseline evaluation and to monitor progress over time.[51,64–66] These tools provide a means to assess memory and concentration, which has proven to be more reliable than routine orientation questions (eg, time, location).[51] Neuropsychological testing of cognitive processing speed, memory performance, and reaction time has proven useful in identifying the presence of concussion in adolescents (sensitivity 71%–88%), but is impractical for use in the acute ED setting.[52] At this time, there is no clearly superior tool, as all require further validation, especially in grade-school athletes.[67] In addition, these screening tools cannot be used alone to diagnose concussion, but should be used as an adjunct to the comprehensive evaluation of a patient with a suspected concussion.

As in all patients with a head injury, the patient with a possible concussion should undergo a careful physical examination, including examination of the head for hematomas or skull fractures, assessment of mental status, and a complete neurologic examination. Although the neurologic examination may be normal, careful attention to balance may reveal subtle deficits.[61] Studies have shown that postural stability deficits may last 72 hours after concussion.[68] Imaging studies should not be used to diagnose concussion, but should be considered to rule out more significant TBI if suspected.

Management

Treatment for patients with concussion is centered on physical and cognitive rest, symptom management, and education of the patient, family, and other significant contacts (eg, coaches, teachers, employers). After a suspected concussion, patients should be withdrawn from physical activities immediately. The phrase, "When in doubt, sit them out!" is crucial in the management of possible pediatric concussions.[69] Children should be prohibited from returning to play until fully evaluated, as discussed previously, and the clinician should ensure that there are no indications of a more serious head injury. RTP guidelines have been developed to provide an individualized course to allow patients adequate recovery time before resuming physical activity to minimize the exacerbation of postconcussive impairments.[51,70] This graduated protocol follows a stepwise increase in activity level as outlined in **Table 4**. Patients should start at the first stage when they are asymptomatic and not taking any medications that may mask or modify the symptoms of concussion. Once the patient remains asymptomatic at the current stage for 24 hours, he or she may progress to the next stage. If concussive symptoms occur, the patient should return to the last asymptomatic step and attempt progression again after an additional 24-hour period without symptoms. As each stage takes 24 hours to complete, patients take approximately 1 week to proceed through the entire rehabilitation protocol.[51] Probable risk factors for prolonged return to play include young age, early posttraumatic headache, fatigue/fogginess and early amnesia, alteration in mental status, or disorientation.[52]

Compared with younger patients, RTP management in adults may be more rapid, with some athletes being allowed to RTP on the same day as the concussion.[71,72] However, collegiate and high school level athletes allowed to RTP on the same day may demonstrate neuropsychological deficits after injury that may not be evident on the sidelines and are more likely to have delayed onset of concussive symptoms.[51,73–75] Therefore, same day RTP is not advised for adolescent or pediatric patients under any circumstances.

Numerous studies have shown that children and adolescents have a longer recovery period, up to 7 to 10 days longer, when compared with college-aged or professional athletes.[76–78] Interestingly, at the time of this writing, 40 states have passed legislation to further emphasize the need for a conservative approach to RTP for these young patients.[79] Many states now require that student athletes are removed from play if they are suspected to have a concussion and are required to obtain written medical authorization before returning to physical activity.[80] In addition, many also require concussion education for trainers, coaches, parents, and athletes.

Physical restrictions should be broad to prevent symptom recurrence and to avoid prolonged recovery. Restrictions should include sports activities, physical education classes, weight training, and even leisure activities, such as bike-riding and skateboarding.[53] Complete cognitive rest should include a break from academic

Table 4
Stepwise return to play

Rehabilitation Stage	Activity Level	Objective
1. No activity	Complete physical and cognitive rest	Recovery
2. Light aerobic activity	Walking, cycling, swimming at 70% maximum heart rate. No resistance training	Increase heart rate
3. Sport-specific exercise	Specific drills, but no head impact	Add movement
4. Noncontact training drills	Specific complex drills. May start light resistance training	Exercise, coordination, cognitive effort
5. Full-contact practice	Normal training (after medical clearance)	Assess skills by coaches; restore confidence
6. Return to play	Normal game play	

Adapted from Schunk JE, Schutzman SA. Pediatric head injury. Pediatr Rev 2012;33(9):398–411.

studies, as well as any other activities that require attention and concentration, such as videogames, text messaging, computer use, and television viewing.[81] Depending on symptom severity, patients may need school accommodations, such as a temporary leave of absence, shortened school day, reduction in workload, or more time to complete assignments.[82] These will be determined by follow-up with the PCP or head injury specialist.

In the acute period, headache after concussion should be managed with acetaminophen. Aspirin and other nonsteroidal anti-inflammatory drugs are typically avoided so as to lessen the theoretical risk of inducing or exacerbating intracranial hemorrhage. However, no controlled trials have demonstrated this risk.[83] Narcotics should be avoided to allow careful serial evaluations of mental status. In addition, prolonged use of narcotics and nonsteroidal anti-inflammatory drugs can lead to rebound headaches, which can further complicate the recovery process.[84–86]

The decision to admit a patient with a concussion should be based on the same criteria as any patient with an acute head injury. Most patients with a concussion, however, can be discharged home. Patients and families must be educated about the importance of monitoring for potential neurologic deterioration in the following hours and days. Clear instructions and guidelines about what concerns necessitate a return to the ED should be discussed and provided in written form.[83,87] These symptoms include persistent vomiting, sleepiness, increased confusion, change in behavior, worsening headache, or seizure.[87] There is debate over the recommendation for periodic wakenings of the concussed patient to evaluate for signs of intracranial bleeding. No documented evidence suggests what severity of injury requires this approach, but some recommend it for patients who have experienced loss of consciousness, prolonged amnesia, or are who continue to experience severe concussive symptoms.[88,89] The patient should be in the care of a responsible adult for at least 24 hours. The patient should be instructed to follow-up with his or her primary care provider for a thorough history and neurologic examination before return to full play. Referral to a pediatric neurologist, neuropsychologist, sports medicine physician, or other specialist with expertise in head injury should be considered for complex or atypical concussions, prolonged symptoms, or for patients who have suffered multiple concussions.

Complications

Most patients with a concussion will have a spontaneous, sequential resolution of their symptoms within 7 to 10 days.[58,73,83,90] Some patients have a prolonged recovery with sustained symptoms known as *postconcussive syndrome (PCS)*. Although there is no clear definition of PCS, some define it as persistent headache, dizziness, cognitive impairment, and psychological symptoms lasting from 6 weeks to 3 months after a concussion.[91,92] The symptomatic treatment of the myriad of symptoms of PCS is quite challenging. Currently, there is no evidence-based pharmacologic treatment to offer the concussed athlete.[93] Subgroups of patients with prolonged recoveries or significant impact on quality of life may benefit from medical therapies. Such treatments should be considered by an experienced practitioner and include tricyclic antidepressants and/or antiepileptic drugs for postconcussive headache and selective serotonin reuptake inhibitors for postconcussive depression.[91,94,95] Patients presenting to the ED with signs and symptoms of PCS should be referred to a pediatric neurologist, neuropsychologist, sports medicine physician, or other specialist with expertise in head injury.

Second impact syndrome (SIS) is a rare but feared complication of concussion. SIS occurs when a patient who has sustained an initial head injury sustains a second impact before the symptoms and pathophysiological changes from the first injury have fully cleared. It is postulated that disordered cerebral autoregulation following cumulative brain injury leads to diffuse cerebral swelling and herniation, ultimately resulting in a 50% to 100% mortality rate.[96,97] Although there is debate over whether SIS is truly due to a second impact or whether it is a catastrophic complication of a single head trauma, practitioners should be aware that pediatric and adolescent patients seem to be at the highest risk of this condition.[98] These patients should be monitored closely for deterioration of neurologic state after one or more concussive events. Strict adherence to RTP guidelines will ensure that patients are not at risk for a second impact during the initial vulnerable period of initial brain injury.

The long-term effects of single or multiple concussions in patients of all ages have been the recent focus of medical literature and general media. *Chronic traumatic encephalopathy (CTE)* is a progressive neurodegenerative disease caused by repetitive head trauma.[99] It is characterized by widespread distribution of hyperphosphorylated tau protein as neurofibrillary tangles in the brain. Originally reported in 1928 with vague "punch drunk" symptoms, recent studies have provided pathologic staging of autopsy specimens with stages of clinical symptomatology.[100] Manifestations include mood disturbances, parkinsonism, ataxia, dysarthric speech, poor concentration, attention and memory loss, and behavioral outbursts.[101] Many popular professional contact sport athletes who have suffered numerous concussions have later struggled with depression, substance abuse, anger, and suicide.[102] Autopsy results from these athletes suggest a link between these manifestations and CTE.[103] Although the magnitude and frequency of head impact needed to cause the neurodegeneration associated with CTE is unclear, it has been neuropathologically diagnosed in an asymptomatic 18-year-old high school football player with a history of concussion.[104,105] More research is needed to further investigate CTE and other long-term effects of concussions, particularly in the young, developing brain.

ABUSIVE HEAD TRAUMA

An important consideration in the evaluation of an infant or young child with head trauma is whether he or she may have sustained an inflicted injury. Up to 30 per 100,000 infants younger than 1 year sustain severe or fatal inflicted brain injuries annually, which makes abusive head trauma (AHT) the most common cause of child abuse deaths.[106,107] Victims of AHT tend to be younger than those with accidental head injuries and have more severe injuries. These injuries may occur as a consequence of shaking, blunt trauma, or a combination of both.[108,109] The diagnosis can be challenging to make because many infants and young children with inflicted head trauma have nonspecific symptoms and, because they are nonverbal, cannot give a history. Missed diagnosis of AHT is common, placing the child at risk for future injury and even death.[110–112] The diagnosis is more likely to be missed in younger infants, those from 2-parent households, nonminority children, and those with nonspecific symptoms,[110] so the clinician must maintain a high level of suspicion when evaluating any head-injured child.

History

The clinician must take a thorough, detailed history of any head-injured child. A history that is inconsistent with the injury is a commonly noted "red flag" for nonaccidental trauma (eg, lack of an explanation for injury, an injury discordant with the proposed mechanism, or a history incompatible with the child's developmental stage).[113] Other factors that have been found to predict inflicted injury are changing histories and injuries blamed on siblings or home resuscitative efforts.[114] Other historical factors more common in victims of abusive head trauma are apnea, respiratory distress, seizures, vomiting, and lethargy.[109,114–117] These symptoms may be mistaken for accidental head trauma or for another illness altogether. These findings highlight the importance of considering AHT in nonambulatory infants with severe head injuries and in infants with nonspecific symptoms.

Physical Examination

On physical examination, the provider should look for other signs of inflicted injury, such as skin findings (eg, bruising, bites, burns, or other patterned markings), abdominal injury, or fractures, although patients with AHT may not have external signs of trauma. Retinal hemorrhages, rib fractures, and long bone and metaphyseal fractures are other findings that should raise suspicion for inflicted injury.[109,115–117]

Imaging Studies

The initial brain imaging study for an infant or child suspected to have AHT is a non-contrast CT scan.[118,119] MRI can later be used to fully assess intracranial injuries of patients with a positive CT scans or patients with negative CT scans but strong clinical concerns.[119] MRI can also be used for infants without symptoms of intracranial injury but with skeletal injuries consistent with shaking, because of its high sensitivity for diagnosing acute and chronic intracranial injury. Shaking without impact does not cause injury to the skull, therefore skull radiographs are not included in the initial evaluation of the head-injured child because they do not identify intracranial injuries. All studies should be reviewed by radiologists experienced in pediatric imaging.

Certain physical and neuroradiological features are helpful in distinguishing abusive head trauma from accidental head trauma (**Table 5**).[116,120,121] Forceful shaking of an infant can stretch and tear bridging cortical veins and axons, leading to subdural hematomas and diffuse axonal injury. In contrast, accidental head trauma is usually caused by blunt trauma, so skull fractures and external injuries are more common.[122,123] Mixed-density subdural hematomas are more common in abusive head trauma, but can also be seen in accidental trauma, so this finding does not necessarily indicate repeated trauma.[122]

Management of Abusive Head Trauma

The initial management of head injury in suspected AHT is similar to the management of other head injuries: the primary priority is to stabilize and treat life-threatening

Table 5
Radiographic and physical characteristics of accidental and abusive head trauma

More Common in Abusive Head Trauma	More Common in Accidental Head Trauma	Do Not Distinguish Between Abusive and Accidental Head Trauma
• Subdural hematoma • Interhemispheric hemorrhage • Cerebral edema • Hypoxic ischemic injury • Multiple hemorrhages • Subdural over convexity • Posterior fossa hemorrhage • Mixed-density hemorrhages • Intracranial injury without skull fracture	• Epidural hematoma • Isolated skull fracture • Scalp swelling or bruising	• Subarachnoid hemorrhage • Focal parenchymal injury

injuries. If there is any suspicion of abusive head trauma, a full workup for nonaccidental trauma should be performed, but this evaluation does not take priority over the management of acute medical issues. The workup includes a careful physical examination, complete blood count, urinalysis, liver and pancreatic enzyme tests, skeletal survey for children younger than 2 years, and fundoscopic examination.[113] Appropriate specialists should be consulted, including child abuse pediatricians, ophthalmologists, and social workers. The history and physical examination should be carefully documented and photos taken as needed. State child protective services should be contacted according to local laws. The patient may need to be admitted to the hospital for management of their acute injuries or to ensure the child's safety while further investigation is performed.

SUMMARY

Children with head injuries frequently present to EDs. Even though most of these children have minor injuries, head injury is the most common cause of traumatic deaths in pediatric patients. The provider must be vigilant to diagnose those who have life-threatening intracranial injuries or are victims of abusive head trauma. The pediatric GCS and decision rules for obtaining head CT imaging help the provider evaluate head-injured infants and children. The goal of the emergency physician is to diagnose and treat the consequences of the primary injury and to limit or prevent secondary injury and to assure proper followup for pediatric patients with minor head injury and concussion.

REFERENCES

1. Faul M, Xu L, Wald M, et al. Traumatic brain injury in the United States: emergency department visits, hospitalizations and deaths 2002-2006. Atlanta (GA): National Center for Injury Prevention and Control, Centers for Disease Control and Prevention; 2010. 2012 (January 3).
2. Schneier AJ, Shields BJ, Hostetler SG, et al. Incidence of pediatric traumatic brain injury and associated hospital resource utilization in the United States. Pediatrics 2006;118(2):483–92.
3. Coronado VG, Xu L, Basavaraju SV, et al. Surveillance for traumatic brain injury-related deaths—United States, 1997-2007. MMWR Surveill Summ 2011;60(5): 1–32.
4. Jennett B, Teasdale G, Braakman R, et al. Predicting outcome in individual patients after severe head injury. Lancet 1976;1(7968):1031–4.
5. James HE. Neurologic evaluation and support in the child with an acute brain insult. Pediatr Ann 1986;15(1):16–22.
6. Cicero MX, Cross KP. Predictive value of initial Glasgow coma scale score in pediatric trauma patients. Pediatr Emerg Care 2013;29(1):43–8.
7. Holmes JF, Palchak MJ, MacFarlane T, et al. Performance of the pediatric Glasgow coma scale in children with blunt head trauma. Acad Emerg Med 2005; 12(9):814–9.
8. Brenner D, Elliston C, Hall E, et al. Estimated risks of radiation-induced fatal cancer from pediatric CT. AJR Am J Roentgenol 2001;176(2):289–96.
9. Brenner DJ, Hall EJ. Computed tomography—an increasing source of radiation exposure. N Engl J Med 2007;357(22):2277–84.
10. Frush DP, Donnelly LF, Rosen NS. Computed tomography and radiation risks: what pediatric health care providers should know. Pediatrics 2003;112(4): 951–7.

11. Hennelly KE, Mannix R, Nigrovic LE, et al. Pediatric traumatic brain injury and radiation risks: a clinical decision analysis. J Pediatr 2013;162(2):392–7.

12. Pearce MS, Salotti JA, Little MP, et al. Radiation exposure from CT scans in childhood and subsequent risk of leukaemia and brain tumours: a retrospective cohort study. Lancet 2012;380(9840):499–505.

13. Lyttle MD, Crowe L, Oakley E, et al. Comparing CATCH, CHALICE and PECARN clinical decision rules for paediatric head injuries. Emerg Med J 2012;29(10): 785–94.

14. Dunning J, Daly JP, Lomas JP, et al. Derivation of the children's head injury algorithm for the prediction of important clinical events decision rule for head injury in children. Arch Dis Child 2006;91(11):885–91.

15. Osmond MH, Klassen TP, Wells GA, et al. CATCH: a clinical decision rule for the use of computed tomography in children with minor head injury. CMAJ 2010; 182(4):341–8.

16. Kuppermann N, Holmes JF, Dayan PS, et al. Identification of children at very low risk of clinically-important brain injuries after head trauma: a prospective cohort study. Lancet 2009;374(9696):1160–70.

17. Nigrovic LE, Lee LK, Hoyle J, et al. Prevalence of clinically important traumatic brain injuries in children with minor blunt head trauma and isolated severe injury mechanisms. Arch Pediatr Adolesc Med 2012;166(4):356–61.

18. Nigrovic LE, Lillis K, Atabaki SM, et al. The prevalence of traumatic brain injuries after minor blunt head trauma in children with ventricular shunts. Ann Emerg Med 2013;61(4):389–93.

19. Lee LK, Dayan PS, Gerardi MJ, et al. Intracranial hemorrhage after blunt head trauma in children with bleeding disorders. J Pediatr 2011;158(6):1003–8.e1–2.

20. Nigrovic LE, Schunk JE, Foerster A, et al. The effect of observation on cranial computed tomography utilization for children after blunt head trauma. Pediatrics 2011;127(6):1067–73.

21. Karpas A, Finkelstein M, Reid S. Which management strategy do parents prefer for their head-injured child: immediate computed tomography scan or observation? Pediatr Emerg Care 2013;29(1):30–5.

22. Hamilton M, Mrazik M, Johnson DW. Incidence of delayed intracranial hemorrhage in children after uncomplicated minor head injuries. Pediatrics 2010; 126(1):e33–9.

23. Ramirez-Schrempp D, Vinci RJ, Liteplo AS. Bedside ultrasound in the diagnosis of skull fractures in the pediatric emergency department. Pediatr Emerg Care 2011;27(4):312–4.

24. Parri N, Crosby BJ, Glass C, et al. Ability of emergency ultrasonography to detect pediatric skull fractures: a prospective, observational study. J Emerg Med 2013;44(1):135–41.

25. Bean A, Jones J. Atropine: re-evaluating its use during paediatric RSI. Emerg Med J 2007;24(5):361–2.

26. Fastle RK, Roback MG. Pediatric rapid sequence intubation: incidence of reflex bradycardia and effects of pretreatment with atropine. Pediatr Emerg Care 2004;20(10):651–5.

27. Robinson N, Clancy M. In patients with head injury undergoing rapid sequence intubation, does pretreatment with intravenous lignocaine/lidocaine lead to an improved neurological outcome? A review of the literature. Emerg Med J 2001;18(6):453–7.

28. Salhi B, Stettner E. In defense of the use of lidocaine in rapid sequence intubation. Ann Emerg Med 2007;49(1):84–6.

29. Vaillancourt C, Kapur AK. Opposition to the use of lidocaine in rapid sequence intubation. Ann Emerg Med 2007;49(1):86–7.

30. Bramwell KJ, Haizlip J, Pribble C, et al. The effect of etomidate on intracranial pressure and systemic blood pressure in pediatric patients with severe traumatic brain injury. Pediatr Emerg Care 2006;22(2):90–3.

31. Kochanek PM, Carney N, Adelson PD, et al. Guidelines for the acute medical management of severe traumatic brain injury in infants, children, and adolescents—second edition. Pediatr Crit Care Med 2012;13(Suppl 1):S1–82.

32. Bar-Joseph G, Guilburd Y, Tamir A, et al. Effectiveness of ketamine in decreasing intracranial pressure in children with intracranial hypertension. J Neurosurg Pediatr 2009;4(1):40–6.

33. Simma B, Burger R, Falk M, et al. A prospective, randomized, and controlled study of fluid management in children with severe head injury: lactated Ringer's solution versus hypertonic saline. Crit Care Med 1998;26(7):1265–70.

34. Kamel H, Navi BB, Nakagawa K, et al. Hypertonic saline versus mannitol for the treatment of elevated intracranial pressure: a meta-analysis of randomized clinical trials. Crit Care Med 2011;39(3):554–9.

35. Luu JL, Wendtland CL, Gross MF, et al. Three-percent saline administration during pediatric critical care transport. Pediatr Emerg Care 2011;27(12):1113–7.

36. Ropper AH. Hyperosmolar therapy for raised intracranial pressure. N Engl J Med 2012;367(8):746–52.

37. Liesemer K, Bratton SL, Zebrack CM, et al. Early post-traumatic seizures in moderate to severe pediatric traumatic brain injury: rates, risk factors, and clinical features. J Neurotrauma 2011;28(5):755–62.

38. Chang BS, Lowenstein DH, Quality Standards Subcommittee of the American Academy of Neurology. Practice parameter: antiepileptic drug prophylaxis in severe traumatic brain injury: report of the Quality Standards Subcommittee of the American Academy of Neurology. Neurology 2003;60(1):10–6.

39. Sturm JJ, Simon HK, Khan NS, et al. The use of ondansetron for nausea and vomiting after head injury and its effect on return rates from the pediatric ED. Am J Emerg Med 2013;31(1):166–72.

40. Hutchison JS, Ward RE, Lacroix J, et al. Hypothermia therapy after traumatic brain injury in children. N Engl J Med 2008;358(23):2447–56.

41. Holmes JF, Borgialli DA, Nadel FM, et al. Do children with blunt head trauma and normal cranial computed tomography scan results require hospitalization for neurologic observation? Ann Emerg Med 2011;58(4):315–22.

42. Almenawer SA, Bogza I, Yarascavitch B, et al. The value of scheduled repeat cranial computed tomography after mild head injury: single-center series and meta-analysis. Neurosurgery 2013;72(1):56–62 [discussion: 63–4].

43. da Silva PS, Reis ME, Aguiar VE. Value of repeat cranial computed tomography in pediatric patients sustaining moderate to severe traumatic brain injury. J Trauma 2008;65(6):1293–7.

44. Tabori U, Kornecki A, Sofer S, et al. Repeat computed tomographic scan within 24–48 hours of admission in children with moderate and severe head trauma. Crit Care Med 2000;28(3):840–4.

45. Washington CW, Grubb RL Jr. Are routine repeat imaging and intensive care unit admission necessary in mild traumatic brain injury? J Neurosurg 2012;116(3):549–57.

46. Stippler M, Smith C, McLean AR, et al. Utility of routine follow-up head CT scanning after mild traumatic brain injury: a systematic review of the literature. Emerg Med J 2012;29(7):528–32.

47. Lee LK. Controversies in the sequelae of pediatric mild traumatic brain injury. Pediatr Emerg Care 2007;23(8):580–3 [quiz: 584–6].
48. Gordon KE, Dooley JM, Fitzpatrick EA, et al. Concussion or mild traumatic brain injury: parents appreciate the nuances of nosology. Pediatr Neurol 2010;43(4): 253–7.
49. Practice parameter: the management of concussion in sports (summary statement). Report of the Quality Standards Subcommittee. Neurology 1997;48(3): 581–5.
50. Cantu R. Guidelines for return to contact sports after a cerebral concussion. Phys Sportsmed 1986;14(10):75–83.
51. McCrory P, Meeuwisse W, Johnston K, et al. Consensus Statement on Concussion in Sport: the 3rd International Conference on Concussion in Sport held in Zurich, November 2008. Br J Sports Med 2009;43(Suppl 1):i76–90.
52. Giza C, Kutcher J, Ashwal S, et al. Summary of evidence-based guideline update: Evaluation and management of concussion in sports: Report of the Guideline Development Subcommittee of the American Academy of Neurology. Neurology 2013. [Epub ahead of print].
53. Halstead ME, Walter KD, Council on Sports Medicine, Fitness. American Academy of Pediatrics. Clinical report—sport-related concussion in children and adolescents. Pediatrics 2010;126(3):597–615.
54. Echlin PS, Tator CH, Cusimano MD, et al. A prospective study of physician-observed concussions during junior ice hockey: implications for incidence rates. Neurosurg Focus 2010;29(5):E4.
55. McCrea M, Hammeke T, Olsen G, et al. Unreported concussion in high school football players: implications for prevention. Clin J Sport Med 2004;14(1): 13–7.
56. Buzzini SR, Guskiewicz KM. Sport-related concussion in the young athlete. Curr Opin Pediatr 2006;18(4):376–82.
57. Meaney DF, Smith DH. Biomechanics of concussion. Clin Sports Med 2011; 30(1):19–31, vii.
58. Giza CC, Hovda DA. The neurometabolic cascade of concussion. J Athl Train 2001;36(3):228–35.
59. Yoshino A, Hovda DA, Kawamata T, et al. Dynamic changes in local cerebral glucose utilization following cerebral conclusion in rats: evidence of a hyper- and subsequent hypometabolic state. Brain Res 1991;561(1):106–19.
60. Sunami K, Nakamura T, Ozawa Y, et al. Hypermetabolic state following experimental head injury. Neurosurg Rev 1989;12(Suppl 1):400–11.
61. Upshaw JE, Gosserand JK, Williams N, et al. Sports-related concussions. Pediatr Emerg Care 2012;28(9):926–32.
62. Blinman TA, Houseknecht E, Snyder C, et al. Postconcussive symptoms in hospitalized pediatric patients after mild traumatic brain injury. J Pediatr Surg 2009; 44(6):1223–8.
63. Schunk JE, Schutzman SA. Pediatric head injury. Pediatr Rev 2012;33(9): 398–411.
64. McCrea M, Kelly JP, Kluge J, et al. Standardized assessment of concussion in football players. Neurology 1997;48(3):586–8.
65. McCrea M, Kelly JP, Randolph C, et al. Standardized assessment of concussion (SAC): on-site mental status evaluation of the athlete. J Head Trauma Rehabil 1998;13(2):27–35.
66. Patricios J, Collins R, Branfield A, et al. The sports concussion note: should SCAT become SCOAT? Br J Sports Med 2012;46(3):198–201.

67. Eckner JT, Kutcher JS. Concussion symptom scales and sideline assessment tools: a critical literature update. Curr Sports Med Rep 2010;9(1):8–15.

68. Guskiewicz KM. Assessment of postural stability following sport-related concussion. Curr Sports Med Rep 2003;2(1):24–30.

69. Aubry M, Cantu R, Dvorak J, et al. Summary and agreement statement of the 1st International Symposium on Concussion in Sport, Vienna 2001. Clin J Sport Med 2002;12(1):6–11.

70. Johnston KM, Bloom GA, Ramsay J, et al. Current concepts in concussion rehabilitation. Curr Sports Med Rep 2004;3(6):316–23.

71. Herring S, Bergfeld J, Boland A, et al. Concussion (mild traumatic brain injury) and the team physician: a consensus statement. Med Sci Sports Exerc 2006; 38(2):395–9.

72. Guskiewicz KM, Bruce SL, Cantu RC, et al. National Athletic Trainers' Association position statement: management of Sport-Related Concussion. J Athl Train 2004;39(3):280–97.

73. Guskiewicz KM, McCrea M, Marshall SW, et al. Cumulative effects associated with recurrent concussion in collegiate football players: the NCAA Concussion Study. JAMA 2003;290(19):2549–55.

74. Collins MW, Field M, Lovell MR, et al. Relationship between postconcussion headache and neuropsychological test performance in high school athletes. Am J Sports Med 2003;31(2):168–73.

75. McCrea M, Guskiewicz KM, Marshall SW, et al. Acute effects and recovery time following concussion in collegiate football players: the NCAA Concussion Study. JAMA 2003;290(19):2556–63.

76. Field M, Collins MW, Lovell MR, et al. Does age play a role in recovery from sports-related concussion? A comparison of high school and collegiate athletes. J Pediatr 2003;142(5):546–53.

77. McClincy MP, Lovell MR, Pardini J, et al. Recovery from sports concussion in high school and collegiate athletes. Brain Inj 2006;20(1):33–9.

78. Pellman EJ, Lovell MR, Viano DC, et al. Concussion in professional football: recovery of NFL and high school athletes assessed by computerized neuropsychological testing—Part 12. Neurosurgery 2006;58(2):263–74 [discussion: 263–74].

79. SportsConcussions.org. State Laws. 2011. Available at: http://www.sports concussions.org/laws.html. Accessed October 28, 2012.

80. Injury Prevention and Control Program, Massachusetts Department of Public Health. Sports Related Concussions and Head Injuries. 2012. Available at: http://www.mass.gov/eohhs/consumer/wellness/injury-prevention/sports-related-concussions-and-head-injuries.html. Accessed November 2, 2012.

81. Grady MF. Concussion in the adolescent athlete. Curr Probl Pediatr Adolesc Health Care 2010;40(7):154–69.

82. Sady MD, Vaughan CG, Gioia GA. School and the concussed youth: recommendations for concussion education and management. Phys Med Rehabil Clin N Am 2011;22(4):701–19, ix.

83. Willer B, Leddy JJ. Management of concussion and post-concussion syndrome. Curr Treat Options Neurol 2006;8(5):415–26.

84. Lane JC, Arciniegas DB. Post-traumatic headache. Curr Treat Options Neurol 2002;4(1):89–104.

85. Lenaerts ME, Couch JR, Couch JR. Posttraumatic headache. Curr Treat Options Neurol 2004;6(6):507–17.

86. Packard RC. Epidemiology and pathogenesis of posttraumatic headache. J Head Trauma Rehabil 1999;14(1):9–21.

87. Fung M, Willer B, Moreland D, et al. A proposal for an evidenced-based emergency department discharge form for mild traumatic brain injury. Brain Inj 2006; 20(9):889–94.

88. Guskiewicz KM, Bruce SL, Cantu RC, et al. Recommendations on management of sport-related concussion: summary of the National Athletic Trainers' Association position statement. Neurosurgery 2004;55(4):891–5 [discussion: 896].

89. de Louw A, Twijnstra A, Leffers P. Lack of uniformity and low compliance concerning wake-up advice following head trauma. Ned Tijdschr Geneeskd 1994; 138(44):2197–9.

90. Iverson GL, Brooks BL, Collins MW, et al. Tracking neuropsychological recovery following concussion in sport. Brain Inj 2006;20(3):245–52.

91. Petraglia AL, Maroon JC, Bailes JE. From the field of play to the field of combat: a review of the pharmacological management of concussion. Neurosurgery 2012;70(6):1520–33 [discussion: 1533].

92. Sedney CL, Orphanos J, Bailes JE. When to consider retiring an athlete after sports-related concussion. Clin Sports Med 2011;30(1):189–200, xi.

93. McCrory P. Should we treat concussion pharmacologically? The need for evidence based pharmacological treatment for the concussed athlete. Br J Sports Med 2002;36(1):3–5.

94. McAllister TW, Arciniegas D. Evaluation and treatment of postconcussive symptoms. NeuroRehabilitation 2002;17(4):265–83.

95. Meehan WP 3rd. Medical therapies for concussion. Clin Sports Med 2011;30(1): 115–24, ix.

96. McCrory PR, Berkovic SF. Second impact syndrome. Neurology 1998;50(3): 677–83.

97. Cantu RC. Second-impact syndrome. Clin Sports Med 1998;17(1):37–44.

98. McCrory P. Does second impact syndrome exist? Clin J Sport Med 2001;11(3): 144–9.

99. Saulle M, Greenwald BD. Chronic traumatic encephalopathy: a review. Rehabil Res Pract 2012;2012:816069.

100. McKee AC, Stein TD, Nowinski CJ, et al. The spectrum of disease in chronic traumatic encephalopathy. Brain 2013;136(Pt 1):43–64.

101. McKee AC, Cantu RC, Nowinski CJ, et al. Chronic traumatic encephalopathy in athletes: progressive tauopathy after repetitive head injury. J Neuropathol Exp Neurol 2009;68(7):709–35.

102. Nowinski C, Ventura J. Head games: football's concussion crisis from the NFL to youth leagues. Boston: Thought Leaders, LLC; 2011.

103. Omalu BI, Bailes J, Hammers JL, et al. Chronic traumatic encephalopathy, suicides and parasuicides in professional American athletes: the role of the forensic pathologist. Am J Forensic Med Pathol 2010;31(2):130–2.

104. Gavett BE, Stern RA, McKee AC. Chronic traumatic encephalopathy: a potential late effect of sport-related concussive and subconcussive head trauma. Clin Sports Med 2011;30(1):179–88, xi.

105. Boston University, Center for the Study of Traumatic Encephalopathy. Case Studies. 2012. Available at www.bu.edu/cste/case-studies. Accessed October 28, 2012.

106. Keenan HT, Runyan DK, Marshall SW, et al. A population-based study of inflicted traumatic brain injury in young children. JAMA 2003;290(5):621–6.

107. U.S. Department of Health and Human Services, Administration for Children and Families, Administration on Children, Youth and Families, Children's Bureau

2012. Child maltreatment 2011. Available at http://www.acfhhs.gov/programs/cb/research-data-technology/statistics-research/child-maltreatment. Accessed January 3, 2013.

108. Christian CW, Block R, Committee on Child Abuse and Neglect, et al. Abusive head trauma in infants and children. Pediatrics 2009;123(5):1409–11.

109. Duhaime AC, Christian CW, Rorke LB, et al. Nonaccidental head injury in infants—the "shaken-baby syndrome". N Engl J Med 1998;338(25):1822–9.

110. Jenny C, Hymel KP, Ritzen A, et al. Analysis of missed cases of abusive head trauma. JAMA 1999;281(7):621–6.

111. Oral R, Yagmur F, Nashelsky M, et al. Fatal abusive head trauma cases: consequence of medical staff missing milder forms of physical abuse. Pediatr Emerg Care 2008;24(12):816–21.

112. Trokel M, Waddimba A, Griffith J, et al. Variation in the diagnosis of child abuse in severely injured infants. Pediatrics 2006;117(3):722–8.

113. Kellogg ND, American Academy of Pediatrics Committee on Child Abuse and Neglect. Evaluation of suspected child physical abuse. Pediatrics 2007;119(6):1232–41.

114. Hettler J, Greenes DS. Can the initial history predict whether a child with a head injury has been abused? Pediatrics 2003;111(3):602–7.

115. Keenan HT, Runyan DK, Marshall SW, et al. A population-based comparison of clinical and outcome characteristics of young children with serious inflicted and noninflicted traumatic brain injury. Pediatrics 2004;114(3):633–9.

116. Maguire S, Pickerd N, Farewell D, et al. Which clinical features distinguish inflicted from non-inflicted brain injury? A systematic review. Arch Dis Child 2009;94(11):860–7.

117. Maguire SA, Kemp AM, Lumb RC, et al. Estimating the probability of abusive head trauma: a pooled analysis. Pediatrics 2011;128(3):e550–64.

118. Section on Radiology, American Academy of Pediatrics. Diagnostic imaging of child abuse. Pediatrics 2009;123(5):1430–5.

119. Kemp A, Rajaram S, Mann M, et al. What neuroimaging should be performed in children in whom inflicted brain injury (iBI) is suspected? A systematic review. Clin Radiol 2009;64(5):473–83.

120. Kemp AM, Jaspan T, Griffiths J, et al. Neuroimaging: what neuroradiological features distinguish abusive from non-abusive head trauma? A systematic review. Arch Dis Child 2011;96(12):1103–12.

121. Piteau SJ, Ward MG, Barrowman NJ, et al. Clinical and radiographic characteristics associated with abusive and nonabusive head trauma: a systematic review. Pediatrics 2012;130(2):315–23.

122. Tung GA, Kumar M, Richardson RC, et al. Comparison of accidental and nonaccidental traumatic head injury in children on noncontrast computed tomography. Pediatrics 2006;118(2):626–33.

123. Adamo MA, Drazin D, Smith C, et al. Comparison of accidental and nonaccidental traumatic brain injuries in infants and toddlers: demographics, neurosurgical interventions, and outcomes. J Neurosurg Pediatr 2009;4(5):414–9.

Cardiac Emergencies

Isabel Araujo Barata, MS, MD

KEYWORDS

• Cardiac emergencies • Pediatrics • Cardiac disease

KEY POINTS

- The diagnosis and management of pediatric cardiac emergencies can be challenging and complicated. Early presentations are usually the result of ductal-dependent lesions and appear with cyanosis and shock.
- Later presentations are the result of volume overload or pump failure and present with signs of congestive heart failure (CHF).
- Acquired diseases also present as CHF or arrhythmias.

Cardiac disease is uncommon in childhood, but a delay in diagnosis may lead to devastating consequences. In addition, pediatric cardiology has expanded greatly in the last decade, with new surgeries and procedures for many congenital cardiac conditions, which clinicians need to be familiar with to manage these children.

Cardiac disease in infancy and childhood can be divided into structural disease, conduction abnormalities, and acquired illnesses. Cardiac lesions can be a combination of many defects; however, structural congenital heart disease (CHD) can be clinically divided into cyanotic and acyanotic categories. The surgical repair of CHD continues to progress, with some lesions now repaired in the neonatal period, and most lesions repaired in the first couple of months of life. However, patients may still appear in the emergency department before palliative surgery, or corrective surgery; these patients can be on multiple medications and require coordinated management with the pediatric cardiologist. Patients may also show postoperative complications such as a dysrhythmia, postpericardiotomy syndrome, or shunt stenosis. Conduction abnormalities can be congenital, the result of a new-onset illness or after a cardiac procedure. Acquired heart disease includes myocarditis, pericarditis, endocarditis, Kawasaki disease (KD), and cardiomyopathies. Timely identification, management, and stabilization of these patients are important goals. This article reviews the more common pediatric cardiac emergencies and their management.

CYANOTIC HEART DISEASE

There are 5 well-known cyanotic congenital heart lesions (also known as the Terrible Ts). They are tetralogy of Fallot (TOF), transposition of the great arteries (TGA), total

Pediatric Emergency Medicine, North Shore University Hospital, 300 Community Drive, Manhasset, NY 11030, USA
E-mail address: ibarata@aol.com

Emerg Med Clin N Am 31 (2013) 677–704
http://dx.doi.org/10.1016/j.emc.2013.04.007
0733-8627/13/$ – see front matter © 2013 Elsevier Inc. All rights reserved.

anomalous pulmonary venous return (TAPVR), tricuspid atresia (TA), and truncus arteriosus.

TOF

Incidence
About 3% to 5% of all infants with a CHD have TOF, with males and females being affected equally.[1]

Anatomy/physiology
TOF consists of 4 basic lesions; a large ventricular septal defect (VSD), right ventricular outflow obstruction (from pulmonic stenosis), an overriding aorta, and right ventricular hypertrophy (RVH). The range of physiology seen with TOF is diverse. The extent of obstruction of the right ventricular outflow track determines the amount of cyanosis present in the patient. Systolic pressures are equally balanced in the right and left ventricle because of the nonrestrictive VSD. There is a left-to-right shunt, a bidirectional shunt, or a right-to-left shunt, depending on the extent of the right ventricular outflow tract obstruction. If the pulmonic stenosis is severe, there is a right-to-left shunt, with subsequent cyanosis and decreased pulmonary blood flow. If there is mild pulmonic stenosis, a left-to-right shunt occurs, resulting in an acyanotic TOF.[2]

Clinical presentation
Patients usually present as neonates with cyanosis, but typically without respiratory distress. In addition to cyanosis, the physical examination may show a systolic thrill at the lower and middle left sternal border. A loud and single S2, an aortic ejection click, and a loud grade 3 to 5/6 systolic ejection murmur in the middle to lower left sternal border are also found. A continuous patent ductus arteriosus (PDA) murmur may also be present.[2] Once the diagnosis is suspected, an electrocardiogram (ECG) and chest radiograph should be obtained. The classic ECG shows right axis deviation (RAD) and RVH with large R waves in the anterior precordial leads and large S waves in the lateral leads.[3] The chest radiograph, of an infant with a cyanotic TOF, shows a boot-shaped cardiac silhouette secondary to upward displacement of the right ventricular apex caused by RVH, and narrowing of the mediastinal shadow caused by the hypoplastic pulmonary outflow tract. The heart size is normal, with decreased pulmonary vascular markings (**Fig. 1**). Infants with acyanotic TOF have a radiograph

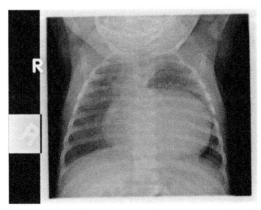

Fig. 1. TOF. Boot-shaped cardiac silhouette secondary to upward displacement of the right ventricular apex caused by RVH, and narrowing of the mediastinal shadow caused by the hypoplastic pulmonary outflow tract. (*Courtesy of* Mark Bittman, MD, New Hyde Park, NY.)

similar to that of moderate VSDs and show cardiomegaly as well as increased pulmonary vascular markings.[2] Diagnosis is confirmed by echocardiography.

Management
First, supplemental oxygen should be given through a humidified system by face mask or nasal cannula. Fluid resuscitation may be given initially, because the child may be intravascularly volume depleted (cautious 5–10 mL/kg aliquots assessing response after each bolus). However, neonates who present with ductal-dependent flow to the lungs need intravenous (IV) prostaglandin E_1 (PGE$_1$) to maintain ductal patency until surgical intervention. Decreasing pulmonary vascular resistance helps in left-to-right shunting and increases pulmonary blood flow. The initial dose of PGE$_1$ is 0.05 μg/kg/min. Apnea and hypotension are potential side effects of PGE$_1$, so airway management is essential. If possible, consultation with pediatric cardiology as well as the critical (neonatal or pediatric) care staff is beneficial.

Initial surgical intervention may be palliative, such as a Blalock-Taussig shunt for patients with significant comorbidities and contraindications to open heart surgery. This shunt creates a systemic-to-pulmonary arterial shunt between the subclavian artery and the ipsilateral pulmonary artery. The modified Blalock-Taussig shunt uses a Gore-Tex shunt and requires less dissection, is not dependent on the vessel length, and has decreased shunt failure. The Rastelli procedure is performed in older patients, and is used in severe TOF with significant right ventricular outflow tract obstruction. There is patch closure of the VSD, with the placement of a conduit from the right ventricle to the pulmonary artery.[4,5] The trend is towards neonatal repair.[6]

Cyanotic or hypoxemic episodes (tet spells) are seen in patients with TOF; hyperpnea, irritability, and increasing cyanosis along with a decreased intensity of the underlying heart murmur. A decrease in systemic vascular resistance or increased resistance to the right ventricular outflow tract increases right-to-left shunting, causing hyperpnea and, then, increased systemic venous return causes increased right-to-left shunting through the VSD. To manage a tet spell the patient should be placed in a knee-chest position and receive oxygen, volume expansion, sedation with morphine or ketamine, and, if needed, vasopressors, such as phenylephrine, to increase systemic vascular resistance and decrease the relative ratio between resistance to pulmonary and systemic output.[2] Oxygen may or may not help because the problem is to improve pulmonary blood flow. Morphine sulfate (0.1–0.2 mg/kg subcutaneously or intramuscularly) stops the hyperpnea. Ketamine (1–3 mg/kg IV) can also increase systemic vascular resistance and provide sedation. Propanolol (0.01–0.2 mg/kg IV over 5 minutes) can be beneficial. Phenylephrine (0.02 mg/kg IV) can help by increasing systemic vascular resistance.

TGA

Incidence
TGA represents around 5% to 8% of CHD and is the most common cyanotic heart lesion in the newborn period.[7]

Anatomy/physiology
In this anomaly, the aorta originates from the morphologic right ventricle, and the main pulmonary artery arises in the morphologic left ventricle. Complete TGA is also known as d-TGA; the d- refers to the dextroposition of the bulboventricular loop. The aorta also tends to be on the right and anterior, and the great arteries are parallel rather than crossing as they do in the normal heart. Because the systemic and pulmonary circulations run in parallel, presence of a VSD, atrial septal defect (ASD), or PDA is essential to survival, because the mixing of the circulations is the only way of providing

oxygenated blood to the systemic system.[8] Associated lesions are VSD found in approximately 20% to 40% of patients, pulmonary outflow tract obstruction, and, less commonly, approximately 5% coarctation of the aorta.[9]

Clinical presentation

If the interventricular septum is intact, these patients are the critically ill. If circulatory mixing is occurring via a PDA, physiologic closure of the ductus causes abrupt cyanosis and clinical deterioration. If there is a VSD or large PDA, the neonate is not so cyanotic but presents with dyspnea and feeding difficulties with congestive heart failure (CHF) and obstructive pulmonary disease.[8] On cardiac examination a loud, single S2 is present as well as a systolic murmur if there is a VSD. The ECG shows RAD and RVH. In an infant with classic TGA, the chest radiograph shows an egg-shaped heart with a narrow mediastinum, in addition to cardiomegaly with increased pulmonary vascular markings (**Fig. 2**). The echocardiogram shows 2 circular structures instead of the circle and sausage pattern of normal great arteries.[8]

Management

The severe arterial hypoxemia does not respond to the administration of oxygen. These patients respond well to PGE$_1$ infusion. Neonates with a VSD or large PDA are not so cyanotic but present with CHF and obstructive pulmonary disease. Early consultation and involvement of both pediatric cardiology and the critical (neonatal or pediatric) care staff is beneficial. Initial surgical intervention for cyanotic babies may be a percutaneous Rashkind atrial balloon septostomy to create an ASD, which may dramatically improve oxygenation until definitive surgery can be performed.[10] Definitive surgery is the arterial switch that corrects TGA at the great artery level. The aortic trunk is attached to the left ventricle and the pulmonic trunk is attached to the right ventricle.[11]

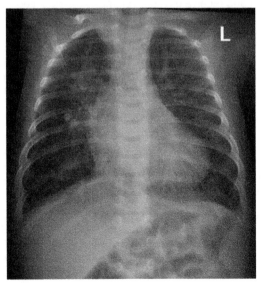

Fig. 2. d-Transposition of great vessels with VSD. Cardiomegaly with a cardiac contour classically described as appearing like an egg on a string. (*Courtesy of* Dr Hani Al Salam, Radiopaedia.org.)

TAPVR

Incidence

TAPVR represents around 1.5% of CHD and has an incidence of 6.8/100,000 live births.[12]

Anatomy/physiology

TAPVR is a congenital lesion, in which the pulmonary veins that normally bring oxygenated blood from the lungs to the left atrium anomalously drain into another structure than the left atrium. TAPVR is generally divided into 4 groups, depending on where the pulmonary veins drain. In the supracardiac type (50%), the common pulmonary vein attaches to the superior vena cava. In the cardiac type (20%), the common pulmonary vein empties into the coronary sinus. In the infracardiac/subdiaphragmatic type (20%), the common pulmonary vein empties into the portal vein, ductus venosus, hepatic vein, or inferior vena cava. A mixed type is seen in 10% of the lesions, which is a combination of any of the types.[13] Although this lesion represents a left-to-right shunt, a right-to-left intracardiac shunt must occur to provide mixing of blood. An ASD or patent foramen ovale is necessary for mixing of the blood.[14,15]

Clinical presentation

The clinical course is dependent on the obstruction to the flow of the anomalous pulmonary venous return or not. If there is obstruction to pulmonary venous return, there is significant cyanosis and respiratory distress. With the blood from both the pulmonary and systemic circulations pumped by the right ventricle, there can be volume overload, with subsequent right ventricular and atrial enlargement. There can be minimal cardiac examination findings, aside from a loud and single S2 and gallop rhythm. A murmur is usually not found. The ECG typically shows RAD and RVH, and the chest radiograph has a normal heart silhouette, with lung fields consistent with pulmonary edema.[16] If there is no obstruction to pulmonary venous return, there is minimal desaturation of the systemic blood; patients present with a history of frequent pneumonias and growth difficulties. In addition to slight cyanosis, patients present with signs of CHF, including tachypnea, tachycardia, and hepatomegaly.[16] There is a hyperactive right ventricular impulse, with a split and fixed S2. A grade 2 to 3/6 systolic ejection murmur is at the upper left sternal border, with a middiastolic rumble at the left lower sternal border. The ECG shows RAD, RVH, and right atrial enlargement. Chest radiography shows significant cardiomegaly, with increased pulmonary vascular markings. The characteristic snowman sign is found in infants older than 4 months (**Fig. 3**).[16]

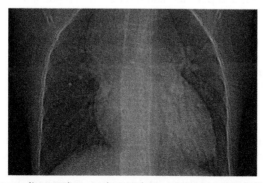

Fig. 3. TAPVR (supracardiac total anomalous pulmonary venous connection). Snowman sign sometimes also referred to as a figure-of-8 sign. (*Courtesy of* Dr Praveen Jha, Radiopaedia. org.)

Management

Unlike many cyanotic lesions in the newborn, management is not ductal dependent and PGE_1 is not indicated. Surgical correction is the first line of treatment, and medical management is to ensure proper acid-base balance, and diuretics if there is CHF. Airway management should take precedence because mechanical ventilation can prevent further respiratory decompensation. Inotropic assistance is important. Dopamine can be started at a continuous infusion at 5 to 10 μg/kg/min. Dobutamine can be started at the same dosing. However, dobutamine should be used with caution in patients younger than 1 year. Amrinone at 0.5 mg/kg IV over 3 minutes and milrinone loading dose of 10 to 50 μg/kg IV over 10 minutes could be another adjunct secondary to their inotropic and vasodilator properties.[17] Pulmonary vasodilators are usually not indicated, because they could exacerbate CHF.

TA

Incidence

TA represents the third most common cause of cyanotic CHD (1%–2% in infancy).[18]

Anatomy/physiology

For this congenital cardiac condition, there is no tricuspid valve and underdevelopment of the right ventricle and pulmonary artery,[19] resulting in decreased pulmonary blood flow. Because there is complete separation of the right atrium and ventricle, to empty, the right atrium needs a right-to-left shunt, so an ASD, VSD, or PDA is necessary for survival. Usually patients are divided into groups: type I, those without TGA; type II, those with transposition; and type III, those with other complex anomalies. The great arteries are transposed in 30% of cases, with a VSD and no pulmonic stenosis. In 50% of cases, there is normal artery anatomy, with a small VSD and pulmonic stenosis. This is a serious lesion that has 50% mortality by 6 months of age without surgical intervention.[20] There is right atrial dilatation and hypertrophy, because all systemic venous return is shunted from the right atrium to the left atrium. Enlargement of the left atrium and ventricle occurs because of the work of handling both systemic and pulmonary returns.

Clinical presentation

All patients with TA have some degree of arterial hypoxemia. The amount of cyanosis is inversely related to the amount of pulmonary blood flow. Severe cyanosis, tachypnea, and poor feeding are common presentations. On cardiac examination, there is a single S2 and the murmur is a grade 2 to 3/6 systolic regurgitant murmur from the VSD and is heard best at the left lower sternal border. There can also be a continuous murmur of a PDA. Hepatomegaly can be found with CHF. The ECG has a superior QRS axis, along with right atrial hypertrophy, left atrial hypertrophy (LAH), and left ventricular hypertrophy (LVH). The chest radiograph shows a normal to slight increase in heart size, along with decreased pulmonary vascular markings.[18]

Management

Airway management should take precedence, because mechanical ventilation can prevent further respiratory decompensation. The key to dealing with this ductal-dependent lesion is to start IV PGE_1. The initial surgical intervention is usually a shunt procedure aimed at improving pulmonary blood flow so that physiologic correction by means of a Fontan-Kreutzer procedure may be performed later.[20]

Truncus Arteriosus

Incidence
Truncus arteriosus is an uncommon cardiac abnormality and is seen in less than 1% of all CHD.[21]

Anatomy/physiology
In truncus arteriosus, a single arterial trunk arises from the ventricle via a single arterial valve to supply the systemic, pulmonary, and coronary circulations. It is also associated with the presence of a VSD, and abnormalities of the coronary arteries.[22,23]

Clinical presentation
The clinical presentation is dependent on the amount of pulmonary blood flow, which is in turn dependent on the presence or absence of pulmonary stenosis or the level of pulmonary arteriolar resistance. With decreased pulmonary blood flow, cyanosis is prevalent. With increased pulmonary blood flow, cyanosis is minimal; however, CHF is more prevalent. The left ventricle has to deal with significant volume overloads. Usually within the first weeks of life, the patient presents with CHF and cyanosis.[24] There is a loud regurgitant 2 to 4/6 systolic murmur at the left sternal border, sometimes associated with a high-pitched diastolic decrescendo murmur or a diastolic rumble. The S2 is single and accentuated. The ECG usually shows bilateral ventricular hypertrophy (**Fig. 4**), and the chest radiograph has cardiomegaly, with increased pulmonary vascular markings.[24]

Management
The priorities are airway management and starting IV PGE_1. Timing of truncus arteriosus repair continues to be a point of discussion. Some surgeons advocate elective

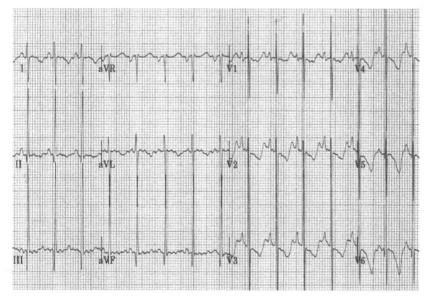

Fig. 4. Truncus arteriosus. The axis of QRS is 90° (roughly isoelectric in I and positive in aVF). This is a rightward axis. The large QRSs in V1 to V6 meet the voltage criteria for both LVH and RVH. This electrocardiogram shows biventricular hypertrophy.

repair of truncus arteriosus without major associated cardiac anomalies during the first 3 months of life;[25,26] others prefer primary neonatal correction.[27–29]

ACYANOTIC HEART DISEASE

Left-to-right shunt lesions include VSDs, ASDs, PDA, and endocardial cushion defects. This group comprises almost 50% of all CHD.[30] Left-to-right shunt lesions have blood shunted from the systemic system into the pulmonary system. CHF results from chamber enlargement, and increased pulmonary vascular pressures. In the neonate, high pulmonary vascular resistance controls the amounts shunted, but once pulmonary vascular resistance starts to decrease in the first few weeks of life, pulmonary blood flow and pressures increase.

ASDs

Incidence
ASD comprise up to 10% of all CHD.[31]

Anatomy/physiology
Any opening in the atrial septum is described as an atrial defect. There are many different types of ASD, such as the typical secundum atrial defect, which is most common and usually single; multiple fenestrations of the septum primum; and sinus venosus defects. The amount of shunting through a large atrial defect is determined by the relative right and left ventricular (LV) compliance. Early in infancy, the right ventricle is less compliant, and left-to-right shunting is minimal. As patients age, the right ventricle becomes more compliant and there is increased left-to-right shunt.

Clinical presentation
About 10% of infants with ASD present with feeding difficulties and failure to gain weight.[32] However, most patients are diagnosed later in life, because patients have nonspecific symptoms, including fatigue and breathlessness. The larger the left-to-right shunt, the greater the risk of developing long-term complications such as atrial fibrillation and pulmonary hypertension. Pulmonary hypertension affects up to 15% of patients with ASD and if not corrected can result in Eisenmenger syndrome (the pressures reverse and it becomes a right-to-left shunt, with decrease in systemic oxygenation). Another condition associated with ASD is stroke.[33] The cardiac examination has a widely split and fixed S2, with a grade 2 to 3/6 systolic ejection murmur at the upper left sternal border, sometimes associated with a middiastolic rumble. ECG findings include RAD and RVH or right bundle branch block (RBBB). Chest radiography shows cardiomegaly with increased pulmonary vascular markings (**Fig. 5**).[34]

Management
Some defects close spontaneously, but larger defects require surgical intervention. The timing of the surgical intervention seems to make a difference because closure after age 40 years is associated with greater frequency of arrhythmias, in particular atrial fibrillation.[35]

VSDs

Incidence
VSDs are the most common type of CHD and present in approximately 25% of all CHD cases.[36,37]

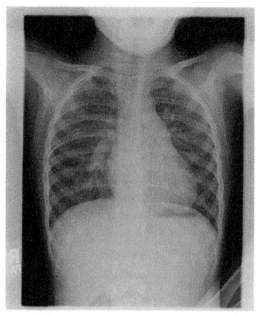

Fig. 5. Atrial septal defect. Cardiomegaly. (*Courtesy of* Mark Bittman, MD, New Hyde Park, NY.)

Anatomy/physiology

Ventricular defects are single or multiple and are classified by their location in the septum; the most common are either membranous or muscular. The extent of the defect determines the degree of cardiac compromise. Large VSDs have volume and pressure overload in the right ventricle as well as volume overload in the left atrium and left ventricle.

Clinical presentation

Large VSDs commonly present with poor weight gain and CHF. Patients with small VSDs are more likely to be asymptomatic; however, the smaller defects produce a louder systolic murmur. Typical examination shows a grade 2 to 5/6 systolic murmur (holosystolic), heard best at the left lower sternal border. A systolic thrill or diastolic rumble can also be present, with a narrowly split S2. ECG findings vary with the size of the defect; moderate VSDs show LAH and LVH, larger VSDs have LVH, RVH, and LAH. The chest radiograph also varies based on the size of the defect and may show cardiomegaly as well as increased pulmonary vascular markings (**Fig. 6**).[38]

Management

Surgical closure is recommended for any subpulmonary defects (except for small ones), perimembranous (subcristal) defects, obvious prolapse, and tricuspid valve involvement shortly after they are diagnosed, if aortic regurgitation is present but mild closure alone is sufficient. Valvuplasty is necessary if regurgitation is at least moderate. Valve replacement is rarely needed, except in older patients. Beyond age 15 years, if regurgitation is mild at most, shunting minimal, and the patient stable, continued medical observation seems reasonable. Sometimes, the additional lesions are the major indication for surgery in these patients.[38]

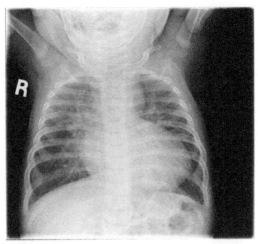

Fig. 6. VSD. Cardiomegaly and pulmonary vascular congestion. (*Courtesy of* Mark Bittman, MD, New Hyde Park, NY.)

PDA

Incidence
PDA is seen in 10% of all CHD. It is the second most common congenital heart defect in adults, making up 10% to 15% of all CHD in adults. There is a female/male ratio of 2:1.[30]

Anatomy/physiology
In patients with PDA, the ductus does not close as it ordinarily would. The ductus connects the descending aorta at the level of the subclavian artery to the left pulmonary artery. In healthy patients, the ductus arteriosus functionally closes within hours after birth and then completely seals around 3 weeks of age, usually at the pulmonary end, often leaving behind a remnant on the aorta called ligamentum arteriosum. In premature infants, the process of ductal closure is the same but is delayed, sometimes for weeks. The incidence of persistent patency of the ductus well past infancy in patients who were premature is greater than it is in the normal population.[39] The degree of the left-to-right shunting is dependent on the lesion length and diameter and pulmonary vascular resistance.

Clinical presentation
CHF is present if the PDA is large. Physical examination is remarkable for a grade 1 to 4/6 continuous machinery like murmur, heard best at the left upper sternal border. A diastolic rumble can also be present as well as bounding peripheral pulses. The ECG is normal when there is a small PDA; it can show LVH and RVH and pulmonary hypertension in large PDAs. Chest radiography shows cardiomegaly and increased pulmonary vascular markings.[39]

Management
Most experts believe that it should be closed either surgically or percutaneously to prevent endarteritis as well as to remove excess flow to the pulmonary circulation.[39]

Endocardial Cushion Defects

Incidence

Endocardial cushion defects represent around 3% of CHD, and almost two-thirds have the complete form. Down syndrome is strongly associated with the complete form of endocardial cushion defects.[30]

Anatomy/physiology

When the endocardial cushion does not develop properly, there are defects to the atrial septum, the ventricular septum, and the atrioventricular (AV) valves. Complete defects involve the entire endocardial cushion and have atrial and ventricular septal lesions and a common AV valve. Incomplete or partial defects have atrial involvement, with an intact ventricular septum. There can also be variations of both complete and incomplete lesions.[40]

Clinical presentation

The presentation for endocardial cushion defects is similar to ventricular or atrial defects or both, with the added possibility of AV valvular regurgitation. A history of failure to thrive and multiple respiratory tract infections is common. Left-to-right shunting is directly dependent on the extent of the defects, with complete lesions presenting with CHF early from volume overload in both the left and right ventricles. Cardiac examination is remarkable for a hyperactive precordium, a systolic thrill, a loud holosystolic regurgitant murmur, and a loud and split S2. The ECG shows a superior QRS axis, with RVH, RBBB, and LVH, along with a prolonged PR interval.[40]

COARCTATION OF THE AORTA

Incidence

Coarctation of the aorta represents 8% to 10% of CHD and is seen in males in a 2:1 ratio.[41]

Anatomy/Physiology

There is congenital narrowing of the descending aorta, which occurs before, at the level of, or after the origin of the left subclavian artery. The extent of the symptoms is dependent on the degree of narrowing, the length of the narrowing, and the presence of other cardiac defects. For a critical coarctation, the PDA is able to temporarily negate the negative effects of the coarctation. When the PDA eventually closes, the development of pulmonary hypertension and subsequent pulmonary venous congestion leads to CHF.[42]

Clinical Presentation

Neonates with critical coarctation often present with shock and metabolic acidosis. The presence of decreased pulses in the lower extremities, compared with the upper extremities, is key in the diagnosis of a coarctation. Disparities between right upper extremity and lower extremity blood pressures and pulse oximeter readings aid in the diagnosis. However, if the patient is in significant shock, pressures can be decreased everywhere.[42] When presenting in CHF, there is a loud gallop, a murmur may or not be present, and pulses are weak. The ECG shows RVH or RBBB (**Fig. 7**). Chest radiography shows cardiomegaly as well as pulmonary edema (**Figs. 8** and **9**). In older children, the appearance of notching of the first rib, also known as the 3 sign, may be present.[42]

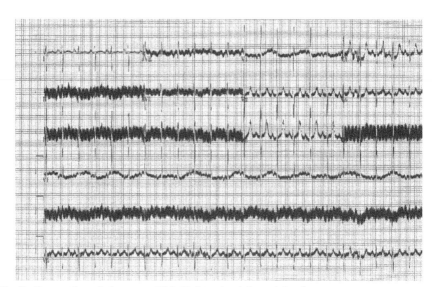

Fig. 7. Coarctation of the aorta ECG. Right axis; right atrial enlargement.

Management

The main aim of initial management is to stabilize the infant's condition so that a diagnosis can be confirmed and a treatment plan can be made. Initial management is to secure ductal patency with PGE_1 infusion. The mainstay is surgical correction with resection and end-to-end anastomosis, prosthetic patch arthroplasty, and interposition grafting.

HYPOPLASTIC LEFT HEART SYNDROME
Incidence

Hypoplastic left heart syndrome (HLHS) is rare, accounting only for 2% to 3% of all CHDs.[43]

Anatomy/Physiology

HLHS is a congenital defect in which the left ventricle, as well as the aortic arch, are underdeveloped or atretic, and atresia of the aortic and mitral valves, or severe

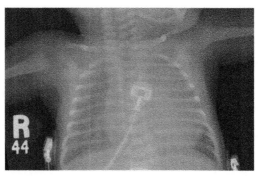

Fig. 8. Coarctation of the aorta. Cardiomegaly and pulmonary vascular congestion (patient had preductal coarctation in segment between innominate artery and left carotid and large VSD).

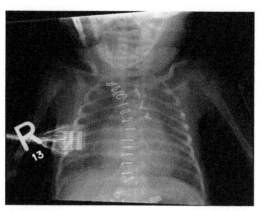

Fig. 9. Coarctation of aorta: Postoperative day 1. Same patient as in **Fig. 8**: Appreciate the difference in heart size.

stenosis, do not allow cardiac output from the left heart, resulting in minimal LV outflow.[44] The right ventricle, via right-to-left flow through the ductus, supports systemic circulation and so is a duct-dependent circulation. Similarly, pulmonary venous return can reach systemic circulation only by traversing the atrial septum (via a patent foramen ovale) to reach the right side of the heart.

Clinical Presentation

These patients typically present in the neonatal period listless, cyanotic, and tachypneic. As the duct closes, this leads to circulatory shock and metabolic acidosis. Increased pulmonary blood flow leads to an increase in left atrial pressure and subsequent pulmonary edema. There is a single heart sound, with a systolic ejection murmur and diminished pulses. The ECG shows right atrial enlargement, RVH, and peaked P waves. The chest radiograph shows cardiomegaly.[45]

Management

The main aim of initial management is to stabilize the infant's condition so that a diagnosis can be confirmed and a treatment plan can be made. Intubation and ventilation are usually necessary to remove the work of breathing and allow for hemodynamic stabilization. Positive-pressure ventilation alleviates pulmonary edema, and permissive hypercapnia can be used to allow the pulmonary vascular resistance to increase and to reduce pulmonary overcirculation. Ductal patency should be secured with PGE_1 infusion. Congestive cardiac failure is treated with diuretics, but if there is worsening tachypnea and acidosis with peripheral constriction, inotropic support (typically dobutamine 5–10 µg/kg/min) might be needed for the volume-loaded right ventricle.[46] These measures stabilize most patients, enabling surgery to be planned over the following days. Patients with restrictive or even intact atrial septum pose a more urgent situation, depending on the severity of the obstruction and subsequent lung injury. The most severe cases are not compatible with life, but those who remain profoundly cyanotic despite ventilatory support need urgent decompression of the left atrium with either balloon atrial septostomy in the catheter laboratory or early surgery. Patients need surgical intervention with initial palliative procedure such as a Norwood operation followed by a bidirectional Glenn procedure and Fontan procedure. The Norwood operation, performed in the neonatal period, is a palliative procedure in

HLHS. The hypoplastic aorta is reconstructed using an aortic or pulmonary artery allograft, the main pulmonary artery is divided, a Gore-Tex shunt is placed on the right to establish pulmonary blood flow, and the atrial septum is excised to provide interatrial mixing. The bidirectional Glenn operation that anastomoses the superior vena cava to the right pulmonary artery is usually performed at 6 months of age. During the Fontan operation, systemic venous return is redirected to the pulmonary artery and is usually performed by 1.5 years of age.[47,48] After a series of operations, the right ventricle functions as the systemic ventricle pumping into a reconstructed aortic arch, and pulmonary blood flow is achieved passively through a Fontan-type circulation.

AORTIC STENOSIS
Incidence

Aortic stenosis is seen in 6% of CHD, with a 5:1 ratio in males.[49]

Anatomy/Physiology

The aortic stenosis can be at the valvular, supravalvular, or subvalvular level, with the degree of obstruction determining the severity of disease in the patient. A congenital bicuspid aortic valve occurs in 1.3% of the population and therefore is one of the most common congenital heart malformations.[43] The physiologic impact of aortic stenosis is obstruction of LV outflow, resulting in increased LV afterload.

Clinical Presentation

Approximately 10% to 15% of patients have severe obstruction presenting with CHF in infancy. The physical examination is remarkable for a systolic thrill in the region of the upper right sternal border, suprasternal notch, or carotid arteries. There can be an ejection click. The murmur is a rough or harsh systolic murmur grade 2 to 4/6 at the right intercostal space or left intercostal space, with transmission to the neck. In cases of severe aortic stenosis, the ECG shows LVH. If there is resultant CHF, the chest radiograph shows cardiomegaly.[45]

Management

Balloon valvuloplasty has generally supplanted open surgical valvotomy as initial treatment of congenital aortic valve stenosis in children and adolescents.[50] Subsequent progression of stenosis or valve regurgitation is expected, with valve replacement considered to be the definitive treatment.

ARRHYTHMIAS

Arrhythmias can be a result of various and often combined abnormalities, such as impulse formation, abnormalities in impulse propagation, and abnormalities in autonomic influence. Cardiac arrhythmias in children are often caused by an underlying congenital heart defect, especially after heart surgery. Certain types of CHD, TOF, corrected d-TGA, TAPVR, large ASDs, VSDs, endocardial cushion defects, aortic and subaortic stenosis, and congenital mitral stenosis are associated with a higher incidence of postsurgical rhythm disturbances. The most common postoperative arrhythmias include supraventricular tachycardia, ventricular tachycardia, sick sinus syndrome, and complete heart block.[51] Other causes of arrhythmias in children include congenital complete heart block, Wolff-Parkinson-White (WPW) syndrome, and long Q-T syndrome. Acquired heart diseases with associated arrhythmias include viral myocarditis, KD, cardiomyopathies, rheumatic carditis, and cardiac tumors. Arrhythmias also may be associated with myriad systemic disorders, including electrolyte derangements, neuromuscular disorders, endocrine disorders, inherited disorders of metabolism, and central nervous system diseases. When children present with new-onset arrhythmias, the possibility of drug and toxic substance ingestion also must be considered.

SUPRAVENTRICULAR TACHYCARDIA
Incidence

Paroxysmal supraventricular tachycardia, previously called paroxysmal atrial tachycardia, is the most common pediatric arrhythmia and occurs in 1 in 250 to 1 in 1000 children.[52]

Anatomy/Physiology

Electrophysiologic studies have shown that supraventricular tachycardia is several arrhythmias. In addition to being caused by abnormal impulse formation, supraventricular tachycardia may also be caused by reentry within the sinoatrial node, atrium, AV nodal approaches, and accessory pathways, including WPW syndrome. Most patients with SVT have normal hearts, with 23% having CHD and 22% with WPW syndrome.[53] WPW is associated with CHD, such as TGA. WPW is a preexcitation syndrome, with an accessory pathway between the atria and ventricles.

Clinical Presentation

Arrhythmias may manifest in several ways, including symptoms of CHF, decreased cerebral perfusion (eg, syncope, dizziness, irritability, inappropriate behavior), decreased coronary perfusion (eg, anginal chest pain), or perception of the arrhythmia (ie, palpitations). Infants may present with a history of irritability, lethargy, or dyspnea, with decreased appetite and vomiting. In more severe cases, mottling and cyanosis may be present, with varying degrees of CHF. Infants with CHF have enlarged livers, but peripheral edema is rare. Older children may report a history of syncope, dizziness, restlessness, fatigue, and dyspnea, or sudden onset of chest pain or palpitations. A typical ECG seen in a pediatric patient with supraventricular tachycardia shows a rapid rate and a narrow QRS complex. P waves can usually be seen, but may be obscured by the ST segment. If P waves are absent, a narrow and regular QRS complex is more likely to be of supraventricular rather than of ventricular origin. Supraventricular tachycardia is characterized by a regular heart rate, which does not fluctuate with agitation, in contrast to sinus tachycardia. The rate of tachycardia in infants ranges from 220 to 320 beats per minute, whereas the rate in older children typically ranges from 150 to 250 beats per minute.

Management

In stable patients, vagal maneuvers (eg, carotid massage, Valsalva maneuver, gag reflex, abdominal compression, rectal stimulation in infants) and pharmacologic cardioversion are indicated as the first line of treatment. However, in hemodynamically unstable patients, synchronized cardioversion should be promptly used. The history and clinical findings should be assessed quickly to determine the most appropriate course of action. Adenosine has become the first-line pharmacologic therapy for supraventricular tachycardia in pediatric patients who present to the emergency department.[54] It has a rapid onset of action, usually within 10 seconds, and a half-life of only several seconds. Because of its short half-life, it is ineffective if administered too slowly. In young patients, adenosine initially should be administered as a rapid IV bolus dose of 0.1 mg/kg, with subsequent dose of 0.2 mg/kg. Patients weighing more than 50 kg may be given an initial dose of 6 mg, with a subsequent dose of

12 mg given 1 to 2 minutes later, if required. If IV access is delayed or if adenosine is not readily available or is unsuccessful in cardioverting a hemodynamically unstable patient, immediate synchronized cardioversion with 0.5 to 1 J/kg should be instituted. If the initial attempt is unsuccessful, the current should be doubled successively until effective or until a dose of 10 J/kg is reached.[55] Because cardioversion may not be successful in the presence of hypoxia or acid-base imbalance, airway support and ventilation may be required to help correct an underlying acidosis. Once the patient's rhythm is converted to sinus rhythm, a pediatric cardiologist should be consulted for further management and evaluation.

COMPLETE HEART BLOCK
Incidence

Complete AV heart block may be congenital or acquired. Congenital complete AV heart block is seen in 1 in 22,000 live births.

Anatomy/Physiology

Congenital heart block may be associated with structural heart defects or with maternal collagen vascular disease. It is speculated that maternal immunoglobins cross the placenta and damage the fetal cardiac conduction system.[56] Acquired complete AV heart block may be secondary to nonsurgical causes, such as inflammatory or infectious diseases,[57] or iatrogenic after cardiac surgery (especially after VSD repair). Postsurgical complete AV heart block may be transient or permanent.[58] Improved knowledge of the location of the conduction system has helped decrease the incidence of postsurgical heart block to less than 1%.

Clinical Presentation

The usual presentation in infancy is CHF. Older children with congenital complete AV heart block tend to present with syncope, diminished exercise tolerance, and fatigue. Congenital heart block presents with bradycardia. The ventricular rate is usually less than 75 beats per minute and rarely more than 100 beats per minute while at rest. Third-degree or complete heart blocks have independent atrial and ventricular activity. There are regular P waves at a normal heart rate for age. The QRS complexes are also regular, but at a slower rate than the P waves. Patients may be evaluated with 24-hour Holter monitoring and echocardiography to assess the possibility of an associated congenital heart lesion or inadequate surgical palliation.

Management

If the patient is symptomatic, isoproterenol, epinephrine, external pacer, or temporary transvenous ventricular pacing are sometimes required. The emergency treatment of congenital or acquired nonsurgical heart block is similar. Priorities are adequate oxygenation and ventilation. Pharmacologic therapy may be tried if treatment of acidosis does not help perfusion. An infusion of isoproterenol (0.02–0.5 μg/kg/min) or epinephrine (0.05–0.5 μg/kg/min) should be started to increase the junctional or ventricular escape rate. Adequate intravascular volume should be maintained during epinephrine infusion, because its vasodilatory effect may result in lowered BP. If cardiac output is inadequate despite pharmacologic measures, an external pacer should be applied while awaiting temporary ventricular pacing.[59]

OTHER HEART BLOCK

AV block is found when there is an interruption of the conduction of the normal sinus impulse and the subsequent ventricular response. In addition to third-degree blocks (complete heart block), there are first-degree and second-degree blocks.

The first-degree block has a prolonged PR interval because of delayed conduction through the AV node. This block is the result of a cardiomyopathy, CHD, postcardiac surgery, or digitalis toxicity or can be found in healthy patients.

In a second-degree block, not all of the P waves are followed by QRS complexes. The Mobitz type I Wenckebach phenomenon has a PR interval that gets progressively longer until the QRS complex is completely decreased. The block is at the AV node level and can be attributed to myocarditis, cardiomyopathy, surgery, CHD, or digitalis toxicity. The Mobitz type II block has similar causes, but the block is at the bundle of His. AV conduction is either all or none. There is potential for a complete block to develop. In 2-to-1 or 3-to-1 blocks, the block is at the level of the AV node, but can also be at the bundle of His. Mobitz II block is rare in children.

Management

First-degree AV block is a well-tolerated condition. Management is aimed at identifying any reversible underlying cause and following the patient closely to be sure that the condition does not progress. Mobitz I block is well tolerated as well and does not always require therapy. For acute symptoms, treatment with IV atropine or isoproterenol usually provides temporary improvement in conduction, but a pacemaker is the safest long-term therapy in symptomatic patients if the underlying cause is not reversible. Mobitz II may have abrupt progression to complete block. When it occurs as the result of surgical trauma, implantation of a pacemaker has been advised.[60]

ACQUIRED DISEASE

Inflammatory diseases of the heart are grouped under carditis. Included in this group are myocarditis, pericarditis, and endocarditis (along with valvulitis).

Myocarditis

Clinical presentation

There are several different causes of myocarditis. Infectious-mediated and autoimmune-mediated, as well as toxin-mediated, processes can contribute to the inflammatory response in the myocardium.[61] Most cases of myocarditis in the United States and Western Europe result from viral infections such as coxsackievirus, influenza, cytomegalovirus, herpes simplex virus, hepatitis C, rubella, varicella, mumps, Epstein-Barr virus, human immunodeficiency virus, and respiratory syncytial virus. Nonviral causes such as protozoans (Chagas disease seen in South America) also cause myocarditis. Less frequently, bacteria, rickettsia, fungal, mycobacteria, and other parasites can be causes; drugs (including antimicrobial medications), hypersensitivity, autoimmune, or collagen vascular diseases such as systemic lupus erythematosus, mixed connective tissue disease, rheumatic fever, rheumatoid arthritis, and scleroderma; or other disorders such as KD and sarcoidosis. In most cases, however, idiopathic myocarditis is encountered.[62] Infants may present with vomiting, decreased activity, poor feeding, and CHF, with tachycardia, tachypnea, a gallop rhythm, and decreased heart tones. There are no specific laboratory tests for myocarditis. Erythrocyte sedimentation rate, white blood cell count, myocardial enzymes, and cardiac troponin are normal or increased. Troponin levels are believed to be more sensitive than cardiac enzymes.[63] ECG abnormalities are common but are nonspecific. There is tachycardia, low QRS voltages, flattened or inverted T waves with ST-T wave changes, and prolongation of the QT interval (**Fig. 10**). Arrhythmias such as premature contractions are also seen. Chest radiography shows cardiomegaly and pulmonary venous congestion, depending on the extent of the disease (**Fig. 11**). Echocardiogram studies show dilatation of the heart chambers and decreased LV function. The echocardiogram also helps to evaluate myocardial contractility and the presence of a pericardial effusion (**Fig. 12**). Radionuclide scanning and endomyocardial biopsies can help in confirming the disease. Mortality in symptomatic neonates with acute viral myocarditis can be significant.[64]

Management
Management of myocarditis revolves around identifying a cause and, if identified, treating that suspected agent, treating the CHF, and controlling the arrhythmias. Supplemental oxygen, diuretics like furosemide, and inotropic agents such as dopamine and dobutamine are mainstays in treatment, along with the use of angiotensin-converting enzyme inhibitors like captopril. Digoxin is used cautiously because of its potential to induce arrhythmias. In KD, high-dose immunoglobulin has been beneficial. Other treatment modalities, such as immunosuppressive agents and corticosteroids (except in severe rheumatic carditis), are not universally accepted. Acute fulminant myocarditis resulting in rapid hemodynamic deterioration is 1 indication for mechanical support by using rapid-response extracorporeal membrane oxygenation.[65]

Pericarditis

Clinical presentation
Inflammation of the pericardium is the hallmark of pericarditis. The most common cause in infancy is a viral cause such as coxsackie, echovirus, adenovirus, or influenza. Viral pericarditis is usually associated with a viral myocarditis, with the myocarditis being the more prominent entity. Acute pericarditis may occur secondary to infectious agents such as *Staphylococcus aureus*, *Streptococcus pneumoniae*, *Haemophilus influenzae*, *Neisseria meningitides*, and streptococci as well as tuberculosis; collagen vascular disease; cardiac surgery; drug therapy; as a manifestation of

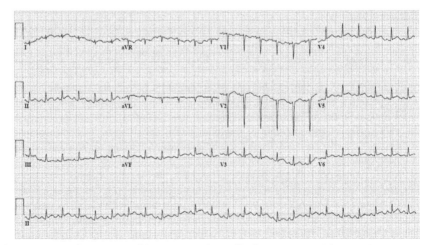

Fig. 10. Myocarditis. 7-year-old patient, tachycardia: heart rate, 143 beats/min; P-R, 57 ms; QRS 62 ms; QT/QTc, 282/435 ms. (*Courtesy of* Robert Bramante, MD and Annabella Salvador, MD, Manhasset, NY.)

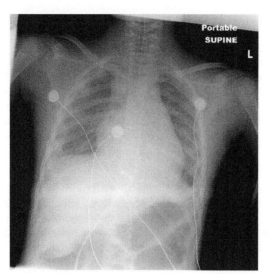

Fig. 11. Myocarditis. Cardiomegaly (same patient as ECG in **Fig. 10**). (*Courtesy of* Robert Bramante, MD and Annabella Salvador, MD, Manhasset, NY.)

rheumatic fever; or in association with chronic renal failure and dialysis. Postpericardiotomy syndrome is seen in patients who have had cardiac surgery involving interruption of the pericardium.[66] The predominant symptom of acute pericarditis is precordial chest pain in as many as 80% of children, exacerbated by breathing, coughing, or motion. Patients are most comfortable in the upright position. In the absence of cardiac tamponade or pneumonitis, respiratory distress is not a common clinical feature. Fever, present in most cases of acute pericarditis, cannot reliably differentiate pericarditis caused by infectious agents, collagen vascular disease, or rheumatic fever. There is usually a predisposing illness in the history, with an upper respiratory infection

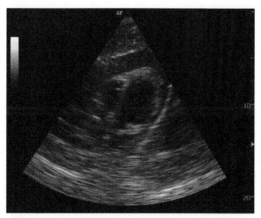

Fig. 12. Myocarditis. Point-of-care ultrasonography: parasternal long view, moderate-sized effusion, no collapse or tamponade; however, the heart showed decreased contractility (same patient as ECG in **Fig. 10** and chest radiograph in **Fig. 11**). (*Courtesy of* Robert Bramante, MD and Annabella Salvador, MD, Manhasset, NY.)

or, in the case of a bacterial pericarditis, a pneumonia, empyema, osteomyelitis, pyelonephritis, or tonsillitis. A pericardial friction rub is diagnostic.[67] A murmur may not be found and the heart is hypodynamic.

On ECG, there is a low-voltage QRS complex. Early in the disease, ST segments are increased everywhere, except in V1 and aVR. Later in the disease, ST segments return to normal and the T waves flatten or invert.[68] A chest radiograph shows cardiomegaly, with the heart in a water-bottle shape. Echocardiogram is the key to establishing the presence of an effusion. In addition, the echo can also evaluate for cardiac tamponade, because it shows the collapse of the right atrial wall or the right ventricular wall in diastole.[66]

Management

In milder cases, nonsteroidal antiinflammatory drugs can be used to treat the discomfort. In more severe cases, especially if an infectious cause is suspected, pericardiocentesis is needed in addition to antibiotics, antivirals, or antifungals, depending on the suspected cause. Multiple blood cultures are also indicated, as well as standard fluid studies. In postpericardiotomy syndrome, which can affect as many as 30% of pediatric patients who undergo cardiovascular surgery involving the pericardium, the patients present with fever, irritability, and a pericardial friction rub from a month to a few months postoperatively.[66]

Endocarditis

Incidence

Infective endocarditis is an uncommon but life-threatening infection. CHD is a significant risk factor in infective endocarditis. In infancy, endocarditis is rare and is associated with open heart surgery.[69]

Anatomy/physiology

It is believed that turbulent flow from pressure gradients leads to endothelial damage and thrombus formation. Transient bacteremia then seeds the damaged areas. With the exception of a secundum ASD, all CHDs and valvular heart diseases are prone to endocarditis, especially if there is any artificial material within the heart (prosthetic heart valve or graft). Common bacterial causes include *Streptococcus viridans*, enterococci, and *Staphylococcus aureus* as well as fungal and bacteria such as *Eikenella* and *Cardiobacterium*.[69]

Clinical presentation

The usual presentation is with fulminant disease and a septic appearance. A heart murmur and fever are always present. Adult patients tend to have more embolic phenomena. Using the Duke Criteria for Infective Endocarditis, a patient must have 2 major criteria or 1 major criterion with 3 minor criteria or 5 minor criteria. Major criteria include 2 separately obtained positive blood cultures growing the typical microorganisms and an echocardiogram with endocardial involvement such as an intracardiac mass on a valve, abscess, partial dehiscence of a prosthetic valve, or new valvular regurgitation. Minor criteria include predisposing conditions, fever, vascular phenomena (emboli, hemorrhages, Janeway lesions), and immunologic phenomena (glomerulonephritis, Osler nodes, Roth spots, rheumatoid factor), microbiological evidence (positive blood culture not meeting major criteria), and echocardiographic findings (not meeting major criteria).[70] Although an echocardiogram identifying valvular vegetation is helpful in the evaluation, the echocardiogram is not 100% sensitive or specific. Because of this, a negative echocardiogram does not exclude endocarditis. Obtaining a positive blood culture makes a definitive diagnosis.

Management

Three or more blood cultures should be taken irrespective of body temperature approximately 1 hour apart. The isolation of a specific microorganism is critical for determining antibiotic therapy. In cases complicated by sepsis, severe valvular dysfunction, conduction disturbances, or embolic events, empirical antimicrobial therapy should be started after blood cultures are obtained. Empirical antibiotic therapy with vancomycin and gentamicin should be initiated in the emergency department.[71] Treatment regimens may take place for weeks to be certain that the microorganism has been eliminated. Prophylactic antibiotics are recommended before dental procedures for patients with prosthetic cardiac valve and previous history of infectious endocarditis. In addition, it is also recommended for patients with CHD with unrepaired cyanotic CHD, including palliative shunts and conduits, or completely repaired congenital heart defect with prosthetic material or device, whether placed by surgery or by catheter intervention, during the first 6 months after the procedure, or repaired CHD with residual defects at the site or adjacent to the site of a prosthetic patch or prosthetic device (which inhibit endothelialization). Another group of patients who need prophylaxis are those who received cardiac transplantation and have developed cardiac valvulopathy.[72]

KD

Incidence

With an annual incidence in the United States of 4 to 15 cases per 100,000 children younger than 5 years, a male/female ratio of 1.5:1, and seasonal peaks in winter and spring, KD has become the leading cause of acquired heart disease in children in the developed world.[73]

Anatomy/Physiology

KD is a self-limiting generalized systemic vasculitis of indeterminate cause. Biochemical and immunologic evidence suggests endothelial cell activation and injury. Studies of KD pathogenesis show a progression of arterial lesions accompanying KD vasculitis and several immunoregulatory changes, including a deficiency of circulating CD8+ suppressor/cytotoxic T cells; an abundance of circulating B cells spontaneously producing immunoglobulins; and circulating, activated monocytes.[73] Stage I (0–9 days) is characterized by perivasculitis of small arteries. Pericarditis, myocarditis, inflammation of the AV conduction system, and endocarditis with valvulitis are also present. Stage II (12–25 days) is characterized by panvasculitis of medium-sized, muscular arteries with aneurysm formation and thrombosis. Myocarditis, pericarditis, and endocarditis with valvulitis may also be present. During stage III (28–31 days), myointimal proliferation in the coronary and other medium-sized arteries is prominent, and acute inflammation disappears from the microvasculature. In stage IV (after 40 days), scarring of arteries with stenosis may occur.[74,75]

Clinical Presentation

KD primarily affects infants and younger children and can occur in endemic or community-wide epidemic forms. The hallmarks of the disease are fever of at least greater than or equal to 5 days duration, and presence of 4 of these features: bilateral nonexudative conjunctivitis, erythema of the mucous membranes (lips, oral mucosa), rash, cervical adenopathy, and extremity changes. Bilateral conjunctival injection involving the bulbar conjunctivae is seen around the time of the fever. There can be erythema; peeling, cracking, or bleeding from the lips and mouth; a strawberry tongue; and diffuse erythema of the mucosa of the oropharynx. The extremity changes include erythema to the palms and soles, with induration and desquamation to the fingers and toes. Sometimes, early desquamation in the perianal region can occur. There can be an extensive erythematous rash, which is usually a nonspecific diffuse maculopapular rash. The cervical lymphadenopathy is generally unilateral, and usually 1 node is greater than 1.5 cm in diameter.[76,77] Although most cases fulfill the principal diagnostic criteria, about 15% of cases have incomplete clinical presentations, with coronary artery complications.[78] Therefore, any infant younger than 6 months with fever duration of 7 days or more, increase of C-reactive protein (CRP) and erythrocyte sedimentation rate (ESR), and no other explanation for the febrile illness should have an echocardiogram. In any child with unexplained fever lasting more than 5 to 7 days with some of these laboratory findings, incomplete KD should be considered and echocardiography should be obtained as well. Furthermore, KD can be diagnosed when 4 or more principal criteria are present on day 4 of illness.[77] Coronary artery aneurysms or ectasia have been found in 15% to 25% of untreated children with KD.[79] Coronary artery aneurysms more than 8 mm in diameter (so-called giant aneurysms) can lead to acute myocardial infarction, which may result in hypotension, arrhythmia, or sudden death.[80] In the acute phase of KD, there can be involvement of all parts of the heart: the pericardium, the myocardium, the endocardium, the valves, and the coronary arteries. The cardiac examination can show tachycardia, a gallop, and a flow murmur or regurgitant pansystolic murmur. Depressed myocardial function can present as cardiogenic shock. The ECG shows nonspecific ST and T wave changes, a prolonged PR interval, or arrhythmia. Laboratory findings include leukocytosis, anemia, and thombocytosis (appears in second week, peaking in third week). Thrombocytopenia in active disease is a risk factor for coronary aneurysms. There is increase of CRP levels or ESR. Serum transaminases can be moderately increased. γ-glutamyl transpeptidase level is increased in most patients. Albumin synthesis declines in the acute phase, and hypoalbuminemia is common. Urinalysis shows so-called sterile pyuria, with white cells (often in the range of 10 to 50/high-power field) noted on microscopic evaluation but not by dipstick.[77]

Management

Any patient suspected of having KD needs to be admitted. The goal of initial management is to reduce inflammation and thus reduce the risk of coronary artery abnormalities. Pharmacologic management of the acute phase of KD includes aspirin and IV immunoglobulin (IVIG). High-dose aspirin at 80 to 100 mg/kg per day is dosed 4 times a day. Length of treatment with aspirin is variable.[81] IVIG is believed to have a generalized antiinflammatory effect and is dosed at 2 g/kg in a single infusion, administered slowly, over 8 to 12 hours, to minimize the chance of hypersensitivity or hyperpyrexia reaction and to prevent solute overloading. Best results are seen when IVIG is started within the first 7 to 10 days of illness.[82,83]

CARDIOMYOPATHIES

Cardiomyopathies affect the heart muscle and are divided into 4 categories by the World Health Organization: hypertrophic, dilated, restrictive, and arrhythmogenic right ventricular cardiomyopathy.[84] However, as a result of new developments in molecular genetics in cardiology and the emergence of ion channelopathies as diseases predisposing to potentially lethal ventricular tachyarrhythmias, a new classification has been proposed by a panel of experts under the auspices of the American Heart Association. This panel recommends that cardiomyopathies be classified as primary ([a] genetic, [b] mixed [genetic and nongenetic], or [c] acquired), and secondary.

Cardiomyopathies are defined as a heterogeneous group of diseases associated with failure of myocardial performance, which may be mechanical (eg, diastolic or systolic dysfunction) or a primary electrical disease prone to life-threatening arrhythmias, associated with ventricular hypertrophy or dilatation from a variety of causes, which are frequently genetic. Cardiomyopathies can be either confined to the heart or be part of a generalized systemic disorder.[85]

Hypertrophic cardiomyopathy (HCM) would be in the primary genetic category, clinically heterogeneous but a common autosomal-dominant genetic heart disease[86] (1:500 of the general population for the disease phenotype recognized by echocardiography), which is probably the most frequently occurring cardiomyopathy. HCM, in the United States, is the most common cause of sudden cardiac death in the young, including trained athletes,[87] and is an important substrate for heart failure disability at any age. There is significant ventricular muscular hypertrophy and increased ventricular contractility, but these factors limit or reduce ventricular filling. The left ventricle is stiff and affects diastolic ventricular filling. The physical examination is notable for a sharp upstroke of the arterial pulse.[88] There can be a systolic ejection murmur or holosystolic murmur. The ECG shows LVH, ST, and T wave changes, deep Q waves, and decreased R waves. The chest radiograph may show a globular heart or cardiomegaly.

Dilated cardiomyopathies (DCM), a mixed form of cardiomyopathy, are a common and largely irreversible form of heart muscle disease, with an estimated prevalence of 1:2500; it is the third most common cause of heart failure and the most frequent cause of heart transplantation. It results from infectious or toxic causes. DCM may manifest clinically at a wide range of ages (most commonly in the third or fourth decade but also in young children) and usually is identified when associated with severe limiting symptoms and disability. DCM has ventricular dilatation with systolic dysfunction. DCM leads to progressive heart failure and a decline in LV contractile function, ventricular and supraventricular arrhythmias, conduction system abnormalities, thromboembolism, and sudden or heart failure–related death.[89] A significant S3 is found on examination.

Restrictive cardiomyopathies (RCM) limit diastolic filling of the ventricles. This is the least common form and results from noncompliant ventricular walls. RCM has multiple causes and may result from myocardial diseases, including noninfiltrative or infiltrative processes, storage diseases, endomyocardial diseases, myocarditis, and after cardiac transplantation.

Arrhythmogenic right ventricular cardiomyopathy/dysplasia (ARVC/D) is an uncommon form of inheritable heart muscle disease (estimated at 1:5000). Even although it is frequently associated with myocarditis (enterovirus or adenovirus in some cases), ARVC/D is not considered an inflammatory cardiomyopathy, but rather a primary genetic cardiomyopathy. ARVC/D involves predominantly the right ventricle with progressive loss of myocytes and fatty or fibrofatty tissue replacement, resulting in regional (segmental) or global abnormalities. In addition, evidence of LV involvement with fibrofatty replacement, chamber enlargement, and myocarditis is reported in up to 75% of patients. It should be considered in individuals with exercise-induced arrhythmias or syncope, 1 or multiple left bundle branch QRS morphology tachycardias, or unexplained right ventricular enlargement on the echocardiogram.[90] ECG shows abnormal repolarization with T wave inversion in leads V_1 to V_3 and small-amplitude potentials at the end of the QRS complex (ε wave); Brugada syndrome–like RBBB and right precordial ST segment increase accompanied by polymorphic ventricular tachycardia have also been reported in a small subpopulation of patients with ARVC/D.[90]

SUMMARY

The diagnosis and management of pediatric cardiac emergencies can be challenging and complicated. Early presentations are usually the result of ductal-dependent lesions and appear with cyanosis and shock. Later presentations are the result of volume overload or pump failure and present with signs of CHF. Acquired diseases also present as CHF or arrhythmias.

REFERENCES

1. Perry LW, Neill CA, Ferencz C, et al. Infants with congenital heart disease: the cases. In: Ferencz C, Rubin JD, Loffredo CA, et al, editors. Perspectives in pediatric cardiology. Epidemiology of congenital heart disease, the Baltimore-Washington Infant Study 1981–1989. Armonk (NY): Futura; 1993. p. 33–62.
2. Siwik ES, Erenberg F, Zahka KG, et al. Tetralogy of Fallot. In: Allen D, Driscoll DJ, Shaddy RE, et al, editors. Moss and Adams' heart disease in infants, children, and adolescents: including the fetus and young adults, vol. 43, 7th edition. Philadelphia: Lippincott Williams & Wilkins; 2008. p. 889–910.
3. Deal BJ, Johnsrude CL, Buck SH, editors. Pediatric ECG interpretation. Malden (MA): Blackwell; 2004. p. 88–122.
4. Ullom RL, Sade RM, Crawford FA Jr, et al. The Blalock-Taussig shunt in infants: standard versus modified. Ann Thorac Surg 1987;44(5):539–43.
5. Fraser CD Jr, McKenzie ED, Cooley DA. Tetralogy of Fallot: surgical management individualized to the patient. Ann Thorac Surg 2001;71:1556–61.
6. Reddy VM, Liddicoat JR, McElhinney DB, et al. Routine primary repair of tetralogy of Fallot in neonates and infants less than three months of age. Ann Thorac Surg 1995;60(Suppl):592–6.
7. Levin DL, Paul MH, Muster AJ, et al. d-Transposition of the great vessels in the neonate: a clinical diagnosis. Arch Intern Med 1977;137:1421–5.
8. Wernovsky G. Transposition of the great arteries. In: Allen D, Driscoll DJ, Shaddy RE, et al, editors. Moss and Adams' heart disease in infants, children, and adolescents: including the fetus and young adults, vol. 51, 7th edition. Philadelphia: Lippincott Williams & Wilkins; 2008. p. 1039–87.
9. Hornung TS, Derrick GP, Deanfield JE, et al. Transposition complexes in the adult: a changing perspective. Cardiol Clin 2002;20:405–20.
10. Rashkind WJ, Miller WW. Creation of an atrial septal defect without thoracotomy: a palliative approach to complete transposition of the great arteries. JAMA 1966;196:991–2.
11. Kang N, de Leval MR, Eliot M, et al. Extending the boundaries of the primary arterial switch operation in patients with transposition of the great arteries and intact ventricular septum. Circulation 1994;110(Suppl II):123.
12. Correa-Villasenor A, Ferencz C, Boughman JA, et al. Total anomalous pulmonary venous return: familial and environmental factors. Teratology 1991;44: 414–28.
13. Gathman GE, Nadas AS. Total anomalous pulmonary venous connection. Clinical and physiologic observation of 75 pediatric patients. Circulation 1970;42:143.
14. Lucas RV, Lock JE, Tandon R, et al. Gross and histologic anatomy of total anomalous pulmonary venous connection. Am J Cardiol 1988;62:292.
15. James CL, Keeling JW, Smith NM, et al. Total anomalous pulmonary venous drainage associated with fatal outcome in infancy. J Thorac Cardiovasc Surg 1994;14(4):665.

16. Keane JF, Fyler DC. Total anomalous pulmonary venous return. In: Keane JF, Lock JE, Fyler DC, editors. Nadas' pediatric cardiology, vol. 48, 2nd edition. Philadelphia: Saunders Elsevier; 2006. p. 773–81.

17. Lee C, Mason LJ. Pediatric cardiac emergencies. Anesthesiol Clin North America 2001;19(2):287–308.

18. Keane JF, Fyler DC. Tricuspid atresia. In: Keane JF, Lock JE, Fyler DC, editors. Nada's pediatric cardiology, vol. 45, 2nd edition. Philadelphia: Saunders Elsevier; 2006. p. 753–9.

19. Van Praagh R, Ando M, Dungan WT. Anatomic types of tricuspid atresia: clinical and developmental implications. Circulation 1971;44:11.

20. Streipe V. Tricuspid atresia. In: Kambam J, editor. Cardiac anesthesia for infants and children. St Louis (MO): Mosby; 1994. p. 258–68.

21. Williams JM, de Leeuw M, Black MD, et al. Factors associated with outcomes of persistent truncus arteriosus. J Am Coll Cardiol 1999;34(2):545–53.

22. Collett RW, Edwards JE. Persistent truncus arteriosus: a classification according to anatomical types. Surg Clin North Am 1948;29:1245.

23. Van Praagh R, Van Praagh S. The anatomy of common aorticopulmonary trunk (truncus arteriosus communis) and its embryologic implications: a study of 57 necropsy cases. Am J Cardiol 1965;16:406–25.

24. Keane JF, Fyler DC. Truncus arteriosus. In: Keane JF, Lock JE, Fyler DC, editors. Nada's pediatric cardiology, vol. 47, 2nd edition. Philadelphia: Saunders Elsevier; 2006. p. 767–71.

25. Brizard CP, Cochrane A, Austin C, et al. Management strategy and long-term outcome for truncus arteriosus. Eur J Cardiothorac Surg 1997;11:687–96.

26. Lacour-Gayet F, Serraf A, Komiya T, et al. Truncus arteriosus: influence of techniques of right ventricular outflow tract reconstruction. J Thorac Cardiovasc Surg 1996;111:849–56.

27. Bove EL, Lupinetti FM, Pridjian AK, et al. Results of a policy of primary repair of truncus arteriosus in the neonate. J Thorac Cardiovasc Surg 1993;105:1057–66.

28. Hanley FL, Heinemann MK, Jonas RA, et al. Repair of truncus arteriosus in the neonate. J Thorac Cardiovasc Surg 1993;105:1047–56.

29. Rajasinghe HA, McElhinney DB, Reddy VM, et al. Long-term follow-up of truncus arteriosus repaired in infancy: a twenty-year experience. J Thorac Cardiovasc Surg 1997;113:869–79.

30. Driscoll DJ. Left to right shunt lesions. Pediatr Clin North Am 1999;46(2):355–68.

31. Dexter L. Atrial septal defect. Br Heart J 1956;18(2):209–25.

32. Studer M, Blackstone E, Kirklin J, et al. Determinants of early and late results of repair of atrioventricular septal (conal) defects. J Thorac Cardiovasc Surg 1982;84(4):523–42.

33. Mas JL, Arquizan C, Lamy C. Recurrent cerebrovascular events associated with patent foramen ovale, atrial septal aneurysm, or both. N Engl J Med 2001;345:1740.

34. Keane JF, Geva T, Fyler DC. Atrial septal defect. In: Keane JF, Lock JE, Fyler DC, editors. Nada's pediatric cardiology, vol. 34, 2nd edition. Philadelphia: Saunders Elsevier; 2006. p. 603–16.

35. Ghosh S, Chatterjee S, Black E, et al. Surgical closure of atrial septal defect in adults: effect of age at operation on outcome. Heart 2002;88(5):485.

36. Kidd L, Driscoll D, Gersony W, et al. Second natural history study of congenital heart defects: results of treatment of patients with ventricular septal defects. Circulation 1993;87(Suppl 2):I38–51.

37. Keith JD, Rowe RD, Vlad P. Heart disease in infancy and childhood. New York: Macmillan; 1967. p. 3.
38. Keane JF, Fyler DC. Ventricular septal defect. In: Keane JF, Lock JE, Fyler DC, editors. Nada's pediatric cardiology, vol. 30, 2nd edition. Philadelphia: Saunders Elsevier; 2006. p. 527–47.
39. Keane JF, Fyler DC. Patent ductus arteriosus. In: Keane JF, Lock JE, Fyler DC, editors. Nada's pediatric cardiology, vol. 35, 2nd edition. Philadelphia: Saunders Elsevier; 2006. p. 617–25.
40. Marx GR, Fyler DC. Endocardial cushion defects. In: Keane JF, Lock JE, Fyler DC, editors. Nada's pediatric cardiology, vol. 38, 2nd edition. Philadelphia: Saunders Elsevier; 2006. p. 663–74.
41. Demircin M, Arsan S, Pasaoglu I, et al. Coarctation of the aorta in infants and neonates: results and assessments of prognostic variables. J Cardiovasc Surg 1995;36(5):459–64.
42. Keane JF, Fyler DC. Coarctation of the aorta. In: Keane JF, Lock JE, Fyler DC, editors. Nada's pediatric cardiology, vol. 36, 2nd edition. Philadelphia: Saunders Elsevier; 2006. p. 627–44.
43. Hoffman JE, Kaplan S. The incidence of congenital heart disease. J Am Coll Cardiol 2002;39:1890.
44. Noonan JA, Nadas AS. The hypoplastic left heart syndrome: an analysis of 101 cases. Pediatr Clin North Am 1958;5:1029–56.
45. Lang P, Fyler DC. Hypoplastic left heart syndrome, mitral atresia, and aortic atresia. In: Keane JF, Lock JE, Fyler DC, editors. Nada's pediatric cardiology, vol. 41, 2nd edition. Philadelphia: Saunders Elsevier; 2006. p. 715–26.
46. Nicolson S, Steven J, Jobes D. Hypoplastic left heart syndrome. In: Lake C, editor. Pediatric anesthesia. 3rd edition. Stamford (CT): Appleton & Lange; 1998. p. 337–52.
47. Norwood WI, Kirklin JK, Sanders SP. Hypoplastic left heart syndrome: experience with palliative surgery. Am J Cardiol 1980;45:78–91.
48. Norwood WI Jr, Jacobs ML, Murphy JD. Fontan procedure for hypoplastic left heart syndrome. Ann Thorac Surg 1992;54:1025–9.
49. Ongley PA, Nadas AS, Paul MH, et al. Aortic stenosis in infants and children. Pediatrics 1958;21:207–21.
50. Lababidi Z. Aortic balloon valvuloplasty. Am Heart J 1983;106:751–2.
51. Vetter V. What every pediatrician needs to know about arrhythmias in children who have had cardiac surgery. Pediatr Ann 1991;20:378.
52. Losek J, Endom E, Losek J, et al. Adenosine and pediatric supraventricular tachycardia in the emergency department: multicenter study and review. Ann Emerg Med 1999;33:185–91.
53. Saul PJ, Scott WA, Brown S, et al. Intravenous amiodarone for incessant tachyarrhythmias in children. A randomized, double-blind, antiarrhythmic drug trial. Circulation 2005;112(22):3470–7.
54. Manole MD, Saladino RA. Emergency department management of the pediatric patient with supraventricular tachycardia. Pediatr Emerg Care 2007;23:176–85.
55. Schamberger MS. Cardiac emergencies in children. Pediatr Ann 1996;25:339–44.
56. Buyon JP, Hiebert R, Copel J, et al. Autoimmune-associated congenital heart block: demographics, mortality, and recurrence rates obtained from a national lupus registry. J Am Coll Cardiol 1998;31:1658.
57. Pinto DS. Cardiac manifestations of Lyme disease. Med Clin North Am 2002;86:285.

58. Weindling SN, Gamble WJ, Mayer JE, et al. Duration of complete atrioventricular block after congenital heart disease surgery. Am J Cardiol 1998;82:525.
59. Sarnaik S, Sarnaik A, Hickey RW. Arrhythmias in children. In: Wolfson AB, editor. Harwood Nuss' clinical practice of emergency medicine, vol. 244, 5th edition. Philadelphia: Lippincott Williams & Wilkins; 2010. p. 1193–5.
60. Walsh EP, Berul CI, Triedman JK. Cardiac arrhythmias. In: Keane JF, Lock JE, Fyler DC, editors. Nada's pediatric cardiology, vol. 29, 2nd edition. Philadelphia: Saunders Elsevier; 2006. p. 477–523.
61. Wynn J, Braunwald E. The cardiomyopathies and myocarditis. In: Braunwald E, editor. Heart disease: a textbook of cardiovascular medicine. Philadelphia: WB Saunders; 1997. p. 1404–63.
62. Towbin JA. Myocarditis. In: Allen HD, Driscoll DJ, Shaddy RE, et al, editors. Moss and Adams' heart disease in infants, children, and adolescents: including the fetus and young adult, vol. 58. Philadelphia: Lippincott Williams & Wilkins; 2008. p. 1208–25.
63. Smith SC, Ladenson JH, Mason JW, et al. Elevations of cardiac troponin I associated with myocarditis: experimental and clinical correlates. Circulation 1997; 95:163–8.
64. English RF, Janosky JE, Ettedgui JA, et al. Outcomes for children with acute myocarditis. Cardiol Young 2004;14:488–93.
65. Duncan BW, Ibrahim AE, Hraska V, et al. Use of rapid-deployment extracorporeal membrane oxygenation for the resuscitation of pediatric patients with heart disease after cardiac arrest. J Thorac Cardiovasc Surg 1998;116(2):305.
66. Breitbart RE. Pericardial disease. In: Keane JF, Lock JE, Fyler DC, editors. Nada's pediatric cardiology, vol. 27, 2nd edition. Philadelphia: Saunders Elsevier; 2006. p. 459–66.
67. Markiewicz W, Brik A, Brook G, et al. Pericardial rub in pericardial effusion: lack of correlation with amount of fluid. Chest 1980;77:643.
68. Kudo Y, Yamasaki F, Doi Y, et al. Clinical correlates of PR-segment depression in asymptomatic patients with pericardial effusion. J Am Coll Cardiol 2002;39: 2000.
69. Baddour LM, Wilson WR, Bayer AS, et al. Infective endocarditis: diagnosis, antimicrobial therapy, and management of complications: a statement for healthcare professionals from the Committee on Rheumatic Fever, Endocarditis, and Kawasaki Disease, Council on Cardiovascular Disease in the Young, and the Councils on Clinical Cardiology, Stroke, and Cardiovascular Surgery and Anesthesia, American Heart Association: endorsed by the Infectious Diseases Society of America. Circulation 2005;111:e394–434.
70. Durack DT, Lukes AS, Bright DK. New criteria for diagnosis of infective endocarditis: utilization of specific echocardiographic findings. Am J Med 1904;96:200–9.
71. Horstkotte D, Follath F, Gottschalk E, et al. Guidelines on prevention, diagnosis and treatment of infective endocarditis executive summary. The Task Force on Infective Endocarditis of the European Society of Cardiology. Eur Heart J 2004;25:267–76.
72. Wilson W, Taubert KA, Gewitz M, et al. Prevention of infective endocarditis. Guidelines from the American Heart Association. Circulation 2007;116(15): 1736–54.
73. Burns JC, Kushner HI, Bastian JF, et al. Kawasaki disease: a brief history. Pediatrics 2000;106:e27.
74. Fujiwara H, Hamashima Y. Pathology of the heart in Kawasaki disease. Pediatrics 1978;61:100–7.

75. Tanaka N, Sekimoto K, Naoe S. Kawasaki disease: relationship with infantile periarteritis nodosa. Arch Pathol Lab Med 1976;100:81–6.
76. Kawasaki T, Kosaki F, Okawa S, et al. A new infantile acute febrile mucocutaneous lymph node syndrome (MLNS) prevailing in Japan. Pediatrics 1974;54: 271–6.
77. Newberger JW, Takahashi M, Gerber MA, et al. Diagnosis, treatment, and long-term management of Kawasaki disease. AHA Scientific Statement. Circulation 2004;110(17):2747–71.
78. Rowley A, Gonzalez-Crussi F, Gidding SS, et al. Incomplete Kawasaki disease with coronary artery involvement. J Pediatr 1985;110:409–13.
79. Genizi J, Miron D, Spiegel R, et al. Kawasaki disease in very young infants: high prevalence of atypical presentation and coronary arteritis. Clin Pediatr 2003; 42(3):263–7.
80. Tatara K, Kusakawa S. Long-term prognosis of giant coronary aneurysm in Kawasaki disease: an angiographic study. J Pediatr 1987;111:705–10.
81. Hsieh KD, Weng KP, Lin CC, et al. Treatment of acute Kawasaki disease: aspirin's role in the febrile stage revisited. Pediatrics 2004;114:e689–93.
82. Newburger JW, Takahashi M, Beiser AS, et al. A single intravenous infusion of gamma globulin as compared with four infusions in the treatment of acute Kawasaki syndrome. N Engl J Med 1991;324:1633–9.
83. Terai M, Shulman ST. Prevalence of coronary artery abnormalities in Kawasaki disease is highly dependent on gamma globulin dose but independent of salicylate dose. J Pediatr 1997;131:888–93.
84. Richardson P, McKenna W, Bristow M, et al. Report of the 1995 World Health Organization/International Society and Federation of Cardiology Task Force on the Definition and Classification of Cardiomyopathies. Circulation 1996;93: 841–2.
85. Maron BJ, Towbin JA, Thiene G, et al. Contemporary definitions and classification of the cardiomyopathies. An American Heart Association Scientific Statement from the Council on Clinical Cardiology, Heart Failure and Transplantation Committee; Quality of Care and Outcomes Research and Functional Genomics and Translational Biology Interdisciplinary Working Groups; and Council on Epidemiology and Prevention. Circulation 2006;113:1807–16.
86. Burch M, Blair E. The inheritance of hypertrophic cardiomyopathy. Pediatr Cardiol 1999;20(5):313–6.
87. Maron BJ, Shirani J, Poliac LC, et al. Sudden death in young competitive athletes: clinical, demographic, and pathological profiles. JAMA 1996;276: 199–204.
88. DeLuca M, Tak T. Hypertrophic cardiomyopathy. Tools for identifying risk and alleviating symptoms. Postgrad Med 2000;107(7):127–40.
89. Luu M, Stevenson WG, Stevenson LW, et al. Diverse mechanisms of unexpected cardiac arrest in advanced heart failure. Circulation 1989;80:1675–80.
90. Thiene G, Nava A, Corrado D, et al. Right ventricular cardiomyopathy and sudden death in young people. N Engl J Med 1988;318:129–33.

Childhood Asthma

A Guide for Pediatric Emergency Medicine Providers

Sarah Kline-Krammes, MD, Nirali H. Patel, MD*,
Shawn Robinson, MD

KEYWORDS

- Asthma • Pediatrics • Emergency department • Asthma exacerbation
- Treatment and management

KEY POINTS

- Although the prevalence of asthma has remained stable, the financial impact of asthma management on the healthcare system remains significant.
- Pediatric asthma scores may facilitate the assessment and management of asthma exacerbations in the emergency room setting.
- The mainstay of treatment for asthma exacerbations include short acting beta agonists, corticosteroids, and ipratropium bromide.
- Patient and family education remains a cornerstone in the prevention and management of future asthma exacerbations.

INTRODUCTION

Asthma is a chronic inflammatory disease of the airways. The immunohistopathologic features of asthma are those of inflammation, and include neutrophils, eosinophils, mast cell activation, and epithelial cell damage.[1] This inflammation causes airway obstruction that is at least partially reversible with medications.

PREVALENCE

Asthma prevalence in children increased steadily from 1980 to 1995, when it peaked at 7.5% (**Fig. 1**). Since 1997, asthma prevalence has remained stable.[2] It affects every state, although the midwest, northeast, and southeast are disproportionately more affected than other regions of the United States. In addition, asthma affects minorities at a higher rate: Hispanic people have the highest risk and are 2.4 times more likely to have asthma compared with the general pediatric population. African-Americans, Native Americans, and Native Aleutians are 1.6 and 1.3 times more likely to be affected

The authors have no financial relationship or conflicts of interest to disclose.
Department of Emergency Medicine, Akron Children's Hospital, 1 Perkins Square, Akron, OH 44308, USA
* Corresponding author.
E-mail address: npatel@chmca.org

Emerg Med Clin N Am 31 (2013) 705–732
http://dx.doi.org/10.1016/j.emc.2013.05.001
0733-8627/13/$ – see front matter © 2013 Elsevier Inc. All rights reserved.

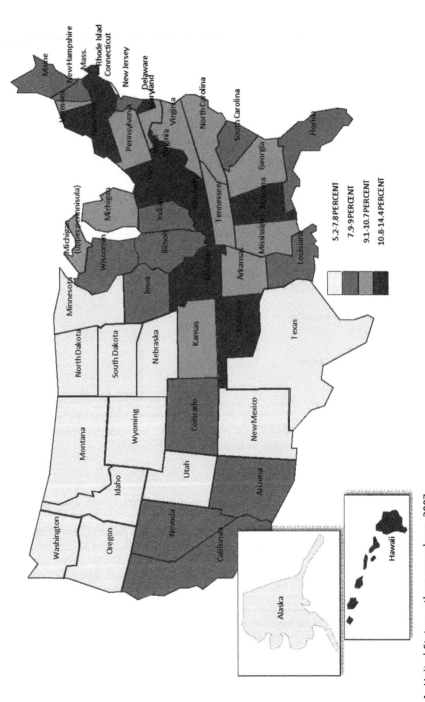

Fig. 1. United States: asthma prevalence 2007.

with asthma. In addition, African-American children are 4 times more likely to die from asthma.[3]

Several theories exist to explain this discrepancy in prevalence. Children are more vulnerable to the effects of air pollution because their immune systems are still maturing and because they have increased minute ventilation per square meter of total body surface area compared with adults.[4] As air pollution of ozone, nitrogen dioxide, sulfur dioxide, and carbon monoxide increases, the odds of developing wheezing in children also increases.[5,6] In addition, the tendency for minorities to reside in densely populated urban regions and have increased exposure to higher levels of air pollution may be a contributing factor for their increase in asthma prevalence.

BURDEN OF DISEASE

The total cost to society of asthma is estimated at $56 billion dollars per year as of 2007. This cost includes morbidity productivity losses of $3.8 billion dollars and mortality productivity losses of $2.1 billion dollars.[7] In pediatrics, the cost of treating asthma is also high, especially if the child requires intubation. Nearly 50% of all children who are intubated for status asthmaticus experience a complication (most commonly aspiration pneumonia, pneumothorax, and pneumomediastinum), and these complications translate to a hospital cost of $117,000 versus $38,000 for a visit with no complications.[8] Most striking is the yearly cost of treating asthma per child. In 2005, the cost per year of health care for a child without asthma was $618. The same yearly cost of health care for a child with asthma was more than 60% higher, costing more than $1000.[9] In addition, asthma is the leading cause of missed school days.[10] Even if a child is not seeking care in a hospital setting, asthma may still affect a child's ability to participate in school and the ability to sleep.[11]

PATHOPHYSIOLOGY

Many studies have documented the relationship of histamine and/or leukotriene release with the inhalation of cold air, leading to bronchoconstriction.[12] However, this does not account for the increased prevalence of asthma in the warmer regions of the southeast United States. A study in 2012 by Hayes and colleagues[13] showed that bronchoconstriction increased among patients with asthma who inhaled hot air versus room air (112% vs 38% respectively) and was mediated by cholinergic reflexes that improved with use of ipratropium, suggesting an underlying seasonal or viral trigger.

Allergic asthma is considered to have a large inflammatory component. Allergens induce a cascade of events leading to interleukin release, mast cell degranulation, mucus hypersecretion, and neutrophilic inflammation, which ultimately contribute to steroid-resistant, severe asthma.[14]

Certain polymorphisms causing structural changes have been associated with an accelerated decrease in lung function with asthma.[15] Xiao and colleagues[16] reported that the bronchial epithelial wall in asthmatics seemed to be damaged such that allergens passed through the epithelial wall, leading to immune activation and asthma exacerbation. Likewise, Lopez-Guisa and colleagues[17] found that interleukin (IL) 3 and IL4 stimulated the production of transforming growth factor B2 and periostin, both of which promote airway remodeling.

Environment may have a contributing role in the development of asthma. Although the prevalence of asthma is increased in areas with high air pollution, a study conducted by Omland and colleagues[18] found that being born and raised on a farm with high allergen exposures reduced the risk of asthma versus being raised in rural, nonfarm environments. They also noted that exposure to dairy confinements, welding smoke, and tobacco smoke were all risk factors for asthma development. They therefore concluded that high exposure to potential allergens early in life may be protective against future development of asthma.

HISTORY

A detailed medical history is an important tool in the assessment of a wheezing child. Many children present to the emergency department (ED) with a first-time episode of wheezing. Although this is a common symptom of asthma, most of these children do not go on to develop asthma. A thorough history is essential in determining causes other than asthma in a first-time wheezing patient. Questions include age of patient, onset of symptoms, and associated symptoms. Sudden onset in symptoms may indicate foreign body aspiration (more common in toddlers with associated choking, cyanosis) or anaphylaxis (with associated urticaria, stridor, and hypotension). Fever with cough or congestion may indicate bronchiolitis (<2 years with first-time wheezing) or lower airway tract infection. More chronic symptoms such as failure to thrive, difficulty feeding, persistent wheezing, or failure to respond to short-acting beta agonists (SABAs) should concern the medical provider for underlying gastroesophageal reflux, cardiac disease/failure, thoracic masses, or cystic fibrosis. Historical clues that help distinguish those that are more suggestive of asthma are included in **Box 1**.[19,20] Patients with a congenital cause for wheezing (vascular rings, cystic lung malformations) usually have a history of wheezing since birth without response to traditional asthma therapies like SABAs and corticosteroids.[21]

When a patient with a history of asthma presents with wheezing, certain historical data can help characterize the underlying severity of asthma. This classification of asthma is based on current symptoms, use of SABAs, and interference with daily activity **(Table 1)**.[1]

Common symptoms of an asthma exacerbation include cough, wheezing, and some degree of respiratory distress. Young children may manifest shortness of breath as decreased activity or vocalizations. To help determine the severity of the exacerbation, it is important to ascertain the current usage of SABAs; compliance with controller medications; and the delivery mode of the medications, including spacer use. Assessment of risk factors of near-fatal asthma is critical because this may change the management of the current exacerbation **(Box 2)**.[22]

Predictors of severe asthma exacerbation remain multifactorial. A study in 2011 noted that experiencing persistent symptoms from asthma was related to having severe exacerbations; receiving inhaled corticosteroids (ICSs) was protective against a severe exacerbation. However, some predictors of a severe exacerbation were independent of persistent symptoms. These factors included young age, history of ED visits or hospitalizations in the past year, and history of greater than or equal to

---

Box 1
History suggestive of asthma

More than 1 episode of wheezing per month

Triggers for wheezing (allergen, exercise, smoke, upper respiratory illness)

Previous bronchodilator use including response to therapy

Family history of asthma (especially in first-degree relative)

Atopy (allergic rhinitis, atopic dermatitis, or food allergy)

3 days of oral steroids in the prior 3 months. Thus, it is important to assess the underlying severity of disease as well as the risk of having a severe exacerbation.[23]

Recent studies have assessed the factors that may be associated with pediatric asthma-related ED visits. Previous studies indicated that age, race, insurance status, and average household income all played a role in predicting ED visits. However, a recent study showed that, after controlling for all variables, the only statistically significant predictor of a pediatric asthma-related ED visit was a previous asthma-related ED visit.[24]

PHYSICAL EXAMINATION

The physical examination of children with asthma brought to the ED begins with a rapid 30-second cardiopulmonary assessment as described by the American Heart Association.[25] This assessment helps with a quick determination of general appearance, airway patency, effectiveness of respiratory effort, and adequacy of circulation. Vitals signs are also helpful in assessment of severity of exacerbation. Children presenting with hypoxia (less than 92%) are more likely to require aggressive treatment and require hospital admission. Severe exacerbations cause tachypnea, tachycardia, and sometimes pulsus paradoxus. Accessory muscle usage is more likely to indicate a severe exacerbation. Severe retractions, especially supraclavicular retractions, indicate a forced expiratory volume less than 50% of predicted. Poor air movement found on chest auscultation is a sign of impending respiratory failure. Patients presenting with agitation or depressed mental status may be approaching respiratory failure.[21,22]

Wheezing is the most common symptom associated with asthma in children aged 5 years and younger. Cough caused by asthma may be recurrent and/or persistent and is usually accompanied by wheezing episodes and breathing difficulties. Shortness of breath that is recurrent or occurs during exercise increases the likelihood of asthma.[19] Cough-variant asthma can present as a dry harsh cough, usually worse at night; these patients often do not wheeze at all.

Physical examination findings can also help distinguish between other causes of cough and wheezing in children. Foreign body aspiration can present as unilateral wheezing. Wheezing secondary to a cardiac cause has hepatomegaly as an associated physical finding. Wheezing along with urticaria and uvular edema suggests anaphylaxis as the cause of wheezing. Wheezing along with signs of upper airway tract infection and fever indicates bronchiolitis.

ASTHMA SCORES

Pediatric asthma scores have been used to help classify severity of exacerbation. Most scores assess suprasternal retractions, air entry, and wheezing, and most also add respiratory rate and oxygen saturation. A study in 2008 showed that the Preschool Respiratory Assessment Measure (PRAM) was applicable to children between 2 and 17 years of age and was a feasible, reliable, valid, and responsive tool to measure asthma severity in a busy pediatric ED.[26] Another tool, the Pediatric Asthma Severity Score (PASS) is a valid, reliable tool to measure asthma in the acute setting in children aged 1 to 18 years in a pediatric ED. The PASS score is limited because it only assesses 3 clinical measures: wheezing, prolonged expiration, and work of breathing. The Pediatric Asthma Score (PAS) is another measurement tool that includes measures of respiratory rate, oxygen saturation, auscultatory findings, retractions, and dyspnea. Kelly and colleagues[27] in 2000 showed that the PAS showed good interobserver agreement and excellent face validity in the ED setting. The PAS allowed providers to have an objective understanding of the severity of each patient being cared

Table 1
Determination of asthma severity in children

	Classifying Asthma Severity and Initiating Therapy in Children							
	Intermittent		Persistent					
			Mild		Moderate		Severe	
Components of Severity	Ages 0–4 y	Ages 5–11 y	Ages 0–4 y	Ages 5–11 y	Ages 0–4 y	Ages 5–11 y	Ages 0–4 y	Ages 5–11 y
Impairment								
Symptoms	≤2 d/wk		>2 d/wk but not daily		Daily		Throughout the day	
Nighttime awakenings	0	≤2/mo	1–2/mo	3–4/mo	3–4/mo	>1/wk but not nightly	>1/wk	Often 7/wk
Short-acting beta-2 agonist use for symptom control	≤2 d/wk		>2 d/wk but not daily		Daily		Several times per day	
Interference with normal activity	None		Minor limitation		Some limitation		Extremely limited	
Lung Function	N/A	Normal FEV$_1$ between exacerbations	N/A	—	N/A	—	N/A	—
FEV$_1$ (predicted) or peak flow (personal best)		>80%		>80%		60%–80%		<60%
FEV$_1$/FVC		>85%		>80%		75%–80%		<75%

Risk	Exacerbations requiring oral systemic corticosteroids (consider severity and interval since last exacerbation)	0–1/y (see notes)	≥2 exacerbations in 6 mo requiring oral systemic corticosteroids, or ≥4 wheezing episodes in 1 y lasting >1 d and risk factors for persistent asthma	—	>2/y (see notes) Relative annual risk may be related to FEV_1	—	—

Notes:

Level of severity is determined by both impairment and risk. Assess impairment domain by caregiver's recall of previous 2 to 4 weeks. Assign severity to the most severe category in which any feature occurs.

Frequency and severity of exacerbations may fluctuate over time for patients in any severity category. There are currently inadequate data to correlate frequencies of exacerbations with different levels of asthma severity. In general, more frequent and severe exacerbations (eg, requiring urgent, unscheduled care; hospitalization; or ICU admission) indicate greater underlying disease severity. For treatment purposes, patients with 2 or more exacerbations described may be considered the same as patients who have persistent asthma, even in the absence of impairment levels consistent with persistent asthma.

Abbreviations: FEV_1, forced expiratory volume in 1 second; FVC, forced vital capacity; ICS, inhaled corticosteroids; ICU, intensive care unit; N/A, not applicable.

From National Heart, Lung, and Blood Institute. Expert panel report 3: guidelines for the diagnosis and management of asthma. US Department of Health and Human Services, National Institutes of Health, National Heart, Lung, and Blood Institute. 2007. NIH Publication Number 08-5486.

Box 2
Characteristics of near-fatal asthma

Characteristics of a near-fatal asthma exacerbation

Doubling of beta agonist usage or using 1 or more metered-dose inhaler canister per month

African-American race

Adolescents

Hospital admission within the past year for asthma

Intensive care unit admission for asthma

Multiple ED visits within the last year for asthma

Oxygen saturations less than 91%

Psychological or psychosocial problems

Difficulty perceiving symptoms of a severe exacerbation

---

for with an asthma exacerbation. This scoring system and corresponding clinical pathway resulted in a decreased length of stay, cost of hospitalization, and improved quality of care when used on the inpatient floors. In the same study, ED nurses preferred the PAS to peak flow measurements.

The PAS has been adapted for use in our institution including the ED, inpatient floors, pediatric intensive care unit (PICU), and transport settings (**Table 2**).

DIFFERENTIAL DIAGNOSIS

Asthma is the most common cause of chronic cough in children, although symptoms of cough, wheeze, and dyspnea can be the presenting symptoms for other diagnoses.

The differential diagnosis for first-time wheezing is broad and requires a thorough history and physical to make the appropriate diagnosis. Although the list can be extensive, it is important for the emergency medicine physician to initially consider and address life-threatening causes of wheezing as well as recognize causes that may need further evaluation. Partial airway obstruction from foreign body aspiration must be considered in toddlers with first-time wheezing that is of sudden onset, with a history of choking or gagging, and findings of unilateral wheezing. Although sudden in onset, anaphylaxis may have associated urticaria as well as a history of exposure to a possible allergen. Respiratory symptoms associated with first-time wheezing in infants may suggest bronchiolitis. History of inhalant use or exposure may indicate a chemical pneumonitis, whereas a history of hemoptysis may indicate pulmonary hemorrhage. Other life-threatening causes of first-time wheezing include cardiac disease and malformation, thoracic masses, or mediastinal masses. These patients often have a history of failure to thrive, feeding difficulties, and physical examination findings of murmur and hepatomegaly in cardiac failure. Wheezing secondary to structural anomalies may present with wheezing since birth, failure of improvement in symptoms following standard asthma treatment, and symptom severity that is associated with positional changes. Tracheomalacia or bronchomalacia caused by tracheal or main stem bronchi collapse manifests as cough and wheezing. In addition, symptoms caused by tracheomalacia improve with prone positioning and worsen with agitation or excitement because of increase in intrathoracic pressures. Right-sided aortic arch also causes mechanical compression of the airway resulting in wheezing.

Table 2 PAS and interpretation			
	1	2	3
Respiratory rate (breaths/minute)			
Age 1–3 y	≤34	35–39	≥40
Age 4–5 y	≤30	31–35	≥36
Age 6–12 y	≤26	27–31	≥31
>12 y	≤23	24–27	≥28
Oxygen requirement (%)	>95 on room air	90–95 on room air	<90 on room air or requiring any amount of O_2
Retractions	None or intercostal	Intercostal and substernal, or nasal flaring (infants)	Intercostal, substernal, and supraclavicular; or nasal flaring and head bobbing (infants)
Dyspnea 1–4 y	Normal feeding, vocalization, and play	Decreased appetite, coughing after play, hyperactivity	Stops eating or drinking, stops playing; or drowsy and confused and/or grunting
Dyspnea >5 y	Counts to ≥10 in 1 breath; or speaks in complete sentences	Counts to 4–6 in 1 breath; or speaks in partial sentences	Counts to ≤3 in 1 breath; or speaks in single words; or grunts
Auscultation	Normal breath sounds, end-expiratory wheezes	Expiratory wheezing	Inspiratory and expiratory wheezing to diminished breath sounds
Total PAS	Mild 5–7	Moderate 8–11	Severe 12–15

Courtesy of Akron Children's Hosptal, Akron, OH.

Gastroesophageal reflux in infants can present as wheezing that is exacerbated by feedings or infant positioning.

Patients who present with chronic cough or wheezing that does not improve with traditional asthma therapy also require a thoughtful differential diagnosis to ensure that the diagnosis is correct. Underlying congenital, immunologic, and infectious causes must be considered. Patients presenting with chronic cough along with multiple respiratory infections and symptoms of malabsorption should be evaluated for cystic fibrosis, primary ciliary dyskinesia, and cardiac disease. Chronic cough may be the presenting symptom of infectious causes such as pertussis or tuberculosis.

Parents often confuse other symptoms for wheezing. Patients with upper airway noises or stridor suggest a viral upper respiratory tract infection or croup as the cause. Vocal cord dysfunction is most common in adolescents and can be misdiagnosed as wheezing, although it is inspiratory stridor associated with chest or throat tightness. Habit cough may present as chronic cough not improving with traditional asthma therapy. Hyperventilation causes dyspnea that can be confused with asthma. Anxiety can also give the sensation of chest tightness resulting in a misdiagnosis of asthma.[28,29] **Box 3** summarizes important differential diagnoses to consider during the presentation of wheezing in the ED.

The distinguishing characteristic of asthma is the response to bronchodilator or corticosteroids when symptomatic. Knowledge of the natural history of asthma and

Box 3	
Differential diagnosis of wheezing	
Congenital	Cystic fibrosis
	Lobar emphysema
	Tracheobronchomalacia
	Tracheal or bronchial stenosis
	Tracheoesophageal fistula
	Vascular ring
	Alpha 1 antitrypsin deficiency
Allergic	Anaphylaxis
	Asthma
Acquired	Foreign body aspiration
	Bronchopulmonary dysplasia
	Mediastinal bronchial compression
	Recurrent aspiration
Infectious	Bronchiolitis
	Viral or bacterial pneumonia
Cardiac	Congestive heart failure
	Pulmonary edema

response to treatment can guide clinicians in determining when to consider alternative diagnoses. Diagnostic testing or chest imaging may be required to help exclude other causes of wheezing or cough.

DIAGNOSTIC EVALUATION

Few diagnostic tools exist that help determine the diagnosis of asthma in the ED setting. In children, asthma is a clinical diagnosis. Diagnostic studies are used to help exclude other causes of wheezing or cough, to help recognize atypical presentations of asthma, and evaluate those patients who do not respond as expected to traditional asthma therapy.

Pulse Oximetry

The clinical assessment of hypoxemia relies on many factors. Under optimal conditions, an arterial blood saturation of approximately 75% is needed before central cyanosis is clinically detectable. Oxygen saturation is a sensitive indicator of disease severity in conditions associated with ventilation/perfusion mismatch like asthma. Oxygen saturations can be used to assess severity of disease and response to treatment. Mild asthma exacerbations are associated with oxygen saturations greater than 95%. Oxygen saturations less than 92% 1 hour after treatment correlate with an increased need for hospitalization.[30] Therefore, pulse oximetry may be a useful tool during the management and disposition planning of an patient with asthma.

Chest Radiograph

For a child with known asthma who is responding as expected to traditional therapy, there is no evidence showing that chest radiographs change the management of asthma in children. Further, they are not helpful as a routine work-up of asthma in children in the ED.[31] Children with an acute asthma exacerbation often have abnormal chest radiographs including hyperinflation, atelectasis, peribronchial thickening, and increased extravascular fluid. These findings do not play a role in directing patient management or assessing severity of exacerbation. A study in 2000 analyzed the clinical predictors of focal infiltrate on chest radiograph. Grunting and pulse oximetry less than or equal to 93% was highly specific when diagnosing pneumonia in a wheezing infant and toddler. First-time wheezing, tachypnea, and fever were not associated with findings of infiltrate on chest radiograph.[32]

Chest radiographs can be used to help exclude other diagnoses of wheezing or cough, especially in patients with first-time wheezing. Acute-onset, unilateral wheezing suggests foreign body aspiration, and patients may show hyperinflation on chest radiographs. Chest radiographs may show a structural abnormality or mass in a patient with chronic wheezing that fails to respond to bronchodilator therapy. Chest radiograph in patients who present in extremis or with impending respiratory failure may help rule out complications from asthma such as pneumothorax or pneumomediastinum as well as other contributing causes for respiratory distress such as superimposed infection or cardiac disease. Although no clear guidelines exist, chest radiographs should be considered in the following instances: asymmetric wheezing, wheezing that fails to respond to bronchodilator therapy, or patients who present in extremis or with impending respiratory failure.

Peak Expiratory Flow Measurements

National guidelines for the treatment of asthma call for measures of peak expiratory flow rate as a valid and reproducible measure of airway obstruction and a guide for treatment plans. They are infrequently done in the ED setting and a 2004 study showed that only 64% of children eligible for peak flow measurements had it attempted in the ED. Most reports state that children less than 5 years old cannot reliably perform this maneuver, which is effort dependent and requires a significant degree of coordination. In the same study, less than half of the patients had a pre–peak flow and post–peak flow measurement obtained with bronchodilator treatment. Children with a more severe exacerbation as judged by asthma score or need for admission were less likely to be judged able to obtain a peak flow measurement.[33]

Peak flow measurements are predicted based on the patient's age, height, and gender. Patients who regularly perform peak flow measurements at home may know their personal best. Peak flow measurements correlate with the forced expiratory volume in 1 second (FEV_1), although there is more variability in peak flow measurements. A peak flow greater than 70% of expected is classified as a mild exacerbation. A peak flow between 40% and 70% is a moderate exacerbation, and less than 40% predicts a severe exacerbation. Both initial peak flow measurement and follow-up measures can help direct management and response to treatments. Patients with a peak flow less than 60% of predicted best after ED treatment are more likely to relapse in the outpatient setting. These measurements add to objective measures of severity of asthma exacerbation but are infrequently performed in the ED.[33]

MANAGEMENT

Children with acute exacerbations should be rapidly assessed and triaged to a location in the ED where observation and frequent reassessment can be performed by medical and nursing staff. Reassessment of patients after each round of treatment is the most important aspect in the management of acute asthma exacerbations.[20] Most children seen in the ED for asthma do not require hospital admission.[21] In 2004, 754,000 children in the United States visited the ED for asthma and approximately 198,000 required hospital admissions.[34] Regardless of disposition, the mainstay of asthma exacerbation treatment in the emergency room are SABAs, systemic corticosteroids, and ipratropium bromide. A summary of medication recommendations established by the National Heart, Lung, and Blood Institute (NHLBI) guidelines are shown in **Table 3**.

Table 3
Drug dosages in asthma exacerbation

Medication	Dosages		Comments
	Child Dose[a]	Adult Dose	
Inhaled SABAs			
Albuterol			
Nebulizer solution (0.63 mg/3 mL, 1.25 mg/3 mL, 2.5 mg/3 mL, 5.0 mg/mL)	0.15 mg/kg (minimum dose 2.5 mg) every 20 min for 3 doses then 0.15–0.3 mg/kg up to 10 mg every 1–4 h as needed, or 0.5 mg/kg/h by continuous nebulization	2.5–5 mg every 20 min for 3 doses, then 2.5–10 mg every 1–4 h as needed, or 10–15 mg/h continuously	Only selective beta-2 agonists are recommended. For optimal delivery, dilute aerosols to minimum of 3 mL at gas flow of 6–8 L/min. Use large-volume nebulizers for continuous administration. May mix with ipratropium nebulizer solution
MDI (90 μg/puff)	4–8 puffs every 20 min for 3 doses, then every 1–4 h inhalation maneuver as needed. Use VHC; add mask in children <4 y old	4–8 puffs every 20 min up to 4 h, then every 1–4 h as needed	In mild to moderate exacerbations, MDI plus VHC is as effective as nebulized therapy with appropriate administration technique and coaching by trained personnel
Bitolterol			
Nebulizer solution (2 mg/mL)	See albuterol dose; thought to be half as potent as albuterol on mg basis	See albuterol dose	Has not been studied in severe asthma exacerbations. Do not mix with other drugs
MDI (370 μg/puff)	See albuterol MDI dose	See albuterol MDI dose	Has not been studied in severe asthma exacerbations
Levalbuterol (R-Albuterol)			
Nebulizer solution (0.63 mg/3 mL, 1.25 mg/0.5 mL, 1.25 mg/3 mL)	0.075 mg/kg (minimum dose 1.25 mg) every 20 min for 3 doses, then 0.075–0.15 mg/kg up to 5 mg every 1–4 h as needed	1.25–2.5 mg every 20 min for 3 doses, then 1.25–5 mg every 1–4 h as needed	Levalbuterol administered in one-half the mg dose of albuterol provides comparable efficacy and safety. Has not been evaluated by continuous nebulization

MDI (45 μg/puff)	See albuterol MDI dose	See albuterol MDI dose	
Pirbuterol			
MDI (200 μg/puff)	See albuterol MDI dose; thought to be half as potent as albuterol on a mg basis	See albuterol MDI dose	Has not been studied in severe asthma exacerbations
Systemic (Injected) Beta-2 Agonists			
Epinephrine 1:1000 (1 mg/mL)	0.01 mg/kg up to 0.3–0.5 mg every 20 min for 3 doses sq	0.3–0.5 mg every 20 min for 3 doses sq	No proven advantage of systemic therapy compared with aerosol
Terbutaline (1 mg/mL)	0.01 mg/kg every 20 min for 3 doses then every 2–6 h as needed sq	0.25 mg every 20 min for 3 doses sq	No proven advantage of systemic therapy compared with aerosol
Anticholinergics			
Ipratropium Bromide			
Nebulizer solution (0.25 mg/mL)	0.25–0.5 mg every 20 min for 3 doses, then as needed	0.5 mg every 20 min for 3 doses then as needed	May mix in same nebulizer with albuterol. Should not be used as first-line therapy; should be added to SABA therapy for severe exacerbations. The addition of ipratropium has not been shown to provide further benefit once the patient is hospitalized
MDI (18 μg/puff)	4–8 puffs every 20 min as needed up to 3 h	8 puffs every 20 min as needed up to 3 h	Should use with VHC and face mask for children <4 y old. Studies have examined ipratropium bromide MDI for up to 3 h
Ipratropium with Albuterol			
Nebulizer solution (each 3-mL vial contains 0.5 mg ipratropium bromide and 2.5 mg albuterol)	1.5–3 mL every 20 min for 3 doses, then as needed	3 mL every 20 min for 3 doses, then as needed	May be used for up to 3 h in the initial management of severe exacerbations. The addition of ipratropium to albuterol has not been shown to provide further benefit once the patient is hospitalized

(continued on next page)

Table 3
(continued)

Medication	Dosages		Comments
	Child Dose[a]	Adult Dose	
MDI (each puff contains 18 µg ipratropium bromide and 90 µg of albuterol)	4–8 puffs every 20 min as needed up to 3 h	8 puffs every 20 min as needed up to 3 h	Should use with VHC and face mask for children <4 y old
Systemic Corticosteroids			
Prednisone Methylprednisolone Prednisolone	1–2 mg/kg in 2 divided doses (maximum 60 mg/d) until PEF is 70% of predicted or personal best	40–80 mg/d in 1 or 2 divided doses until PEF reaches 70% of predicted or personal best	For outpatient "burst," use 40–60 mg in single or 2 divided doses for total of 5–10 d in adults (children, 1–2 mg/kg/d maximum 60 mg/d for 3–10 d)

Notes:

There is no known advantage for higher doses of corticosteroids in severe asthma exacerbations, nor is there any advantage for intravenous administration compared with oral therapy provided gastrointestinal transit time or absorption is not impaired.

The total course of systemic corticosteroids for an asthma exacerbation requiring an ED visit or hospitalization may last from 3 to 10 days. For corticosteroid courses of less than 1 week, there is no need to taper the dose. For slightly longer courses (eg, up to 10 days), there probably is no need to taper, especially if patients are concurrently taking ICSs.

ICSs can be started at any point in the treatment of an asthma exacerbation.

Abbreviations: MDI, metered-dose inhaler; PEF, peak expiratory flow; sq, subcutaneous; VHC, valved holding chamber.

[a] Children ≤12 years of age.

From National Heart, Lung, and Blood Institute. Expert panel report 3: guidelines for the diagnosis and management of asthma. US Department of Health and Human Services, National Institutes of Health, National Heart, Lung, and Blood Institute. 2007. NIH Publication Number 08-5486.

OXYGEN

Children, and especially infants, are at risk for respiratory failure and develop hypoxemia more rapidly than adults. Therefore, monitoring of oxygen saturation is necessary.[1,20,35] NHLBI guidelines recommend oxygen administration to maintain saturations greater than 90% (greater than 95% in pregnant women and in patients who have coexistent heart disease). Sao_2 is to be monitored until a clear response to bronchodilator therapy has occurred.[1] Indiscriminate high-flow oxygen despite good saturations can lead to poorer outcomes.[20,36]

SABAS

SABA is the most effective treatment of relieving bronchospasm and reversing airway obstruction. The most commonly used SABA in the United States is the beta-2 selective drug albuterol.[37] Through its sympathomimetic effects, it exerts bronchodilating effects by relaxing airway smooth muscle and thus relieving bronchospasm. Secondary effects are enhancement of water output from bronchial mucous glands and improvement of mucociliary clearance.

Albuterol is available in 2 forms: albuterol or levalbuterol. Albuterol is a 50:50 mixture of R-enantiomers and S-enantiomers. The R-enantiomer is pharmacologically active and shows more potent binding to beta-2 receptors than the S-enantiomer. The S-enantiomer is pharmacologically inactive, has a longer elimination half-life, and may induce paradoxical bronchospasm, contributing to airway irritation.[20] Levalbuterol consists solely of the R-enantiomer and is thought to provide maximum bronchodilating benefits and to minimize adverse side effects, including tachycardia and hypokalemia.[20,38,39] Studies have shown mixed results, with some trials showing benefits in pulmonary function, reduction in hospital admission rate, and reduced side effects, whereas other studies have shown no difference.[20,39–45] Current guidelines do not recommend using one rather than the other.

Albuterol has 2 common mechanisms of delivery: a metered-dose inhaler (MDI) with a spacer or nebulized solution typically via small-volume constant output jet nebulizers (SVN). A newer mechanism of delivery is breath-actuated nebulizer treatments, which are nebulizers that initiate aerosol production with the onset of inhalation, limiting the loss of aerosol during exhalation. A randomized control study conducted in the ED found that a breath-actuated nebulizer improved clinical asthma score, decreased respiratory rate, and decreased hospital admissions, but did not significantly affect length of stay in the ED.[46] In mild to moderate asthma, an MDI with spacer has been shown to be at least equivalent, if not better, in efficacy to a nebulizer and is more cost-effective.[20,47–51] Factors that influence delivery mechanism include patient cooperation, response to treatment via MDI, severity of exacerbation, and local protocols.[20] Children less than 24 months old are thought to have a more difficult time with MDI and spacer. However, a double-blind, randomized, placebo-controlled clinical trial by Delgado and colleagues[52] showed that MDI with spacers may be as efficacious as nebulizers in the ED treatment of wheezing in children from 2 to 24 months of age. Another double-blind, randomized equivalence trial of MDI with spacer versus nebulizer treatment in children 12 to 60 months of age found that the efficacy of albuterol administered via MDI and spacer was equivalent to nebulizer.[53] The type of delivery system used may be determined by institution policy as well as provider preference and comfort.

Albuterol can be given as intermittent therapy every 20 minutes (up to 3 doses) or continuously for an hour depending on severity. Response to medication on reevaluation determines further frequency. Following reassessment, SABA can be administered by MDI and spacer, 2 to 4 puffs, continuous or spaced to hourly based on severity (**Fig. 2**) or asthma score. Albuterol administered via nebulizer can be given at 0.15 to 0.3 mg/kg with a minimum of 2.5 mg and a maximum of 5 mg. The volume of albuterol is then diluted with normal saline for a total of 5 mL fluid per nebulized mask.[20] With continuous nebulization, the recommended dose of albuterol is 0.5 mg/kg/h with the total hourly dose not to exceed 10 to 15 mg/h.[1,20] Approximately 2% to 10% of albuterol given by nebulized treatment

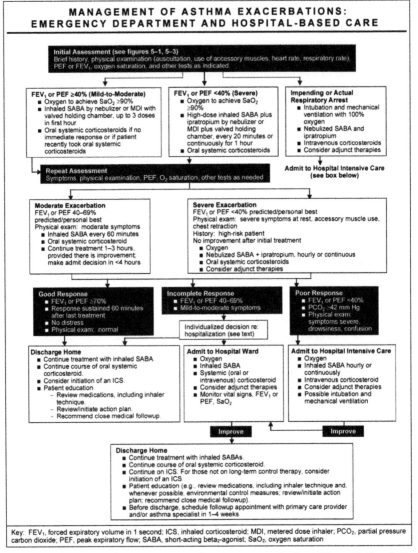

Fig. 2. ED evaluation and management of asthma exacerbation. (*From* National Heart, Lung, and Blood Institute. Expert panel report 3: guidelines for the diagnosis and management of asthma. US Department of Health and Human Services, National Institutes of Health, National Heart, Lung, and Blood Institute. 2007. NIH Publication Number 08-5486.)

reaches the lung. An MDI gives 90 μg/puff, but the delivery is considered to be more efficient.[37]

Side effects of albuterol are common, but minor in severity. Sinus tachycardia is the most common side effect, but rarely causes serious problems. Other cardiovascular-related effects include palpitations, hypertension, and, rarely, ventricular dysrhythmias. Central nervous system side effects are secondary to stimulation and include tremors, hyperactivity, and nausea with vomiting. Metabolic side effects include hypokalemia and hyperglycemia. Periodic serum potassium levels should be monitored with long-term continuous use of SABA treatment.

SYSTEMIC CORTICOSTEROIDS

The overriding physiologic derangement in asthma is airway inflammation and corticosteroids are among the mainstays of treatment. Glucocorticoids suppress cytokine production, granulocyte-macrophage colony-stimulating factor, and inducible nitric oxide synthase activation (all important components of the underlying inflammatory cells), decrease airway mucous production, and attenuate microvascular permeability.[21] The guidelines indicate use of steroid in asthma exacerbation when the patient does not completely respond to one inhaled beta agonist treatment, even if the patient is having a mild exacerbation.[1] Systemic corticosteroids have been shown to decrease the need for hospital admission as well as the length of stay.[20,54–56] A time series controlled trial on nurse initiation of oral systemic steroids in triage for moderate to severe asthma exacerbation in children 2 to 17 years of age showed earlier clinical improvement, decreased hospital admission rates, and earlier time to discharge in triage-administered steroids compared with systemic oral corticosteroid administration following physician assessment.[57]

Systemic corticosteroids may be given either orally or intravenously. Studies have showed that the effects of oral and intravenous (IV) steroids are equivalent.[37,58] Advantages of oral dosing include ease of administration and decreased cost. IV steroids are indicated when a patient cannot tolerate oral medication, is too ill to take oral medication, or has intestinal issues affecting absorption of medication.[1,20,35] Patients who vomit within 30 minutes of an oral dose should have dosing repeated.[37] Side effects of systemic corticosteroids are more prevalent in the critically ill child because of duration and dose of medication, and include hyperglycemia, hypertension, and occasionally agitation related to steroid-induced psychosis.

Systemic corticosteroids begin to exert their effect in 1 to 3 hours and reach maximal effect within 4 to 8 hours.[21] Oral prednisone or prednisolone is administered at a dose of 1 to 2 mg/kg once daily (maximum of 60 mg/d),[20,59,60] typically for 3 to 5 days. The total course of systemic corticosteroids for an asthma exacerbation requiring an ED visit of hospitalization may last longer. For corticosteroid courses of less than 1 week, there is no need to taper the dose. For slightly longer courses (eg, up to 10 days), there probably is no need to taper, especially if patients are concurrently taking ICSs.[1] IV steroids can be given as methylprednisolone, 2 mg/kg/d.[21] An alternative to prednisone is dexamethasone. Dexamethasone is well absorbed orally and has the same bioavailability as when given parenterally, with the action lasting up to 72 hours after a single dose.[61] Studies suggest that a 2-day course of oral dexamethasone at a dose of 0.6 mg/kg daily (maximum 16 mg) is as effective and well tolerated as a 5-day course of oral prednisone in adults and children.[20,62–64] In addition, Qureshi and colleagues[65] found that 2 doses of oral dexamethasone had fewer side effects with similar efficacy and better compliance compared with 5 doses of oral prednisone in children with acute asthma. High doses of ICS may be considered in conjunction with oral corticosteroids in the ED. The data on ICS use in children are inconsistent and may be a result of dosing inconsistency.[1,66] One trial reporting greater efficacy for oral corticosteroids used a single high dose of an ICS (2 mg fluticasone), whereas a trial giving multiple doses of budesonide (1.2 mg total) reported increased efficacy for the inhaled route.[67,68] Although the data are suggestive, a meta-analysis concluded that evidence was insufficient for firm conclusions.[69] ICSs in the ED management of acute asthma exacerbations are currently not recommended as a replacement for oral systemic corticosteroids because of lack of efficacy when used alone.[37,54,55,67,69–71]

IPRATROPIUM BROMIDE

Ipratropium bromide, an anticholinergic agent, is also used in the treatment of severe asthma exacerbation. Ipratropium promotes bronchodilation without inhibiting mucociliary clearance, as with atropine. It also acts as a parasympatholytic, antagonizing acetylcholine effects and ultimately impairing bronchial smooth muscle contraction.[21] Adding multiple high doses of ipratropium bromide (0.5 mg nebulizer solution or 8 puffs by MDI in adults; 0.25–0.5 mg nebulizer solution or 4–8 puffs by MDI in children) to a selective SABA produces additional bronchodilation, resulting in fewer hospital admissions, particularly in patients who have severe airflow obstruction.[1,72,73] It can be administered every 30 minutes for up to 3 doses. The most common adverse effects are dry mouth, bitter taste, flushing, tachycardia, and dizziness.[21] However, because of inability to cross membranes from the lung to the systemic circulation, there is no significant effect on the systemic system, including heart rate, even at high doses.[37,74]

IV FLUIDS

Children presenting with severe or life-threatening asthma exacerbation are often dehydrated secondary to poor oral intake as well as increased insensible losses from increased minute ventilation. Appropriate fluid resuscitation is necessary; however, care should be used in avoiding overhydration, which may place these children at risk for pulmonary edema secondary to microvascular permeability, increased left ventricular afterload, and alveolar fluid migration associated with the inflammatory lung process.[21] Oral routes of hydration are preferable except in exacerbations with the possibility of noninvasive ventilator support or endotracheal intubation.[1]

MAGNESIUM SULFATE

Magnesium sulfate is a bronchodilator that should be used in severe asthma. Magnesium sulfate acts through its role as a calcium channel blocker, ultimately inhibiting calcium-mediated smooth muscle contraction and facilitating bronchodilation.[21] Recommendations for use of IV magnesium sulfate include those whose FEV_1 fails to improve to more than 60% of predicted in 1 hour following therapy,[60] exacerbations that remain in the severe category after 1 hour of intensive conventional therapy, or life-threatening asthma.[1] It has shown improved clinical asthma scores with minimal side effects.[20,75,76] It is also inexpensive, easily administered intravenously, and well tolerated.[37] A randomized control study also showed that IV magnesium sulfate therapy within the first hour of hospitalization in children aged 2 to 15 years classified as acute severe asthma had a reduced requirement for mechanical ventilation support and had a statistically significant shorter PICU and hospital stay.[77] However, not all individual studies have found positive results.[1,78–80] The treatment has no apparent value in patients who have exacerbations of lesser severity, and one study found that IV magnesium sulfate improved pulmonary function only in patients whose initial FEV_1 was less than 25% predicted, and the treatment did not improve hospital admission rates.[81] If administered, a single IV dose of 25 to 75 mg/kg (maximum of 2 g) magnesium sulfate can be given over 20 to 30 minutes.[1,20,35]

Nebulized magnesium is also available. A recent meta-analysis of 6 trials suggests that the use of nebulized magnesium sulfate in combination with SABA may result in further improvements in pulmonary function. A Cochrane Review found that 1 study from 3 trials suggested possible improvement in pulmonary function in those with severe exacerbations (FEV_1 <50% predicted). However, heterogeneity among the trials precluded definite conclusions. In addition, there is currently no good evidence that inhaled $MgSO_4$ can be used as a substitute for inhaled SABA. When used in addition to inhaled SABA (with or without inhaled ipratropium), there is currently no overall clear evidence of improved pulmonary function or reduced hospital admissions.[82] Inhaled magnesium sulfate may be used as a diluent in place of normal saline (usually 2.5 mL of a 250 mmol/L solution) combined with albuterol and ipratropium bromide in the same mask.[20,82] Magnesium levels do not need to be monitored if a 1 time dose is given, but may be followed if repeated doses are considered.[37] Side effects include hypotension, central nervous system depression, muscle weakness, and flushing. More serious side effects include cardiac arrhythmias, including complete heart block, respiratory failure caused by severe muscle weakness, and sudden cardiopulmonary arrest, but these are usually in the setting of very high serum magnesium levels.[21]

IV BETA AGONIST

IV and subcutaneous administration of beta agonists in the management of acute severe asthma are controversial. It has been postulated that children presenting with acute severe asthma exacerbation do not optimally benefit from inhaled SABA therapy because of the inability of the medication to penetrate constricted airways.[83] Systemic administration of a beta agonist may help dilate obstructed airways and improve the efficacy of inhaled beta agonist in severe asthma exacerbations. A double-blind, randomized controlled study in Australia showed more rapid improvement in patients who received a single bolus of IV albuterol in addition to nebulized albuterol than in those who received nebulized albuterol alone.[37,84]

IV terbutaline, a selective beta-2 agonist, is available in the United States for IV or subcutaneous administration. It may be used in children with no IV access as an adjunct to inhaled SABA. Subcutaneous dosing is 0.01 mg/kg/dose with a maximum dose of 0.3 mg. This dose may be repeated every 15 to 20 minutes for up to 3 doses. IV terbutaline is started with a loading dose of 10 µg/kg over 10 min followed by continuous infusion at 0.1 to 10 µg/kg/min. The side effects include a risk of myocardial ischemia caused by selective beta agonist activity. Between 10% and 50% of asthmatics can have increased troponin I levels during terbutaline therapy. However, data are limited and monitoring cardiac-specific enzymes (creatine phosphokinase or troponin) may be of value in children who receive more than 1 dose of terbutaline.[21]

Nonselective beta agonists such as ephedrine, epinephrine, and isoproterenol are rarely used because of their high side effect profile and availability of more selective IV or subcutaneous agents.[21] The NHLBI guidelines do not recommend use of IV isoproterenol in the treatment of asthma because of the danger of myocardial toxicity.[85]

At present, the NHLBI guidelines do not consider systemic beta agonist therapy to have advantage compared with inhaled SABA.[1] A meta-analysis addressing this issue concluded that there was no evidence supporting the use of IV beta agonists compared with aerosol administration in the treatment of acute severe asthma.[86] Data are also sparse on the benefit of adding an IV beta-2 agonist to high-dose nebulized therapy.[84] Systemic beta-2 agonists should be only considered in patients with life-threatening asthma exacerbations who have failed to respond to maximal inhaled therapy and systemic corticosteroids.[37]

LEUKOTRIENE RECEPTOR ANTAGONISTS

Leukotriene receptor antagonists (LTRAs) (montelukast, zafirlukast) have been shown to decrease symptoms of mild to moderate asthma exacerbations.[20] Leukotriene pathways are activated in acute asthma, as shown in increases of urinary leukotriene excretion.[87–89] LTRAs block the production of these natural mediators that are involved in bronchoconstriction.[37] LTRAs are considered to have potential additive benefit in combination with inhaled SABA and corticosteroids. There is some evidence in the adult literature that IV administration may be effective in acute, severe asthma[20,87] and this may be another route of rapid bronchodilation in life-threatening asthma.[1] A randomized, double-blind, parallel-group pilot study of IV montelukast versus placebo in adults with moderate to severe asthma exacerbation showed significant improvement in FEV_1 within 10 minutes of administration of montelukast. There was also a trend toward reduction of inhaled beta agonist use compared with the placebo.[87] Although its role in acute asthma is now being explored, there are insufficient data to recommend it as a possible adjunct treatment.[1]

HELIOX

Heliox, a blend of helium and oxygen (80% helium/20% oxygen), is less dense than air and improves air flow resistance in small airways by reducing turbulent flow and enhancing laminar gas flow,[90] increasing carbon dioxide elimination, increasing expiratory flow, decreasing work of breathing, and enhancing particle deposition of aerosolized medication in distal lung segments.[91–93] However, hypoxemia is one of the limits of this therapy.[37] A Cochrane Review concluded that existing evidence did not support the therapeutic use of heliox-driven albuterol in all patients presenting to the ED with status asthmaticus. However, the review only included 3 pediatric trials with a total of 82 patients.[94] Of these, a prospective, randomized controlled, single-blind study conducted by Kim and colleagues[95] in children 2 to 18 years of age with moderate to severe asthma showed that continuously nebulized albuterol delivery by heliox early in the course of care was associated with a greater degree of clinical improvement than delivery by oxygen. There was also a statistically significant difference in discharge rates at the 12-hour treatment point between the two groups. However, there was no statistically significant difference in ED discharge or PICU admission rates. Other pediatric studies have shown that there was no clinical benefit compared with standard therapy in the initial treatment of moderate to severe asthma in the ED,[91] nor was there decreased length of hospital stay or time to clinical improvement.[90] At this time, heliox is to be considered in patients with life-threatening asthma or those who are considered to have severe asthma after 1 hour of conventional therapy.[1]

NONINVASIVE MECHANICAL VENTILATION

Mortality in mechanically ventilated children with life-threatening asthma is increased compared with children who do not need mechanical ventilation. Noninvasive positive pressure ventilation (NIPPV) is an alternative to conventional mechanical ventilation and is used in 3% to 5% of critically ill asthmatic children.[21] NIPPV is considered to be a temporizing measure that may help avoid intubation and improve outcomes in children with status asthmaticus.[20,96–100] A Cochrane Review highlighted one trial that showed the benefit of NIPPV in hospitalization rates, number of patients discharged, FEV_1, forced vital capacity, and respiratory rates compared with medical therapy alone. However, they still concluded that data were insufficient and that NIPPV was still controversial therapy in severe asthma.[101] More recently, multiple pediatric trials have shown NIPPV to be well tolerated, safe, and to have minimal complications in pediatric patients.[97,102,103] A recent study also showed that bilevel positive airway pressure ventilation, a form of NIPPV, was well tolerated in pediatric patients weighing less than 20 kg with no major complications, including death or pneumothorax.[104] NIPPV in the pediatric patient does require pediatric specific equipment (mask, ventilator), and pediatric respiratory therapists who can monitor the circuit.[104] If NIPPV is available, a trial may be warranted before the institution of conventional mechanical ventilation.

INTUBATION

Tracheal intubation in the management of asthma exacerbation is absolutely indicated for patients who present with apnea or coma.[1] However, intubation should be strongly considered for the following conditions: refractory hypoxemia, significant respiratory acidosis unresponsive to pharmacotherapy,[21] worsening mental status,[37] and exhaustion.[1] Ventilation goals should include maintaining adequate oxygenation, allowing for permissive hypercarbia (moderate respiratory acidosis), and minute ventilation adjustment (peak pressure, tidal volume, and rate) to maintain an arterial pH of 7.2. Strategies should attempt to minimize hyperinflation and air trapping, which can be accomplished by using slow ventilator rates with prolonged expiratory phase, minimal end-expiratory pressure, and short inspiratory time. In addition, adjustment to ventilator rate, inspiratory and expiratory time, or positive end-expiratory pressure can be made to facilitate full expiration between breaths.[21]

DISPOSITION

Adequate evaluation of the severity of asthma exacerbation is important for the initial management of patients, as well as for assessing the clinical response[105] and subsequent disposition. Clinicians often have varying degrees of experience in determining the severity of an asthma exacerbation. More objective tools such as peak flow and spirometry require trained personnel as well as a patient who has adequate coordination and comprehension.[105] This requirement makes such tools more difficult to use in the pediatric population, especially in infants and toddlers. To standardize asthma management in the ED, the PAS score has been used. The authors' institution's PAS-based management is shown in **Fig. 3** for reference.

No single measure is best for assessing severity or predicting hospital admission. Lung function measures (FEV_1 or peak expiratory flow) may be useful for children 5 years of age, but these measures may not be obtainable during an exacerbation. Pulse oximetry may be useful for assessing the initial severity; a repeated measure of pulse oximetry of less than 92% to 94% after 1 hour predicts the need for hospitalization. Children who have signs and symptoms after 1 to 2 hours of initial treatment and who continue to meet the criteria for a moderate or severe exacerbation have greater than an 84% chance of requiring hospitalization.[1] If patients are being discharged, a written asthma action plan should be considered. Most guidelines

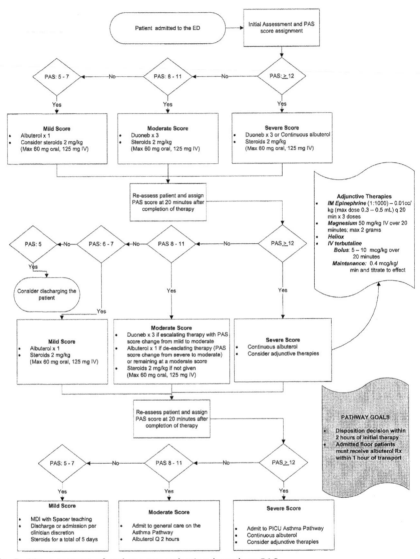

Fig. 3. Management of asthma exacerbation based on PAS.

recommend the provision of a written discharge plan with instructions for medication and follow-up.[1,26,60,106] Although there are limited data to firmly conclude that provision of an action plan is superior to none, there is clear evidence suggesting that symptom-based plans are superior to peak flow–based plans in children and adolescents.[107] Use of written action plans significantly reduced acute care visits per child compared with control subjects. Children using plans also missed less school, had less nocturnal awakening, and had improved symptom scores.

Patients who have severe exacerbations and are slow to respond to therapy may benefit from admission to an intensive care unit (ICU), where they can be monitored closely and intubated if indicated.[1,21]

SUMMARY

Pediatric asthma plays a significant role in health care costs as well as quality of life. Early treatment of asthma exacerbation is the best strategy for management and includes patient education, an asthma action plan, early recognition of worsening symptoms, and intensification of treatment. Despite this, asthma exacerbations may require urgent medical attention. In these cases, beta agonists, systemic corticosteroids, and ipratropium bromide remain the cornerstones of treatment. With life-threatening asthma, various adjunct therapy including IV magnesium, IV beta agonists, heliox, and NIPPV may be considered. Although morbidity secondary to asthma is significant, overall mortality remains low.

REFERENCES

1. National Heart, Lung, and Blood Institute. Expert panel report 3: guidelines for the diagnosis and management of asthma. Washington, DC: US Department of Health and Human Services, National Institutes of Health, National Heart, Lung, and Blood Institute; 2007. NIH Publication Number 08-5486.
2. Akinbami LJ, Moorman JE, Garbe PL, et al. Status of childhood asthma in the United States, 1980-2007. Pediatrics 2009;123(Suppl 3):S131–45.
3. Mayrides M, Levy R. Ethnic disparities in the burden and treatment of asthma. Reston (VA): Allergy and Asthma Foundation of America and the National Pharmaceutical Council; 2005.
4. Moya J, Bearer CF, Etzel RA. Children's behavior and physiology and how it affects exposure to environmental contaminants. Pediatrics 2004;113(Suppl 4):996–1006.
5. Kim BJ, Kwon JW, Seo JH, et al. Association of ozone exposure with asthma, allergic rhinitis, and allergic sensitization. Ann Allergy Asthma Immunol 2011; 107(3):214–9.e1.
6. McConnell R, Berhane K, Gilliland F, et al. Asthma in exercising children exposed to ozone: a cohort study. Lancet 2002;359(9304):386–91.
7. Barnett SB, Nurmagambetov TA. Costs of asthma in the United States: 2002–2007. J Allergy Clin Immunol 2011;127(1):145–52.
8. Carroll CL, Zucker AR. The increased cost of complications in children with status asthmaticus. Pediatr Pulmonol 2007;42(10):914–9.
9. Wang LY, Zhong Y, Wheeler L. Direct and indirect costs of asthma in school-age children. Prev Chronic Dis 2005;2(1):A11.
10. Asthma's impact on children and adolescents. Atlanta (GA): National Center for Environmental Health Centers for Disease Control and Prevention; 2005.
11. Merkle SL, Wheeler LS, Gerald LB, et al. Introduction: learning from each other about managing asthma in schools. J Sch Health 2006;76(6):202–4.
12. Anderson SD, Daviskas E. The mechanism of exercise-induced asthma is…. J Allergy Clin Immunol 2000;106(3):453–9.
13. Hayes D Jr, Collins PB, Khosravi M, et al. Bronchoconstriction triggered by breathing hot humid air in patients with asthma: role of cholinergic reflex. Am J Respir Crit Care Med 2012;185(11):1190–6.
14. Levine SJ, Wenzel SE. Narrative review: the role of Th2 immune pathway modulation in the treatment of severe asthma and its phenotypes. Ann Intern Med 2010;152(4):232–7.
15. Koppelman GH, Sayers I. Evidence of a genetic contribution to lung function decline in asthma. J Allergy Clin Immunol 2011;128(3):479–84.
16. Xiao C, Puddicombe SM, Field S, et al. Defective epithelial barrier function in asthma. J Allergy Clin Immunol 2011;128(3):549–56.e1–12.

17. Lopez-Guisa JM, Powers C, File D, et al. Airway epithelial cells from asthmatic children differentially express proremodeling factors. J Allergy Clin Immunol 2012;129(4):990–7.e6.

18. Omland O, Hjort C, Pedersen OF, et al. New-onset asthma and the effect of environment and occupation among farming and nonfarming rural subjects. J Allergy Clin Immunol 2011;128(4):761–5.

19. Pedersen SE, Hurd SS, Lemanske RF, et al. Global strategy for the diagnosis and management of asthma in children 5 years and younger. Pediatr Pulmonol 2011;46(1):1–17.

20. Choi J, Lee GL. Common pediatric respiratory emergencies. Emerg Med Clin North Am 2012;30(2):529–63, x.

21. Bigham M. Status asthmacticus. In: Rogers M, Nichols D, editors. Textbook of pediatric intensive care. 4th edition. Philadelphia: Williams & Wilkins; 2012.

22. Partridge R, Abramo T. Acute asthma in the pediatric emergency department. Pediatric Emergency Medicine Practice. Available at: ebmedicine.net. 2008. Accessed October 22, 2012.

23. Wu AC, Tantisira K, Li L, et al. Predictors of symptoms are different from predictors of severe exacerbations from asthma in children. Chest 2011;140(1):100–7.

24. Tolomeo C, Savrin C, Heinzer M, et al. Predictors of asthma-related pediatric emergency department visits and hospitalizations. J Asthma 2009;46(8):829–34.

25. Chameides L, editor. Pediatric Advanced Life Support Manual. Dallas (TX): American Heart Association; 2011.

26. Ducharme FM, Chalut D, Plotnick L, et al. The pediatric respiratory assessment measure: a valid clinical score for assessing acute asthma severity from toddlers to teenagers. J Pediatr 2008;152(4):476–80, 480.e1.

27. Kelly CS, Andersen CL, Pestian JP, et al. Improved outcomes for hospitalized asthmatic children using a clinical pathway. Ann Allergy Asthma Immunol 2000;84(5):509–16.

28. Slaughter MC. Not quite asthma: differential diagnosis of dyspnea, cough, and wheezing. Allergy Asthma Proc 2007;28(3):271–81.

29. Weinberger M, Abu-Hasan M. Pseudo-asthma: when cough, wheezing, and dyspnea are not asthma. Pediatrics 2007;120(4):855–64.

30. Fouzas S, Priftis KN, Anthracopoulos MB. Pulse oximetry in pediatric practice. Pediatrics 2011;128(4):740–52.

31. Hederos CA, Janson S, Andersson H, et al. Chest X-ray investigation in newly discovered asthma. Pediatr Allergy Immunol 2004;15(2):163–5.

32. Mahabee-Gittens EM, Dowd MD, Beck JA, et al. Clinical factors associated with focal infiltrates in wheezing infants and toddlers. Clin Pediatr (Phila) 2000;39(7):387–93.

33. Gorelick MH, Stevens MW, Schultz T, et al. Difficulty in obtaining peak expiratory flow measurements in children with acute asthma. Pediatr Emerg Care 2004;20(1):22–6.

34. Akinbami L. Asthma prevalence, health care use and mortality 2003-2005. Available at: http://www.cdc.gov/nchs/data/hestat/asthma03-05/asthma03-05.htm. Accessed October 22, 2012.

35. British Thoracic Society Scottish Intercollegiate Guidelines Network. British guideline on the management of asthma. Thorax 2008;63(Suppl 4):iv1–121.

36. Rodrigo GJ, Rodriquez Verde M, Peregalli V, et al. Effects of short-term 28% and 100% oxygen on $PaCO_2$ and peak expiratory flow rate in acute asthma: a randomized trial. Chest 2003;124(4):1312–7.

37. Baren JM, Zorc JJ. Contemporary approach to the emergency department management of pediatric asthma. Emerg Med Clin North Am 2002;20:115–38.
38. Asmus MJ, Hendeles L. Levalbuterol nebulizer solution: is it worth five times the cost of albuterol? Pharmacotherapy 2000;20(2):123–9.
39. Milgrom H, Skoner DP, Bensch G, et al. Low-dose levalbuterol in children with asthma: safety and efficacy in comparison with placebo and racemic albuterol. J Allergy Clin Immunol 2001;108(6):938–45.
40. Nelson HS, Bensch G, Pleskow WW, et al. Improved bronchodilation with levalbuterol compared with racemic albuterol in patients with asthma. J Allergy Clin Immunol 1998;102(6 Pt 1):943–52.
41. Gawchik SM, Saccar CL, Noonan M, et al. The safety and efficacy of nebulized levalbuterol compared with racemic albuterol and placebo in the treatment of asthma in pediatric patients. J Allergy Clin Immunol 1999;103(4):615–21.
42. Carl JC, Myers TR, Kirchner HL, et al. Comparison of racemic albuterol and levalbuterol for treatment of acute asthma. J Pediatr 2003;143(6):731–6.
43. Tripp K, McVicar WK, Nair P, et al. A cumulative dose study of levalbuterol and racemic albuterol administered by hydrofluoroalkane-134a metered-dose inhaler in asthmatic subjects. J Allergy Clin Immunol 2008;122(3):544–9.
44. Lam S, Chen J. Changes in heart rate associated with nebulized racemic albuterol and levalbuterol in intensive care patients. Am J Health Syst Pharm 2003; 60(19):1971–5.
45. Wilkinson M, Bulloch B, Garcia-Filion P, et al. Efficacy of racemic albuterol versus levalbuterol used as a continuous nebulization for the treatment of acute asthma exacerbations: a randomized, double-blind, clinical trial. J Asthma 2011;48(2):188–93.
46. Sabato K, Ward P, Hawk W, et al. Randomized controlled trial of a breath-actuated nebulizer in pediatric asthma patients in the emergency department. Respir Care 2011;56(6):761–70.
47. Cates CJ, Crilly JA, Rowe BH. Holding chambers (spacers) versus nebulisers for beta-agonist treatment of acute asthma. Cochrane Database Syst Rev 2006;(2):CD000052.
48. Closa RM, Ceballos JM, Gómez-Papí A, et al. Efficacy of bronchodilators administered by nebulizers versus spacer devices in infants with acute wheezing. Pediatr Pulmonol 1998;26(5):344–8.
49. Wildhaber JH, Devadason SG, Hayden MJ, et al. Aerosol delivery to wheezy infants: a comparison between a nebulizer and two small volume spacers. Pediatr Pulmonol 1997;23(3):212–6.
50. Rubilar L, Castro-Rodriguez JA, Girardi G. Randomized trial of salbutamol via metered-dose inhaler with spacer versus nebulizer for acute wheezing in children less than 2 years of age. Pediatr Pulmonol 2000;29(4):264–9.
51. Doan Q, Shefrin A, Johnson D. Cost-effectiveness of metered-dose inhalers for asthma exacerbations in the pediatric emergency department. Pediatrics 2011; 127(5):e1105–11.
52. Delgado A, Chou KJ, Silver EJ, et al. Nebulizers vs metered-dose inhalers with spacers for bronchodilator therapy to treat wheezing in children aged 2 to 24 months in a pediatric emergency department. Arch Pediatr Adolesc Med 2003;157(1):76–80.
53. Ploin D, Chapuis FR, Stamm D, et al. High-dose albuterol by metered-dose inhaler plus a spacer device versus nebulization in preschool children with recurrent wheezing: a double-blind, randomized equivalence trial. Pediatrics 2000;106(2 Pt 1):311–7.

54. Row B, Edmonds M, Spooner C, et al. Corticosteroid therapy for acute asthma. Respir Med 2004;43(5):321–31.
55. Fiel SB, Vincken W. Systemic corticosteroid therapy for acute asthma exacerbations. J Asthma 2006;43(5):321–31.
56. Smith M, Iqbal S, Elliott TM, et al. Corticosteroids for hospitalised children with acute asthma. Cochrane Database Syst Rev 2003;(2):CD002886.
57. Zemek R, Plint A, Osmond MH, et al. Triage nurse initiation of corticosteroids in pediatric asthma is associated with improved emergency department efficiency. Pediatrics 2012;129(4):671–80.
58. Rowe BH, Keller JL, Oxman AD. Effectiveness of steroid therapy in acute exacerbations of asthma: a meta-analysis. Am J Emerg Med 1992;10(4):301–10.
59. American Lung Association EaSU. Trends in asthma morbidity and mortality. Available at: http://www.lung.org/finding-cures/our-research/trend-reports/asthma-trend-report.pdf. Accessed October 22, 2012.
60. Global Initiative for Asthma. Global strategy for asthma management and prevention. Bethesda (MD): Global Initiative for Asthma; 2010.
61. Derendorf H, Hochhaus G, Möllmann H, et al. Receptor-based pharmacokinetic-pharmacodynamic analysis of corticosteroids. J Clin Pharmacol 1993;33(2):115–23.
62. Kravitz J, Dominici P, Ufberg J, et al. Two days of dexamethasone versus 5 days of prednisone in the treatment of acute asthma: a randomized controlled trial. Ann Emerg Med 2011;58(2):200–4.
63. Greenberg RA, Kerby G, Roosevelt GE. A comparison of oral dexamethasone with oral prednisone in pediatric asthma exacerbations treated in the emergency department. Clin Pediatr (Phila) 2008;47(8):817–23.
64. Shefrin AE, Goldman RD. Use of dexamethasone and prednisone in acute asthma exacerbations in pediatric patients. Can Fam Physician 2009;55(7):704–6.
65. Qureshi F, Zaritsky A, Poirier MP. Comparative efficacy of oral dexamethasone versus oral prednisone in acute pediatric asthma. J Pediatr 2001;139(1):20–6.
66. Rowe BH, Bota GW, Fabris L, et al. Inhaled budesonide in addition to oral corticosteroids to prevent asthma relapse following discharge from the emergency department: a randomized controlled trial. JAMA 1999;281(22):2119–26.
67. Schuh S, Reisman J, Alshehri M, et al. A comparison of inhaled fluticasone and oral prednisone for children with severe acute asthma. N Engl J Med 2000;343(10):689–94.
68. Singhi S, Banerjee S, Nanjundaswamy H. Inhaled budesonide in acute asthma. J Paediatr Child Health 1999;35(5):483–7.
69. Edmonds ML, Camargo CA, Pollack CV, et al. Early use of inhaled corticosteroids in the emergency department treatment of acute asthma. Cochrane Database Syst Rev 2003;(3):CD002308.
70. FitzGerald JM, Becker A, Sears MR, et al. Doubling the dose of budesonide versus maintenance treatment in asthma exacerbations. Thorax 2004;59(7):550–6.
71. Schuh S, Dick PT, Stephens D, et al. High-dose inhaled fluticasone does not replace oral prednisolone in children with mild to moderate acute asthma. Pediatrics 2006;118(2):644–50.
72. Rodrigo GJ, Castro-Rodriguez JA. Anticholinergics in the treatment of children and adults with acute asthma: a systematic review with meta-analysis. Thorax 2005;60(9):740–6.

73. Plotnick LH, Ducharme FM. Combined inhaled anticholinergics and beta2-agonists for initial treatment of acute asthma in children. Cochrane Database Syst Rev 2000;(4):CD000060.
74. Anderson W. Hemodynamic and nonbronchial effects of ipratropium bromide. Am J Med 1986;81:45–52.
75. Rowe BH, Bretzlaff JA, Bourdon C, et al. Intravenous magnesium sulfate treatment for acute asthma in the emergency department: a systematic review of the literature. Ann Emerg Med 2000;36(3):181–90.
76. Rowe BH, Bretzlaff JA, Bourdon C, et al. Magnesium sulfate for treating exacerbations of acute asthma in the emergency department. Cochrane Database Syst Rev 2000;(2):CD001490.
77. Torres S, Sticco N, Bosch JJ, et al. Effectiveness of magnesium sulfate as initial treatment of acute severe asthma in children, conducted in a tertiary-level university hospital: a randomized, controlled trial. Arch Argent Pediatr 2012; 110(4):291–6.
78. Boonyavorakul C, Thakkinstian A, Charoenpan P. Intravenous magnesium sulfate in acute severe asthma. Respirology 2000;5(3):221–5.
79. Porter RS, Nester BA, Braitman LE, et al. Intravenous magnesium is ineffective in adult asthma, a randomized trial. Eur J Emerg Med 2001;8(1):9–15.
80. Scarfone RJ, Loiselle JM, Joffe MD, et al. A randomized trial of magnesium in the emergency department treatment of children with asthma. Ann Emerg Med 2000;36(6):572–8.
81. Silverman RA, Osborn H, Runge J, et al. IV magnesium sulfate in the treatment of acute severe asthma: a multicenter randomized controlled trial. Chest 2002; 122(2):489–97.
82. Blitz M, Blitz S, Hughes R, et al. Aerosolized magnesium sulfate for acute asthma: a systematic review. Chest 2005;128(1):337–44.
83. Bogie AL, Towne D, Luckett PM, et al. Comparison of intravenous terbutaline versus normal saline in pediatric patients on continuous high-dose nebulized albuterol for status asthmaticus. Pediatr Emerg Care 2007;23(6):355–61.
84. Browne GJ, Penna AS, Phung X, et al. Randomised trial of intravenous salbutamol in early management of acute severe asthma in children. Lancet 1997; 349(9048):301–5.
85. Maguire JF, O'Rourke PP, Colan SD, et al. Cardiotoxicity during treatment of severe childhood asthma. Pediatrics 1991;88(6):1180–6.
86. Travers A, Jones AP, Kelly K, et al. Intravenous beta2-agonists for acute asthma in the emergency department. Cochrane Database Syst Rev 2001;(2):CD002988.
87. Camargo CA, Smithline HA, Malice MP, et al. A randomized controlled trial of intravenous montelukast in acute asthma. Am J Respir Crit Care Med 2003; 167(4):528–33.
88. Drazen JM, O'Brien J, Sparrow D, et al. Recovery of leukotriene E4 from the urine of patients with airway obstruction. Am Rev Respir Dis 1992;146(1): 104–8.
89. Sampson AP, Castling DP, Green CP, et al. Persistent increase in plasma and urinary leukotrienes after acute asthma. Arch Dis Child 1995;73(3):221–5.
90. Bigham MT, Jacobs BR, Monaco MA, et al. Helium/oxygen-driven albuterol nebulization in the management of children with status asthmaticus: a randomized, placebo-controlled trial. Pediatr Crit Care Med 2010;11(3):356–61.
91. Rivera ML, Kim TY, Stewart GM, et al. Albuterol nebulized in heliox in the initial ED treatment of pediatric asthma: a blinded, randomized controlled trial. Am J Emerg Med 2006;24(1):38–42.

92. Berkenbosch J, Grueber R, Graff G, et al. Patterns of helium-oxygen (heliox) usage in the critical care environment. J Intensive Care Med 2004;19(6):335–44.
93. Kudukis TM, Manthous CA, Schmidt GA, et al. Inhaled helium-oxygen revisited: effect of inhaled helium-oxygen during the treatment of status asthmaticus in children. J Pediatr 1997;130(2):217–24.
94. Rodrigo G, Pollack C, Rodrigo C, et al. Heliox for nonintubated acute asthma patients. Cochrane Database Syst Rev 2006;(4):CD002884.
95. Kim IK, Phrampus E, Venkataraman S, et al. Helium/oxygen-driven albuterol nebulization in the treatment of children with moderate to severe asthma exacerbations: a randomized, controlled trial. Pediatrics 2005;116(5):1127–33.
96. Bernet V, Hug MI, Frey B. Predictive factors for the success of noninvasive mask ventilation in infants and children with acute respiratory failure. Pediatr Crit Care Med 2005;6(6):660–4.
97. Carroll CL, Schramm CM. Noninvasive positive pressure ventilation for the treatment of status asthmaticus in children. Ann Allergy Asthma Immunol 2006;96(3): 454–9.
98. Essouri S, Chevret L, Durand P, et al. Noninvasive positive pressure ventilation: five years of experience in a pediatric intensive care unit. Pediatr Crit Care Med 2006;7(4):329–34.
99. Padman R, Lawless ST, Kettrick RG. Noninvasive ventilation via bilevel positive airway pressure support in pediatric practice. Crit Care Med 1998;26(1):169–73.
100. Thill PJ, McGuire JK, Baden HP, et al. Noninvasive positive-pressure ventilation in children with lower airway obstruction. Pediatr Crit Care Med 2004;5(4): 337–42.
101. Ram FS, Wellington S, Rowe BH, et al. Non-invasive positive pressure ventilation for treatment of respiratory failure due to severe acute exacerbations of asthma. Cochrane Database Syst Rev 2005;(1):CD004360.
102. Mayordomo-Colunga J, Medina A, Rey C, et al. Non-invasive ventilation in pediatric status asthmaticus: a prospective observational study. Pediatr Pulmonol 2011;46(10):949–55.
103. Beers SL, Abramo TJ, Bracken A, et al. Bilevel positive airway pressure in the treatment of status asthmaticus in pediatrics. Am J Emerg Med 2007;25(1):6–9.
104. Williams AM, Abramo TJ, Shah MV, et al. Safety and clinical findings of BiPAP utilization in children 20 kg or less for asthma exacerbations. Intensive Care Med 2011;37(8):1338–43.
105. Gouin S, Robidas I, Gravel J, et al. Prospective evaluation of two clinical scores for acute asthma in children 18 months to 7 years of age. Acad Emerg Med 2010;17(6):598–603.
106. Ducharme FM, Zemek RL, Chalut D, et al. Written action plan in pediatric emergency room improves asthma prescribing, adherence, and control. Am J Respir Crit Care Med 2011;183(2):195–203.
107. Zemek RL, Bhogal SK, Ducharme FM. Systematic review of randomized controlled trials examining written action plans in children: what is the plan? Arch Pediatr Adolesc Med 2008;162(2):157–63.

Pediatric Seizures

Maneesha Agarwal, MD, Sean M. Fox, MD*

KEYWORDS

- Seizures • Febrile seizures • New-onset seizures • Neonatal seizures • Pediatric
- Ketogenic diet • Status epilepticus

KEY POINTS

- Neonatal seizures may often be subtle but still have a high correlation with significant pathologic conditions.
- Because patients who have had a simple febrile seizure are at no greater risk for having meningitis than those who have a fever without a seizure, the evaluation of a simple febrile seizure should focus on an age-appropriate evaluation of the fever, and the management should include appropriate anticipatory guidance and education for the family.
- Complex febrile seizures include a vast spectrum of disease; therefore, the evaluation should be tailored to the individual case but with greater suspicion for potential central nervous system infection.
- Patients who have had a first-time afebrile seizure should have neuroimaging (with the preferred modality being magnetic resonance imaging), which can be performed as an outpatient if appropriate follow-up has been arranged.
- Emergent neuroimaging should be obtained in the emergency department after a new-onset seizure for those patients who have specific risk factors (eg, bleeding disorder, sickle cell disease, human immunodeficiency virus, head injury, ventriculoperitoneal shunt, age less than 6 months, focal seizure, prolonged postictal period, status epilepticus, and so forth).
- Status epilepticus becomes more refractory as seizure activity persists, so it should be aggressively treated. Standard algorithms for the management are still applicable, but new routes for administration of benzodiazepines and new second-line and third-line medications may be considered for use.

INTRODUCTION

Seizures represent the most common neurologic emergency of childhood and can be terrifying for patients and families. Although there are a variety of potential causes for seizures, the common pathophysiology entails abnormal electrical discharge of neurons; the extent of this aberrant electrical activity and subsequent manifestation of

Disclosures: None.
Department of Emergency Medicine, Carolinas Medical Center, 3rd Floor Medical Education Building, 1000 Blythe Boulevard, Charlotte, NC 28203, USA
* Corresponding author.
E-mail address: sean.fox@carolinas.org

Emerg Med Clin N Am 31 (2013) 733–754
http://dx.doi.org/10.1016/j.emc.2013.04.001
0733-8627/13/$ – see front matter © 2013 Elsevier Inc. All rights reserved.

the seizure may range from subtle, nonconvulsive events to stereotypic movements to dramatic generalized convulsions. Additionally, the severity of a seizure can be varied, ranging from self-limited episodes without any hemodynamic compromise to prolonged events that may ultimately prove to be fatal in as many as 3% to 4% of patients.[1,2]

Seizures will affect 4% to 10% of children at some point during their lifetime, which translates to approximately 150,000 children in the United States experiencing a new-onset seizure annually.[3] About 10% of these new-onset pediatric seizures may present to the emergency department in status epilepticus.[4] Fortunately, of patients presenting with a new-onset seizure, only 30 000 will go on to develop epilepsy,[3] whereas the remainder will have manifested seizures secondary to other causes, such as fever, infection, or trauma. Those newly diagnosed with epilepsy will add to the 326,000 children residing in the United States who already carry a diagnosis of epilepsy undergoing various treatments ranging from medications to special diets to surgical interventions.[5] Given these numbers, it is critical for every emergency physician to be adept in the acute management of pediatric seizures and possess basic knowledge pertaining to pediatric epilepsy, its management, and potential complications.

SEIZURE MIMICS

Appropriate diagnosis of a seizure is critical to management. However, it is important to recognize that events that result in an altered level of consciousness or abnormal movements may not actually represent a seizure. A detailed history of the event by eyewitnesses (who may not always accompany patients to the emergency department) and a thorough physical examination of patients may yield an alternative diagnosis from a seizure. The differential diagnosis of seizurelike activity is broad but must be considered in all patients, even in those who carry a diagnosis of epilepsy (**Box 1**).

Infants and toddlers, who have developing nervous systems, may present with a myriad of diagnoses unique to their age group that may be interpreted by the family as a seizure. Parents can misinterpret the normal neonatal reflexes, particularly the startle reflex, as seizure activity. Additionally, they may exhibit jitteriness, which is characterized by symmetric tremor of the extremities with facial sparing; unlike seizure activity, these common movements can be stopped with gentle restraint.[6,7] During sleep, migrating myoclonic movements that do not disturb or wake the child may represent self-limited benign sleep myoclonus.[8] Additionally, shuddering attacks can cause concern with parents and consist of rapid shivering of the head, shoulder, and trunk as if cold water were dripping down the child's spine. These attacks may also have start in infancy and can persist through early childhood.[9] Severe gastroesophageal reflex may manifest as Sandifer syndrome, which has also been misconstrued as seizures because of its associated back arching, crying, and writhing.

In addition, some common childhood behaviors can also mimic seizure activity. Breath-holding spells is a well-documented entity that can be seen in 5% of all children between 6 months and 5 years of age. They can have varied presentations, and some can seem to be associated with seizurelike activity. Breath-holding spells are associated with emotional stimuli or minor trauma and are brief, self-resolving, and without a postictal phase. They have an excellent prognosis with spontaneous remission with age.[10] In some children, families may also potentially interpret the rhythmic movements of self-gratification or stimulation as seizure activity.[11] Sleep disturbances, such as pavor nocturnus (night terrors), represent another category of seizure mimics in young children.

Box 1
Differential diagnosis of seizures

- Arrhythmia
- Benign myoclonus of sleep
- Breath-holding spells
- Dystonic reaction
- Hyperekplexia
- Jitteriness
- Migrainous syndromes (confusional, basilar)
- Opsoclonus-myoclonus-ataxia syndrome (neuroblastoma)
- Paroxysmal movement disorders
- Psychiatric disorders (attention-deficit hyperactivity disorder, hysteria, rage attacks)
- Psychogenic nonepileptic seizures (pseudoseizures)
- Sandifer syndrome
- Self-gratification disorder
- Shuddering attacks
- Sleep disorders (pavor nocturnus/night terrors, somnambulism/sleepwalking, narcolepsy)
- Spasmus nutans
- Syncope
- Tics, stereotypies

Although some entities that mimic seizure activity can be caused by benign causes, others are associated with more concerning causes. Hyperekplexia (when infants have marked startling at sudden sounds or touch) may be so profound that it results in total body stiffening and apnea. Spasmus nutans is another entity that presents in children 4 to 12 months of age with pendular nystagmus, head nodding, and some head tilt or unusual head positioning. The rare syndrome of opsoclonus-myoclonus-ataxia that is associated with neuroblastoma may also be misconstrued as seizure activity.[8]

As children age, the differential diagnosis of seizurelike activity becomes similar to that of adults. New-onset narcolepsy, particular with regard to cataplexy, may raise concern for atonic (drop) seizures. Syncope may also be confused with seizures; in one study of patients with controlled initiation of ventricular arrhythmia, 65% of all patients had convulsive movements without an electrographic correlate of seizure activity.[12] Arrhythmia must be considered in any patient presenting with a concern for a new seizure.

One diagnosis that is difficult to differentiate from seizures is psychogenic nonepileptic seizures (PNES). This disorder may begin to present in early adolescence. These seizures are involuntary, physical expressions in response to psychological conflict from emotional, physical, or social distress.[13,14] Patients with PNES are overwhelmingly female, typically with psychiatric comorbidities, such as posttraumatic stress disorder, anxiety, or depression, and have had prior exposure to individuals with a history of seizures that serve as a model for seizurelike activity. Characteristics that are more suggestive of seizures include tongue biting, injury, bowel or bladder incontinence, significant vital sign instability, cyanosis, altered pupillary responses, and postictal state.[15] Prolonged events in excess of 15 to 30 minutes; bizarre motor activity along the lines of thrashing, arching, or flailing; occurrence of events only in the presence of an audience; incorporation of verbal cues from bystanders; and brief or odd postictal states with crying or baby talking are more likely to represent PNES.[14] It can be particularly difficult to distinguish between PNES and true seizures because, in part, many individuals may suffer from both PNES and epilepsy. In some populations, accurate diagnosis may be delayed by a mean of 7 years with patients receiving aggressive antiepileptic therapy and other interventions for difficult-to-control epilepsy or recurrent cases of "refractory status epilepticus."[13]

NEONATAL SEIZURES

Although the previously mentioned entities and others can be inappropriately misconstrued as seizure activity, true seizures that occur in neonates ($\leq$28 days of age) can often be misidentified as being benign. Neonatal seizures are not often as dramatic and clinically evident as seizures in older children and adults. Generalized tonic-clonic activity is rarely seen in neonates; instead, the neonate's immature nervous system and pattern of myelination generally leads to more subtle presentations of seizures.[16,17] Ocular movements, lip smacking, bicycling movements, and even apnea can be seizure presentations in neonates. Subtle seizure types account for approximately 50% of all neonatal seizures.[18] Other clonic or tonic seizure types are possible but are seen less commonly. The myoclonic seizure type can be easily perceived as representing a Moro reflex and can be of a benign origin or indicate a more ominous sign of significant brain damage.[16,18] Additionally, alterations in vital signs (eg, hypertension, tachycardia) of an unclear cause can also represent neonatal seizures.[19]

Although the presentations of neonatal seizures may be subtle, the cause is often associated with significant morbidity and mortality. Ninety percent of seizures in fullterm newborns are caused by an identifiable cause.[20] The immature nervous system of neonates not only leads to a restricted repertoire from which patients can demonstrate illness to their families and physicians but also makes it more susceptible to having seizures because of any perturbation in its physiology. This circumstance leads to a broad differential diagnosis list for neonatal seizures. From an emergency medicine standpoint, one substantial cause to consider is infection. There should be a low threshold to initiate the workup of possible meningoencephalitis in neonates who are presenting with seizures. The commonly considered organisms (group B streptococci, *Escherichia coli*, and *Listeria*) may be the culprits; but other entities must also be considered, whether newly acquired or congenital, like toxoplasmosis, rubella, cytomegalovirus, and herpes simplex virus.[16]

Fortunately, although infection is extremely important to consider on the differential of neonatal seizures, it is not the most common cause. Hypoxic-ischemic encephalopathy (HIE) is the most common cause of neonatal seizures and usually manifests within the first 48 hours of life.[18] Intracranial hemorrhage should be considered also because it accounts for 10% of neonatal seizures.[16] Birth trauma can lead to subarachnoid or subdural hemorrhage and, because of the subtle nature of the neonatal seizures, may not be noticed until after hospital discharge. Premature infants are particularly at risk for intracranial hemorrhage, and all children are at risk for sustaining injury caused by nonaccidental trauma. Aside from hemorrhage, congenital intracranial anomalies, such as tuberous sclerosis, pachygyria, or lissencephaly, can also lead to seizures in neonates.[19]

Although intracranial abnormalities is intuitively linked to seizures, there are other important entities to consider in neonates who are seizing. Metabolic disturbances and derangements should be considered in neonates with seizures. Hypoglycemia, hypocalcemia, hypomagnesemia, hypernatremia, and hyponatremia are all known to cause seizures and can result from a variety of conditions, from errors in mixing formula to inborn errors of metabolism.[16] Although the indiscriminant investigation of electrolytes is often unnecessary in older patients, chemistry panels can prove to be useful in this at-risk neonatal population,[21] particularly in those who are actively seizing. Seizures caused by inborn errors of metabolism are poorly responsive to conventional therapies for seizures.[20] The specific inborn errors of metabolism that can lead to neonatal seizures are beyond the scope of this review but do warrant consideration as a whole when evaluating a child with neonatal seizures because additional blood, cerebrospinal fluid (CSF), and urine should ideally be obtained and held to assist with making the definitive diagnosis during the hospitalization.

The evaluation and management of neonates with seizures should initially focus on the life-threatening and treatable causes while keeping a perspective about what is common as well as rare. A thorough history and physical examination may help direct the evaluation (eg, fevers, bulging fontanelle, dysmorphic features, hepatosplenomegaly, bruising), but a normal examination does not eliminate the need for concern. After airway, breathing, and circulation issues have been addressed, obtaining a glucose level is imperative. Although infection is not the most common cause of neonatal seizures, the authors think that its potential existence should be addressed rapidly and appropriate cultures obtained and antimicrobials initiated. Metabolic laboratory investigation is also warranted, and the consideration of possible inborn errors of metabolism before the initiation of therapies can aid in making the diagnosis. Emergent neurologic imaging should also be considered to investigate for intracranial pathologies like hemorrhage or congenital anomalies. In neonates, although ultrasound may provide valuable information regarding interventricular or parenchymal hemorrhage, computed tomography (CT) imaging is superior in identifying the extent of intracranial hemorrhage, cortical lesions, subarachnoid blood, and other pathologies and is generally viewed as the preferred imaging modality.[18,22] If patients are clinically stable and there is rapid availability, however, magnetic resonance imaging (MRI) will typically reveal even more detailed and useful information.[23]

Therapeutic medication options for actively seizing neonates still start with benzodiazepines; however, should seizures persist beyond benzodiazepine therapy, phenobarbital is generally favored over phenytoin in neonates.[16,24] Weight-based doses for these medicines are the same as for older children (**Table 1**). Obvious electrolyte abnormalities, such as hyponatremia, should also be promptly corrected. For status epilepticus that is resistant to traditional therapies, pyridoxine dependency may be the culprit, and empiric pyridoxine administration of 50 to 100 mg intravenously may prove to be useful.[16,19]

FEBRILE SEIZURES

Febrile seizures represent an entity unique to pediatric populations that requires special discussion. They are estimated to occur in approximately 2% to 5% of the US pediatric population, with a peak incidence at 18 months.[25] Given the dramatic presentation, often in a previously well child, these patients are almost universally brought to the emergency department for evaluation; thus, it is critical that every

Table 1
Medications to treat status epilepticus

First-Line Medications: Benzodiazepines	
Lorazepam	IV/IM 0.05–0.1 mg/kg (max: 4 mg per dose)
Diazepam	IV 0.2–0.3 mg/kg (max: 10 mg per dose) PR 0.5–1.0 mg/kg
Midazolam	IV 0.05–0.1 mg/kg (max: 6 mg per dose less than 6 y; 10 mg per dose 6 y and older) IM 0.1–0.2 mg/kg (max: 5 mg per dose) IN 0.2–0.3 mg/kg (max: 7.5 mg per dose) Buccal 0.15–0.3 mg/kg (max: 20 mg per dose)
Second-Line Medications	
Phenytoin	IV 15–20 mg/kg (no faster than 1 mg/kg/min)
Fosphenytoin	IV/IM 15–20 PE/kg (no faster than 3 PE/kg/min)
Phenobarbital	IV 15–20 mg/kg (no faster than 1 mg/kg/min)
Valproate	IV 20–40 mg/kg load; can follow with 3–6 mg/kg/min infusion
Levetiracetam	IV 20–30 mg/kg load
Dextrose	IV 2–4 mL/kg of 25% dextrose
Pyridoxine	IV 50–100 mg per dose
Infusions for Refractory Status Epilepticus	
Midazolam	IV 0.1–0.3 mg/kg load followed by 0.05–0.4 mg/kg/h
Propofol	IV 2.0–3.5 mg/kg load followed by 125–300 μg/kg/min
Pentobarbital	IV 0.5–1.0 mg/kg load followed by 1–6 mg/kg/h
Ketamine	IV 1–2 mg/kg load followed by 5–20 μg/kg/min
Lidocaine	IV 1–2 mg/kg load followed by 4–6 mg/kg/h

Abbreviations: IM, intramuscular; IN, intranasal; IV, intravenous; max, maximum; PE, phenytoin equivalents; PR, rectally.
   Data from Refs.[10,22,111,138]

practicing emergency medicine physician be well versed in the diagnosis, evaluation, management, and anticipated outcomes in this condition.

The generally accepted definition of febrile seizures in the United States set forth by the American Academy of Pediatrics (AAP) "is a seizure accompanied by a fever (temperature ≥100.4°F or 38°C by any method), without central nervous system infection, that occurs in infants and children 6 through 60 months of age."[26] Febrile seizures are further defined as either simple or complex; this classification helps better delineate workup and outcomes. Simple febrile seizures consist of primary generalized tonic-clonic seizures lasting for less than 15 minutes. The postictal period is generally brief, often resolving by the time of evaluation in the emergency department and the child returns to his or her neurologic baseline. Evidence of focality, duration of 15 minutes or more, or recurrence within 24 hours characterize complex febrile seizures (AAP 2011)[27]; about 35% of febrile seizures are thought to be complex and 5% may actually present in febrile status epilepticus.[25] In fact, febrile status epilepticus is thought to account for about one-third of all instances of pediatric status epilepticus cases and is by far the most common cause of status epilepticus in this age group.[1,4]

The exact pathophysiology of febrile seizures remains unclear, with competing theories pertaining to the rate of increase of fever versus the peak temperature. There is also new data suggesting a possible correlation with iron deficiency anemia.[27,28] Evidence does exist that there is a genetic predisposition, with a positive family history of febrile seizures in about 25% to 40% of patients.[10,25] Additionally, febrile seizures have been associated with specific causes, such as human herpesvirus 6,[29,30] influenza A,[31] and even some routine childhood immunizations.[32–34]

The appropriate management of a child with a febrile seizure focuses on 3 key principles: acute management if the child is still seizing, diagnosis and management of the source of the fever, and anticipatory guidance to parents. It is in the last 2 principles that defining the febrile seizure as simple or complex impacts the care and messages delivered.

As with any seizing patient, acute management of a child with a febrile seizure focuses on the initial management of the airway, breathing, and circulation. Further management of ongoing seizure activity is discussed later; treatment is similar to afebrile seizures, with the addition of antipyretic therapy to control the fever.

From an emergency medicine perspective, the combination of fever and seizure provokes a concern for meningitis. Fortunately, it is known that if the child fits the definition of a simple febrile seizure, then he or she is not at any increased risk for meningitis.[35,36] Comprehensive review of the extensive medical literature on febrile seizures has been used to generate a clinical practice guideline by the AAP.[26] Research, both before and after the release of the newer immunizations for *Haemophilus influenzae* type b and *Streptococcus pneumoniae*, document that the risk of bacteremia, urinary tract infection, and meningitis are similar between children presenting with a simple febrile seizure versus those who present with a fever without seizure.[36–40] Thus, it is recommended that the evaluation of simple febrile seizures essentially become the evaluation of fever alone. Even with aggressive evaluation for a source, approximately 30% of children with a febrile seizure will have no focal illness or specific viral or bacterial cause identified.[38] There is no role or evidence to support routine neuroimaging, specific blood work, or obtaining an electroencephalogram (EEG).[36] It is important, however, to ensure that patients are appropriately diagnosed as having a simple febrile seizure before relying on this information.

While evaluating a child who has presented with a seizure and does fit the definition of simple febrile seizure, often the parental concern will still focus on meningitis. It is important and useful to convey that bacterial meningitis does not typically present with seizure as its sole manifestation.[41] Additionally, in a large study of more than 700 children aged 6 to 18 months with simple febrile seizures, no child had bacterial meningitis.[35] Thus, in the child with a simple febrile seizure, empiric antibiotics are not advantageous and the lumbar puncture is not mandatory. Lumbar puncture is worth consideration if patients are younger than 12 months with a less reliable physical examination, incompletely immunized, or pretreated with antibiotics that might mask the signs and symptoms of meningitis. Certainly, any child with symptoms concerning for meningitis (such as nuchal rigidity, persistent postictal period, altered mental status, or bulging fontanelle) warrants a lumbar puncture for CSF analysis. If CSF is obtained, recent studies suggest pleocytosis should not be attributed to the seizure and instead managed appropriately.[42,43]

In contrast to the well-supported guidelines for the evaluation and management of simple febrile seizure, complex febrile seizures do not have any definitive management guidelines because of the significant clinical heterogeneity within the definition of complex febrile seizures. For example, the febrile 3-year-old child with clear herpangina who has had 2 seizures within a 24-hour period as well as the 18-month-old child who presents with febrile status epilepticus both are classified as complex febrile seizures. Certainly though, these 2 cases represent extremely different clinical scenarios. With each case of complex febrile seizures, a strategy for obtaining laboratory values, cultures, neuroimaging, neurology consultation, and admission needs to be tailored for the individual based on the available history and physical examination and at the discretion of the treating physicians.

Despite the lack of clear, definitive guidelines for complex febrile seizures, there is some evidence pertaining to the risk of meningitis and the potential benefit of neuroimaging. In a recent study of more than 500 patients presenting with a complex febrile seizure, 3 patients were ultimately diagnosed with bacterial meningitis; 2 patients had abnormal findings on examination, and 1 patient was presumptively treated for bacterial meningitis based on a lack of CSF but positive blood culture.[44] In the instance of febrile status epilepticus, which is included within the broader category of complex febrile seizures, there is a definite increased risk of meningitis compared with those with simple febrile seizures, with an estimated risk of bacterial meningitis of 12% to 18%.[1,45] Thus, in the case of complex febrile seizures, a lumbar puncture should be strongly considered and any pleocytosis should be appropriately interpreted.

Again, with the complex febrile seizure cohort including a diverse set of conditions, the utility of neuroimaging needs to be addressed on an individual case basis. The child with clinical herpangina and 2 simple febrile seizures in a 24-hour period may not benefit greatly from a CT scan of the brain, whereas the child in febrile status epilepticus may. Routine imaging should not be performed for patients with complex febrile seizures, but rather the clinical scenario should help determine who is at greater risk of having an intracranial abnormality. Abnormalities are generally noted only in patients with an abnormal physical examination.[46,47]

Parental concern surrounding this event will often be appropriately high; thus, it is imperative that for every child who meets criteria for discharge after suffering a febrile seizure, the emergency physician provides appropriate anticipatory guidance to the parents. Guidance should be provided on the risk of recurrence, appropriate precautions in the event of another seizure, subsequent risk of epilepsy, and the generally excellent prognosis for children who suffer febrile seizures despite the lack of therapies to prevent further seizure activity. The risk of recurrence of a febrile seizure is about 33%, with about 10% having multiple seizures.[25] Specific risk factors that increase the risk of recurrence include age less than 18 months, a family history of febrile seizures, a shorter duration of fever before seizing, and lower temperature at onset of seizing. The presence of multiple risk factors increases the likelihood of seizure recurrence further.[25,48,49] Although seizure recurrence is not uncommon, the risk of epilepsy after a child suffers a febrile seizure is the same as the general population at 1%.[50] The risk may increase to 10% in some studies, especially in the context of a preexisting neurodevelopmental abnormality, family history of epilepsy, patient history of complex febrile seizure, multiple complex features to the seizure, and brief duration of fever.[25,51]

Unfortunately, extensive research on preventing the recurrence of febrile seizures or the subsequent development of epilepsy has been unfruitful. Routine antipyretic therapy during febrile illnesses has not demonstrated any benefit in prevention.[52–54] Intermittent and routine antiepileptic therapy with benzodiazepines, phenytoin, phenobarbital, valproate, and other agents have varying levels of efficacy; however, the range of adverse side effects outweigh any potential benefit.[49,55–57] Fortunately, research also indicates that febrile seizures, even when prolonged, are not associated with any negative impact on cognitive function.[58,59] Thus, the AAP does not recommend routine use of antipyretics or antiepileptics in patients with from febrile seizures.[50] Under extenuating circumstances (eg, febrile status epilepticus, distance from emergency health care, severe parental anxiety), one could consider discharging patients home with a prescription for rectal diazepam for use in case of a prolonged febrile seizure with appropriate instruction in its use. Fortunately, for most cases of simple febrile seizures, education and reassurance will be all that is required.

NEW-ONSET AFEBRILE SEIZURES

Every year, between 25,000 and 40,000 children in the United States will have an initial afebrile seizure[60]; thus, it is also critical for emergency physicians to understand the basic evaluation of a new-onset afebrile seizure. It is important for one to remember that a seizure does not always equal epilepsy and instead signifies some sort of brain dysfunction that has resulted in abnormal electrical activity in the brain[61]; thus, a broad differential diagnosis beyond epilepsy is required when considering the child who has suffered an afebrile seizure. Naturally, after acute stabilization of patients, a thorough history and physical examination are critical initial steps in the evaluation. A detailed description of the event is critical to categorizing the event as a seizure and further delineation into categories, such as simple, partial, or partial with secondary general-ization. A history of focality to the seizure, prior abnormal neurodevelopment, altered fluid intake, recent immigration after years in a developing country, and possible sub-stance exposure or the findings of abnormal skin lesions, hepatosplenomegaly, or retinal hemorrhages all help delineate whether the seizure represents a de novo pre-sentation of epilepsy versus a symptom of another process, such as a brain tumor, hyponatremia, intracranial infection, ingestion, neurocutaneous syndrome (eg, tuber-ous sclerosis), inborn error of metabolism, or nonaccidental trauma.

Just as the differential diagnosis list for afebrile seizure is diverse, the potential eval-uation is vast. There is no standardized laboratory panel for children presenting with an initial afebrile seizure that can be recommended. As documented in the American Academy of Neurology practice parameter on the evaluation of afebrile seizures in children, the yield of routine laboratory studies is abysmally low.[60] Instead, laboratory investigation should be tailored to the individual case as suggested by the patients' history and physical examination. It is prudent to have a low threshold to obtain a bedside glucose because hypoglycemia represents an easily correctable cause of seizure. A basic electrolyte panel may be particularly useful in younger patients because electrolyte abnormalities have been noted more frequently in this popula-tion.[21,62] Other studies that may warrant consideration based on the individual pa-tient's history and physical examination include complete blood counts, toxicology screens, ammonia levels, serum organic acids, and urine amino acids. Lumbar punc-ture may also be considered if there is clinical concern for meningoencephalitis, although the yield of routine CSF studies is extremely low in patients with a normal mental status and physical examination.

Potential structural anomalies and abnormalities also need to be contemplated during the initial evaluation of patients with a new-onset afebrile seizure. There are clear recommendations for neuroimaging in most cases of new-onset afebrile seizures,[63] and emergent CT imaging is available in most emergency departments. However, there is growing concern about the detrimental effects of radiation on the pediatric brain.[64,65] Additionally, it has been found that the information gleaned from the head CT performed after an afebrile seizure seldom results in a change in manage-ment or in any acute intervention.[60,66] Studies are also suggestive of the superiority of MRI regarding identifying lesions compared with CT; in one study, 33% of patients with an initially normal CT scan had abnormal findings identified on MRI.[23] Thus, MRI is the preferred modality for definitive neuroimaging.[60,63] Unfortunately, MRI is less readily available on an emergency basis and may require additional resources for sedation in younger patients. Given the risks and benefits of various modalities of neuroimaging, a uniform approach cannot be recommended. It is thought best to discuss the risks, benefits, and limitations of the imaging modalities against the risk for emergent intracranial pathologic conditions with patients' families and the neurologist on an individual basis.

The desire to obtain the most prudent studies must be balanced with the physician's suspicion for important, emergent pathologic conditions. There are factors that may heighten suspicion for pathologic conditions that might require immediate intervention, such as a stroke or increased intracranial pressure, and, thus, lower the threshold for obtaining emergent neuroimaging (**Box 2**). Unfortunately, the very young (less than 6 months of age) are more difficult to obtain a reliable neurologic examination on; some advocate for obtaining emergent neuroimaging in these patients after a new-onset afebrile seizure.[67] Additionally, a prolonged seizure (>15 minutes), persistent postictal focal deficit, or aberration from neurologic baseline should increase concern for focal disease processes.[60,67] Additionally, patients with a predisposing condition like sickle cell disease, bleeding disorder, cerebrovascular disease, neurocutaneous disorder, malignancy, human immunodeficiency virus, hemihypertrophy, hydrocephalus, travel to an area endemic for cysticercosis, or a closed-head injury should increase suspicion for significant abnormalities.[67,68] Focal seizures in children younger than 33 months should also lower the threshold for obtaining emergent neuroimaging.[68] Otherwise, in the absence of the aforementioned concerning factors, children with a reassuring neurologic examination and an appropriate, established

---

Box 2
Factors lower threshold to obtain emergent neuroimaging for first-time afebrile seizure

Findings

- Less than 6 months of age
- Abnormal physical examination
- Prolonged seizure (>15 minutes)
- Persistent postictal period
- Altered mental status
- Persistent focal neurologic deficit
- Focal seizure in child less than 33 months of age
- Closed-head injury
- Travel to endemic area for cysticercosis

Concurrent medical conditions

- Bleeding disorder
- Cerebrovascular disease
- Hemihypertrophy
- Human immunodeficiency virus
- Hydrocephalus/ventriculoperitoneal shunt
- Malignancy
- Neurocutaneous disorder
- Sickle cell disease

Data from Refs.[60,67,68]

outpatient follow-up plan may be appropriate for out-patient MRI rather than CT before discharge from the emergency department.[67]

Before discharge, the family should be informed that the outpatient evaluation would likely also include additionally studies. An EEG is indicated in all children with an afebrile seizure, although the best time to obtain this study remains unclear.[60] Nonspecific abnormalities secondary to the seizure are commonly seen in the few days after a seizure; thus, there is no role for routine EEG before discharge for patients with an initial afebrile seizure who have returned completely to neurologic baseline. However, it is critical that these patients have appropriate outpatient follow-up for EEG within a timely fashion because EEG abnormalities may in fact be the best predictor of seizure recurrence.[69]

Generally speaking, the outcomes of children with a new-onset afebrile seizure are quite good. The overall recurrence rate of seizures is about 54%, with most recurrences occurring within 2 years of the initial seizure; thus, almost half of all children with an initial afebrile seizure will not develop epilepsy. The risk of subsequent epilepsy is increased in patients with an abnormal EEG and history of abnormal neurodevelopment.[70,71] Unfortunately, there are no known therapies that alter a patient's potential progression to epilepsy after an initial afebrile seizure. Because there have been no detrimental effects noted in delaying seizure therapy until after a second seizure, the initiation of antiepileptic medication is not recommended after an initial afebrile seizure, with possible exceptions as discussed earlier in febrile seizures for prescribing rectal diazepam.[72] Antiepileptic medication initiation is best left to the physician who will follow patients long-term and monitor for potential complications. Even among patients who go on to develop epilepsy, outcomes are not completely unfavorable. In one longitudinal cohort of children with epilepsy, around 70% of children were able to achieve remission from seizures and 60% were able to discontinue antiepileptic treatment, whereas only 10% had intractable epilepsy.[73]

STATUS EPILEPTICUS

Most patients who present to the emergency department for evaluation of a seizure are no longer seizing. However, patients who are actively seizing will generate immediate attention; seizure activity may easily recur or develop in any emergency department patient. The annual incidence of pediatric status epilepticus is more than 80,000.[74] This entity accounts for approximately 10% of all patients with new-onset pediatric seizures presenting to the emergency department[4] and is most common in children less than 2 years of age.[75,76] Although there are many potential precipitants of status epilepticus ranging from central nervous system infection to trauma to congenital anomalies to toxins, febrile seizures are the most common cause of status epilepticus in children, accounting for approximately one-third of all episodes[1,77,78]; this is in contrast to adults whereby cerebrovascular accidents represent the most common cause of status epilepticus.[79] Fortunately, the quoted mortality rate for pediatric status epilepticus is quite low, ranging from 3% to 5%.[80,81]

Historically, status epilepticus has been defined as continuous seizure activity for 30 minutes or 2 or more seizures occurring without full recovery of consciousness between episodes.[77] However, there has been a recent trend to categorize seizures lasting longer than 5 to 10 minutes as status epilepticus because there is evidence that seizures are less likely to spontaneously cease after this time frame.[82] From an emergency medicine perspective, the categorization is less vital because it is the patients' clinical condition that mandates the management of the patients.

Although the exact categorical label may still be debated, resolving the seizures as expeditiously as possible is beneficial. With short-duration seizures, the increased metabolic demands of the brain are met with increased cerebral blood flow; however, as the seizure continues, autoregulation can fail and the blood flow to tenuous areas can be compromised, potentially leading to irreversible cerebral damage.[77] Persistent neuronal excitation may also mediate neuronal injury.[83] Furthermore, prolonged seizures can be associated with hyperthermia, myoglobinuria, hyperuricemia, renal impairment, multiple metabolic derangements, aspiration, respiratory failure, hepatic failure, and persistent neurodevelopmental abnormalities.[77,84,85] Finally, there is excellent evidence suggesting that seizures become more refractory to therapy the longer they persist.[75,86,87] In an effort to minimize the chance that the seizure will progress to a refractory state, aggressive therapy should be initiated as soon as possible.

As with all efforts to stabilize patients during emergent conditions, the initial steps should focus on maintaining a patent airway, ensuring there is adequate ventilation, and assessing patients for appropriate circulation. Actively seizing patients can have derangements in one or all of these important systems. Although more aggressive maneuvers may be necessary, often a simple jaw thrust will be adequate to help maintain a patent airway. Supplemental oxygen is advisable if respirations become compromised, and suctioning should be readied in case of emesis. The use of bite blocks to protect the tongue has fallen out of favor given the risk of aspiration.

Although it is reasonable to observe patients briefly before administering medicines in case the seizure spontaneously ceases, there is good evidence that seizures that persist beyond 5 minutes are unlikely to stop[82]; thus, at this point, it is beneficial to administer medications to halt the seizure. Benzodiazepines are considered first line therapy for essentially all seizure disorders; they work by modulating the gamma-aminobutyric acid (GABA) receptor.[88] All medicines in this class carry the risk of respiratory depression and hypotension, necessitating close monitoring for these complications, especially when multiple doses or other medications are given. Each benzodiazepine has unique characteristics and dosing (see **Table 1**). Diazepam is commonly used given its rapid onset secondary to its highly lipophilic properties enabling rapid penetration across the blood-brain barrier. It is also frequently prescribed to patients with known seizure disorders for home administration rectally; it can also be used in this manner in the emergency department if intravenous access has not been established.[89] More recently, midazolam has started to gain favor in the prehospital and emergency department environments because of its ease of use and efficacy via intranasal, intramuscular, and buccal routes.[90-99] Because vascular access is often difficult in pediatric patients (particularly ones who are ill), intramuscular, intranasal, or buccal routes should be considered early in the management. However, when intravenous access is established, lorazepam is the most commonly used benzodiazepine because of its efficacy and duration of action of 6 to 12 hours.[77]

Continued seizure activity despite successive doses of benzodiazepine should lead to the administration of medications that work by a different mechanism (see **Table 1**). Phenytoin and fosphenytoin have traditionally been selected as second-line agents and affect voltage-gated sodium channels. Unfortunately, phenytoin cannot be administered rapidly because of the associated hypotension, widening of the QT interval, and dysrhythmias owing to its diluents. There is also the risk of purple glove syndrome.[77,100,101] Unlike phenytoin, fosphenytoin can be administered more rapidly, safely, and even given intramuscularly; however, it is a prodrug of phenytoin and takes longer to have an effect.[77,102]

Phenobarbital has long held position as a third-line medication in the treatment of status epilepticus. Although it also works on GABA receptors, it does so via a different mechanism from benzodiazepines. It takes longer to terminate seizure activity but has a prolonged therapeutic effect. Although there is no definitive evidence, it is a commonly held belief that phenobarbital is more strongly associated with respiratory depression, potential need for intubation, and hypotension compared with phenytoin. Interestingly, phenobarbital is commonly favored over benzodiazepines as a first-line or second-line therapy for the treatment of neonatal seizures and should be potentially considered for use earlier when managing younger patients.[24,103]

Newer medications have recently demonstrated promise and potential value in the acute management of status epilepticus. Valproate has shown benefit as a second-line medication, with particular utility in patients already maintained on this medication or who have nonconvulsive or partial status epilepticus.[104–110] It also lacks adverse effects on the cardiovascular or respiratory systems but does have potential risks of hepatic dysfunction, parkinsonism, pancreatitis, and thrombocytopenia.[102,111] Levetiracetam has been shown to be safe in children as young as 6 months of age; it is generally well tolerated, and side effects are reversible with cessation of the medication.[112] Levetiracetam also offers the advantage of being able to be converted easily over to oral medications later in the patients' management. Preliminary evidence suggests that levetiracetam may be safely administered intravenously as therapy for status epilepticus, although further research is necessary to recommend routine use of this medication.[110,113–115]

Unfortunately, refractory status epilepticus occurs in 25% of patients with status epilepticus.[116] If patients have continued to seize despite the previous interventions, the seizure is considered to be refractory[117] and patients are at an increased risk for adverse events. Before this period, patients may or may not have required intubation to protect airway patency; however, the management of refractory status epilepticus will require intubation because most therapies will essentially induce general anesthesia and coma. In this scenario, emergent EEG monitoring is of vital importance to guide further therapy because paralytics will mask potential continued convulsions. There are no clear guidelines on what is the most advantageous therapy, but standard options include continuous infusions of midazolam, propofol, pentobarbital, ketamine, and lidocaine. Additional therapies that have growing evidence and may eventually have a standardized role in the management of status epilepticus include lacosamide, magnesium, topiramate, isoflurane, steroids, therapeutic hypothermia, electroconvulsive therapy, vagal nerve stimulation, and emergent surgery.[116,118–122]

Any discussion of status epilepticus would be incomplete without the consideration of nonconvulsive status epilepticus. This entity is thought to account for approximately 25% of all cases of status epilepticus and is more common in patients with certain epilepsy syndromes.[123] The classic subtypes include absence status epilepticus and complex partial status epilepticus. About a quarter of cases of nonconvulsive status epilepticus follow convulsive status epilepticus and represent burnt out or subtle generalized status epilepticus.[123,124] These patients may have a range of altered mental status ranging from mild confusion to psychosis to coma with subtle physical movements, such as twitches or automatisms.[124] Nonconvulsive status epilepticus should be considered in patients with an inexplicable, sudden change in mental status or behavior, clinical concern for encephalopathy, unexplained coma, or delayed recovery of mental status after a seizure.[123–125] EEG monitoring is paramount to be able to make the appropriate diagnosis and management of this entity. Treatment is the same as for convulsive status epilepticus with the possible consideration of valproate as a second-line medication.[124]

ADDITIONAL PEDIATRIC SEIZURE SYNDROMES AND UNIQUE THERAPIES

Although the authors have already discussed febrile seizures, which constitute the largest category of seizures unique to the pediatric population, there are many other seizure syndromes unique to pediatric patients. It is useful for the emergency medicine physician to possess a basic knowledge about a few of these particular syndromes. These entities range from benign, self-limited conditions to neurologically devastating diseases and are further discussed in **Table 2**.

Despite the recent advent of new antiepileptic drugs and generally good prognosis for patients with epilepsy, about 10% of children will have intractable epilepsy.[73,126] Poorly controlled seizures are the primary risk factor for sudden unexpected death in epilepsy, increasing the risk of this event from 1 in 1000 to 1 in 150.[2,127–129] In these cases, novel therapies, including implantable devices, specific diets, and surgery, may be required. Rudimentary knowledge of some of these more aggressive therapies is warranted.

The only implantable device currently approved for use in the United States is the vagal nerve stimulator (VNS). This device consists of an implanted device in a subcutaneous pocket, either under the clavicle or in abdominal tissue in smaller patients; a microprocessor and battery are attached to the left vagus nerve via leads. The VNS is typically set to deliver a stimulus designed to terminate seizures when a small handheld magnet is held directly over the device for a few seconds; thus, activation of a VNS may be useful in the management of seizures in patients who possess this technology. If mandated, MRI generally can be completed regardless of VNS placement; but this is best coordinated between neurosurgery and radiology. There is a 3% to 5% risk of infection of the VNS, and lead fractures may occur after direct trauma to the neck. Patients may also present with complaints of twitching, coughing, dysphagia, or other sensations secondary to VNS firing. Continual device activation may occur rarely, and taping the magnet over the patients' VNS should turn it off until neurosurgical evaluation can be obtained. Otherwise VNS are generally helpful in reducing seizure frequency by about half in 50% of all patients.[130,131]

Another therapy that patients with intractable epilepsy may use is the ketogenic diet. Essentially a starvation state is used to induce ketosis, generally resulting in up to a 30% to 40% reduction in seizures in numerous types of epilepsies, with even better results in some individual patients.[132] Within a few weeks of initiation, patients may present with complications, such as dehydration, hypoglycemia, and other metabolic derangements. However, long-term complications are typically limited to osteopenia, nephrolithiasis, and cardiomyopathy. Occasionally, these patients will present to the emergency department with ongoing seizure activity, potentially with hypoglycemia. In this situation, correcting hypoglycemia may actually be harmful and worsen seizure activity by breaking the patients' ketotic state. Thus, dextrose infusion must be reserved for patients with severe hypoglycemia, and other typical seizure therapies should be maximized. Additionally, in cases of refractory status epilepticus, it may be wise to avoid propofol because these patients are at a higher risk of propofol infusion syndrome.[22,133,134]

Occasionally, patients will have seizures of such severity that they may require experimental therapies or even surgery. At present, there are numerous devices,[135] medications, alternative diets, and other therapies under investigation. Surgeries may be particularly beneficial in focal epilepsies and the most intractable diseases. These surgeries, such as hemispherectomy, corpus callosotomy, and anterior temporal lobe resection, may be associated with delayed complications, such as bleeding, hematoma formation, and obstructive hydrocephalus[136]; however, they

Table 2
Seizure syndromes unique to pediatric patients

Benign Convulsions Associated with Gastroenteritis	6–60 mo Peaks 13–24 mo	Afebrile, brief, generalized seizures accompanying symptoms of gastroenteritis without metabolic derangement, fever, or *Shigella* infection; associated strongly with rotavirus, although seen with other viral causes; seizures may cluster, be difficult to treat; spontaneously remits at conclusion of illness[139–141]
Benign Familial Neonatal Convulsions	Initial days of life Remits within 1 y	Presentation may include behavioral arrest, eye deviation, tonic stiffening, myoclonic jerks; associated with positive family history; some may develop subsequent epilepsy[16]
Benign Idiopathic Neonatal Convulsions	Initial days of life Remits within 15 d	Also called "fifth day fits"; presentation may include clonic movements, apnea; associated with positive family history; may account for up to 5% of all seizures in term infants[16]
Absence Seizures	5–10 y Remits by 14 y	Associated with sudden cessation of activity, possible eye fluttering, brief duration (about 30 s), and no postictal period; seizures may be triggered by hyperventilation; 70% of patients spontaneously remit; 40% of patients may have associated generalized tonic-clonic seizures[22,142]
Benign Rolandic Epilepsy	3–13 y Remits by early adulthood	Typically associated with nighttime clonus (especially facial) while sleeping, which may secondarily generalize; associated with autosomal dominant inheritance[22,143]
Juvenile Myoclonic Epilepsy of Janz	12–15 y	Typically associated with myoclonic jerks on awaking, although also many have generalized tonic-clonic or absence seizures; triggered by stress, lack of sleep, alcohol; associated with autosomal dominant inheritance; generally requires ongoing treatment[22,143]
Infantile Spasms	4–18 mo Peaks 4–6 mo	Sudden jerking of extremities, head, neck, and trunk, occasionally with associated cry, typically occurring in clusters; associated with other neurologic conditions (such as tuberous sclerosis, HIE, congenital infections); 95% of patients also have mental retardation; treated with steroids, vigabatrin; spasms typically spontaneously remit, but most patients develop new seizures[143–145]
Lennox-Gastaut Syndrome	3–5 y	Patients suffer from multiple seizure types including tonic, absence, atonic, myoclonic, and status epilepticus; associated with static encephalopathy, mental retardation, intractability despite multiple medications or use of rare therapies, such as surgery, special diets[22,145]

Data from Refs.[16,22,139–145]

may ultimately be the most effective measure in providing relief to patients with intractable epilepsy.[137]

SUMMARY

Pediatric seizures are common and have many characteristics that distinguish them from seizures in adults. Appropriate diagnosis of seizures may be challenging given numerous seizure mimics and the subtle presentation of neonatal seizures. Making an appropriate diagnosis as to the presence of a seizure and any potential cause is critical to delivering appropriate care. Although some entities may be relatively benign, such as febrile seizures, status epilepticus and refractory seizure syndromes can produce significant morbidity and mortality. Fortunately, the outcomes of seizures in pediatric patients are generally excellent; there has been ongoing development of additional therapies, including medications, diets, devices, and surgeries.

REFERENCES

1. Chin RF, Neville BG, Peckham C, et al. Incidence, cause, and short-term outcome of convulsive status epilepticus in childhood: prospective population-based study. Lancet 2006;368:222–9.
2. Nesbitt V, Kirkpatrick M, Pearson G, et al. Risk and causes of death in children with a seizure disorder. Dev Med Child Neurol 2012;54:612–7.
3. Hauser WA. The prevalence and incidence of convulsive disorders in children. Epilepsia 1994;35(Suppl 2):S1–6.
4. Singh RK, Stephens S, Berl MM, et al. Prospective study of new-onset seizures presenting as status epilepticus in childhood. Neurology 2010;74:636–42.
5. Epilepsy Foundation. Living with epilepsy: parents and caregivers. Available at: http://www.epilepsyfoundation.org/livingwithepilepsy/parentsandcaregivers/index.cfm. Accessed December 20, 2012.
6. Evans D, Levene M. Neonatal seizures. Arch Dis Child Fetal Neonatal Ed 1998;78:F70–5.
7. Parker S, Zuckerman B, Bauchner H, et al. Jitteriness in full term neonates: prevalence and correlates. Pediatrics 1990;85:17–23.
8. Alam S, Lux AL. Epilepsies in infancy. Arch Dis Child 2012;97:985–92.
9. Tibussek D, Karenfort M, Mayatepek E, et al. Clinical reasoning: shuddering attacks in infancy. Neurology 2008;70:e38–41.
10. Blumstein MD, Friedman MJ. Childhood seizures. Emerg Med Clin North Am 2007;25:1061–86.
11. Patel H, Dunn DW, Austin JK, et al. Psychogenic nonepileptic seizures (pseudoseizures). Pediatr Rev 2011;32:e66–72.
12. Aminoff MJ, Cheinman MM, Griffin JC, et al. Electrocerebral accompaniments of syncope associated with malignant ventricular arrhythmias. Ann Intern Med 1988;108:791–6.
13. Brown RJ, Syed TU, Benbadis S, et al. Psychogenic nonepileptic seizures. Epilepsy Behav 2011;22:85–93.
14. Selbst SM, Clancy R. Pseudoseizures in the pediatric emergency department. Pediatr Emerg Care 1996;12:185–8.
15. Sahaya K, Dholakia SA, Sahota PK. Psychogenic non-epileptic seizures: a challenging entity. J Clin Neurosci 2011;18:1602–7.
16. Zupanc ML. Neonatal seizures. Pediatr Clin North Am 2004;51:961–78.
17. Stafstrom CE. Neonatal seizures. Pediatr Rev 1995;16:248–55.

18. Panayiotopoulos CP. Chapter 5: neonatal seizures and neonatal syndromes. In: The epilepsies: seizures, syndromes, and management. Oxfordshire (United Kingdom): Bladon Medical Publishing; 2005. Available at: http://www.ncbi. nlm.nih.gov/books/NBK2599/.
19. Bernes SM, Kaplan AM. Evolution of neonatal seizures. Pediatr Clin North Am 1994;41:1069–104.
20. Ficicioglu C, Bearden D. Isolated neonatal seizures: when to suspect inborn errors of metabolism. Pediatr Neurol 2011;45:283–91.
21. Scarfone RJ, Pond K, Thompson K, et al. Utility of laboratory testing for infants with seizures. Pediatr Emerg Care 2000;16:309–12.
22. Sharieff GQ, Hendry PL. Afebrile pediatric seizures. Emerg Med Clin North Am 2011;29:95–108.
23. Hsieh DT, Chang T, Tsuchida TN, et al. New-onset afebrile seizures in infants: role of neuroimaging. Neurology 2010;74:150–6.
24. Rennie JM, Boylan GB. Neonatal seizures and their treatment. Curr Opin Neurol 2003;16:177–81.
25. Shinnar S, Glauser T. Febrile seizures. J Child Neurol 2002;17(Suppl 1):S44–52.
26. Hartfield DS, Tan J, Yager JY, et al. The association between iron deficiency and febrile seizures in childhood. Clin Pediatr (Phila) 2009;48:420–6.
27. American Academy of Pediatrics. Neurodiagnostic evaluation of the child with a simple febrile seizure. Pediatrics 2011;127:389–94.
28. Ozaydin E, Arhan E, Cetinkaya B, et al. Differences in iron deficiency anemia and mean platelet volume between children with simple and complex febrile seizures. Seizure 2012;21:211–4.
29. Barone SR, Kaplan MH, Krilov LR. Human herpesvirus-6 infection in children with first febrile seizures. J Pediatr 1995;127:95–7.
30. Epstein LG, Shinnar S, Hesdorffer DC, et al. Human herpesvirus 6 and 7 in febrile status epilepticus: the FEBSTAT study. Epilepsia 2012;56:1481–8.
31. Chiu SS, Tse CY, Lau YL, et al. Influenza A infection is an important cause of febrile seizures. Pediatrics 2001;108:E63.
32. Barlow WE, Davis RL, Glasser JW, et al. The risk of seizures after receipt of whole-cell pertussis or measles, mumps, and rubella vaccine. N Engl J Med 2001;345:656–61.
33. Leroy Z, Broder K, Menschik D, et al. Febrile seizures after 2010-2011 influenza vaccine in young children, United States: a vaccine safety signal from the vaccine adverse event reporting system. Vaccine 2012;30:2020–3.
34. Sun Y, Christensen J, Hviid A, et al. Risk of febrile seizures and epilepsy after vaccination with diphtheria, tetanus, acellular pertussis, inactivated poliovirus, and Haemophilus influenzae type B. JAMA 2012;307:823–31.
35. Kimia AA, Capraro AJ, Hummel D, et al. Utility of lumbar puncture for first simple febrile seizure among children 6 to 18 months of age. Pediatrics 2009;123:6–12.
36. Teach SJ, Geil PA. Incidence of bacteremia, urinary tract infections, and unsuspected bacterial meningitis in children with febrile seizures. Pediatr Emerg Care 1999;15:9–12.
37. Chamberlain JM, Gorman RL. Occult bacteremia in children with simple febrile seizures. Am J Dis Child 1988;142:1073–6.
38. Colvin JM, Jaffe DM, Muenzer JT. Evaluation of the precision of emergency department diagnoses in young children with fever. Clin Pediatr (Phila) 2012;51:51–7.
39. Shah SS, Alpern ER, Zwerling L, et al. Low risk of bacteremia in children with febrile seizures. Arch Pediatr Adolesc Med 2002;156:469–72.

40. Trainor JL, Hampers LC, Krug SE, et al. Children with first-time simple febrile seizures are at low risk of serious bacterial illness. Acad Emerg Med 2001;8:781–7.
41. Green SM, Rothrock SG, Clem KJ, et al. Can seizures be the sole manifestation of meningitis in febrile children? Pediatrics 1993;92:527–34.
42. Frank LM, Shinnar S, Hesdorffer DC, et al. Cerebrospinal fluid findings in children with fever-associated status epilepticus: results of the consequences of prolonged febrile seizures (FEBSTAT) study. J Pediatr 2012;161:1169–71.
43. Haeusler GM, Tebruegge M, Curtis N. Question 1. Do febrile convulsions cause CSF pleocytosis? Arch Dis Child 2012;97:172–5.
44. Kimia A, Ben-Joseph EP, Rudloe T, et al. Yield of lumbar puncture among children who present with their first complex febrile seizure. Pediatrics 2010;126:62–9.
45. Chin RF, Neville BG, Scott RC. Meningitis is a common cause of convulsive status epilepticus with fever. Arch Dis Child 2005;90:66–9.
46. Kimia AA, Ben-Joseph E, Prabhu S, et al. Yield of emergent neuroimaging among children presenting with a first complex febrile seizure. Pediatr Emerg Care 2012;28:316–21.
47. Teng D, Dayan P, Tyler S, et al. Risk of intracranial pathologic conditions requiring emergency intervention after a first complex febrile seizure episode among children. Pediatrics 2006;117:304–8.
48. Berg AT, Shinnar S, Darefsky AS, et al. Predictors of recurrent febrile seizures. A prospective cohort study. Arch Pediatr Adolesc Med 1997;151:371–8.
49. Offringa M, Newton R. Prophylactic drug management for febrile seizures in children. Cochrane Database Syst Rev 2012;(4):CD003031.
50. American Academy of Pediatrics. Febrile seizures: clinical practice guideline for the long-term management of the child with simple febrile seizures. Pediatrics 2008;121:1281–6.
51. Neligan A, Bell GS, Giavasi C, et al. Long-term risk of developing epilepsy after febrile seizures: a prospective cohort study. Neurology 2012;78:1166–70.
52. Schnaiderman D, Lahat E, Sheefer T, et al. Antipyretic effectiveness of acetaminophen in febrile seizures: ongoing prophylaxis versus sporadic usage. Eur J Pediatr 1993;152:747–9.
53. Strengell T, Uhari M, Tarkka R, et al. Antipyretic agents for preventing recurrences of febrile seizures: randomized controlled trial. Arch Pediatr Adolesc Med 2009;163:799–804.
54. van Stuijvenberg M, Derksen-Lubsen G, Steyerberg EW, et al. Randomized, controlled trial of ibuprofen syrup administered during febrile illnesses to prevent febrile seizure recurrences. Pediatrics 1998;102:E51.
55. Knudsen FU. Recurrence risk after first febrile seizure and effect of short term diazepam prophylaxis. Arch Dis Child 1985;60:1045–9.
56. Rosman NP, Colton T, Labazzo J, et al. A controlled trial of diazepam administered during febrile illnesses to prevent recurrence of febrile seizures. N Engl J Med 1993;329:79–84.
57. Uhari M, Rantala H, Vainionpaa L, et al. Effect of acetaminophen and of low intermittent doses of diazepam on prevention of recurrences of febrile seizures. J Pediatr 1995;126:991–5.
58. Ellenberg JH, Nelson KB. Febrile seizures and later intellectual performance. Arch Neurol 1978;35:17–21.
59. Norgaard M, Ehrenstein V, Mahon BE, et al. Febrile seizures and cognitive function in young adult life: a prevalence study in Danish conscripts. J Pediatr 2009;155:404–9.

60. Hirtz D, Ashwal S, Berg A, et al. Practice parameter: evaluating a first non-febrile seizure in children: report of the quality standards subcommittee of the American Academy of Neurology, the Child Neurology Society, and the American Epilepsy Society. Neurology 2000;55:616–23.

61. Scheuer ML, Pedley TA. The evaluation and treatment of seizures. N Engl J Med 1990;323:1468–74.

62. Farrar HC, Chande VT, Fitzpatrick DF, et al. Hyponatremia as the cause of seizures in infants: a retrospective analysis of incidence, severity, and clinical predictors. Ann Emerg Med 1995;26:42–8.

63. Gaillard WD, Chiron C, Cross JH, et al. Guidelines for imaging infants and children with recent-onset epilepsy. Epilepsia 2009;50:2147–53.

64. Brenner DJ, Hall EJ. Computed tomography–an increasing source of radiation exposure. N Engl J Med 2007;357:2277–84.

65. Pearce MS, Salotti JA, Little MP, et al. Radiation exposure from CT scans in childhood and subsequent risk of leukaemia and brain tumours: a retrospective cohort study. Lancet 2012;380:499–505.

66. Garvey MA, Gaillard WD, Rusin JA, et al. Emergency brain computed tomography in children with seizures: who is most likely to benefit? J Pediatr 1998;133:664–9.

67. Warden CR, Brownstein DR, Del Beccaro MA. Predictors of abnormal findings of computed tomography of the head in pediatric patients presenting with seizures. Ann Emerg Med 1997;29:518–23.

68. Sharma S, Riviello JJ, Harper MB, et al. The role of emergent neuroimaging in children with new-onset afebrile seizures. Pediatrics 2003;111:1–5.

69. Shinnar S, Kang H, Berg AT, et al. EEG abnormalities in children with a first unprovoked seizure. Epilepsia 1994;35:471–6.

70. Shinnar S, Berg AT, Moshe SL, et al. The risk of seizure recurrence after a first unprovoked afebrile seizure in childhood: an extended follow-up. Pediatrics 1996;98:216–25.

71. Stroink H, Brouwer OF, Arts WF, et al. The first unprovoked, untreated seizure in childhood: a hospital based study of the accuracy of the diagnosis, rate of recurrence, and long term outcome after recurrence. Dutch study of epilepsy in childhood. J Neurol Neurosurg Psychiatry 1998;64:595–600.

72. Hirtz D, Berg A, Bettis D, et al. Practice parameter: treatment of the child with a first unprovoked seizure: report of the Quality Standards Subcommittee of the American Academy of Neurology and the Practice Committee of the Child Neurology Society. Neurology 2003;60:166–75.

73. Geerts A, Arts WF, Stroink H, et al. Course and outcome of childhood epilepsy: a 15-year follow-up of the Dutch Study of Epilepsy in Childhood. Epilepsia 2010; 51:1189–97.

74. Roberts MR. Status epilepticus in children. Emeg Med Clin North Am 1995;13: 489–507.

75. Prasad AN, Seshia SS. Status epilepticus in pediatric practice: neonate to adolescent. Adv Neurol 2006;97:229–43.

76. Shinnar S, Pellock JM, Moshe SL, et al. In whom does status epilepticus occur: age-related differences in children. Epilepsia 1997;38:907–14.

77. Haafiz A, Kissoon N. Status epilepticus: current concepts. Pediatr Emerg Care 1999;15:119–29.

78. Lewena S, Pennington V, Acworth K, et al. Emergency management of pediatric convulsive status epilepticus. Pediatr Emerg Care 2009;25:83–7.

79. DeLorenzo RJ, Towne AR, Pellock JM, et al. Status epilepticus in children, adults, and the elderly. Epilepsia 1992;33(Suppl 4):S15–25.

80. Maytal J, Shinnar S, Moshe SL, et al. Low morbidity and mortality of status epilepticus in children. Pediatrics 1989;83:323–31.
81. Raspall-Chaure M, Chin RF, Neville BG, et al. Outcome of paediatric convulsive status epilepticus: a systematic review. Lancet Neurol 2006;5:769–79.
82. Shinnar S, Berg AT, Moshe SL, et al. How long do new onset seizures in children last? Ann Neurol 2001;49:659–64.
83. Huff JS, Fountain NB. Pathophysiology and definitions of seizures and status epilepticus. Emerg Med Clin North Am 2011;29:1–13.
84. Michael GE, O'Connor RE. The diagnosis and management of seizures and status epilepticus in the prehospital setting. Emerg Med Clin North Am 2011;29:29–39.
85. Roy H, Lippe S, Lussier F, et al. Developmental outcome after a single episode of status epilepticus. Epilepsy Behav 2011;21:430–6.
86. Chin RF, Neville BG, Peckham C, et al. Treatment of community-onset, childhood convulsive status epilepticus: a prospective, population-based study. Lancet Neurol 2008;7:696–703.
87. Hesdorffer DC, Benn EK, Bagiella E, et al. Distribution of febrile seizure duration and associations with development. Ann Neurol 2011;70:93–100.
88. Anderson M. Benzodiazepines for prolonged seizures. Arch Dis Child Educ Pract Ed 2010;95:183–9.
89. Chiang LM, Wang HS, Shen HH, et al. Rectal diazepam solution is as good as rectal administration of intravenous diazepam in the first-aid cessation of seizures in children with intractable epilepsy. Pediatr Neonatol 2011;52:30–3.
90. Wolfe TR, Macfarlane TC. Intranasal midazolam therapy for pediatric status epilepticus. Am J Emerg Med 2006;24:343–6.
91. Scott RC, Besag FM, Neville BG. Buccal midazolam and rectal diazepam for treatment of prolonged seizures in childhood and adolescence: a randomised trial. Lancet 1999;353:623–6.
92. Nakken KO, Lossius MI. Buccal midazolam or rectal diazepam for treatment of residential adult patients with serial seizures or status epilepticus. Acta Neurol Scand 2011;124:99–103.
93. Ashrafi MR, Khosroshahi N, Karimi P, et al. Efficacy and usability of buccal midazolam in controlling acute prolonged convulsive seizures in children. Eur J Paediatr Neurol 2010;14:434–8.
94. Rainbow J, Browne GJ, Lam LT. Controlling seizures in the prehospital setting: diazepam or midazolam? J Paediatr Child Health 2002;38:582–6.
95. Chamberlain JM, Altieri MA, Futterman C, et al. A prospective, randomized study comparing intramuscular midazolam with intravenous diazepam for the treatment of seizures in children. Pediatr Emerg Care 1997;13:92–4.
96. Fitzgerald BJ, Okos AJ, Miller JW. Treatment of out-of-hospital status epilepticus with diazepam rectal gel. Seizure 2003;12:52–5.
97. Holsti M, Sill BL, Firth SD. Prehospital intranasal midazolam for the treatment of pediatric seizures. Pediatr Emerg Care 2007;23:148–53.
98. MCMullan J, Sasson C, Pancioli A, et al. Midazolam versus diazepam for the treatment of status epilepticus in children and young adults: a meta-analysis. Acad Emerg Med 2010;17:575–82.
99. Appleton R, Macleod S, Martland T. Drug management for acute tonic-clonic convulsions including convulsive status epilepticus in children. Cochrane Database Syst Rev 2008;(3):CD001905.
100. Fischer JH, Patel TV, Fischer PA. Fosphenytoin: clinical pharmacokinetics and comparative advantages in the acute treatment of seizures. Clin Pharmacokinet 2003;42:33–58.

101. Prince NJ, Hill C. Purple glove syndrome following intravenous phenytoin administration. Arch Dis Child 2011;96:734.
102. Foreman B, Hirsch LJ. Epilepsy emergencies: diagnosis and management. Neurol Clin 2012;30:11–41.
103. Bartha AI, Shen J, Katz KH, et al. Neonatal seizures: multicenter variability in current treatment practices. Pediatr Neurol 2007;37:85–90.
104. Yamamoto LG, Yim GK. The role of intravenous valproic acid in status epilepticus. Pediatr Emerg Care 2000;16:296–8.
105. Hovinga CA, Chicella MF, Rose DF. Use of intravenous valproate in three pediatric patients with nonconvulsive or convulsive SE. Ann Pharmacother 1999;33:579–84.
106. Trinka E. The use of valprooate and new antiepileptic drugs in status epilepticus. Epilepsia 2007;48(Suppl 8):49–51.
107. Trinka E. What is the relative value of the standard anticonvulsants: phenytoin and fosphenytoin, phenobarbital, valproate, and levetiracetam? Epilepsia 2009;50(Suppl 12):40–3.
108. Trinka E. What is the evidence to use new intravenous AEDs in status epilepticus? Epilepsia 2011;52(Suppl 8):35–8.
109. Uberall MA, Trollmann R, Wunsiedler U, et al. Intravenous valproate in pediatric epilepsy patients with refractory status epilepticus. Neurology 2000;54:2188–9.
110. Holtkamp M. Treatment strategies for refractory status epilepticus. Curr Opin Crit Care 2011;17:94–100.
111. Shorvon S. The treatment of status epilepticus. Curr Opin Neurol 2011;24:165–70.
112. Verrotti A, D'Adamo E, Parisi P, et al. Levetiracetam in childhood epilepsy. Paediatr Drugs 2010;12:177–86.
113. Misra UK, Kalita J, Maurya PK. Levetiracetam versus lorazepam in status epilepticus: a randomized, open labeled pilot study. J Neurol 2012;259:645–8.
114. Zelano J, Kumlien E. Levetiracetam as alternative stage two antiepileptic drug in status epilepticus: a systematic review. Seizure 2012;21:233–6.
115. Ng YT, Hastriter EV, Cardenas JF, et al. Intravenous levetiracetam in children with seizures: a prospective safety study. J Child Neurol 2010;25:551–5.
116. Fernandez A, Claassen J. Refractory status epilepticus. Curr Opin Crit Care 2012;18:127–31.
117. Lowenstein DH, Alldredge BK. Status epilepticus. N Engl J Med 1998;338:970–6.
118. Akyildiz BN, Kumandas S. Treatment of pediatric refractory status epilepticus with topiramate. Childs Nerv Syst 2011;27:1425–30.
119. Harrison AM, Lugo RA, Schunk JE. Treatment of convulsive status epilepticus with propofol. Pediatr Emerg Care 1997;13:420–2.
120. Hofler J, Unterberger I, Dobesberger J, et al. Intravenous lacosamide in status epilepticus and seizure clusters. Epilepsia 2011;52:e148–52.
121. Walker MC. The potential of brain stimulation in status epilepticus. Epilepsia 2011;52(Suppl 8):61–3.
122. Shorvon S. Super-refractory status epilepticus: an approach to therapy in this difficult clinical situation. Epilepsia 2011;52(Suppl 8):53–6.
123. Galimi R. Nonconvulsive status epilepticus in pediatric populations: diagnosis and management. Minerva Pediatr 2012;64:347–55.
124. Chang AK, Shinnar S. Nonconvulsive status epilepticus. Emerg Med Clin North Am 2011;29:65–72.
125. Greiner HM, Holland K, Leach JL, et al. Nonconvulsive status epilepticus: the encephalopathic pediatric patient. Pediatrics 2012;129:e748–55.

126. Kossoff EH. Intractable childhood epilepsy: choosing between the treatments. Semin Pediatr Neurol 2011;18:145–9.
127. Hirsch LJ, Donner EJ, So EL, et al. Abbreviated report of the NIH/NINDS workshop on sudden unexpected death in epilepsy. Neurology 2011;76:1932–8.
128. Shorvon S, Tomson T. Sudden unexpected death in epilepsy. Lancet 2011;378: 2028–38.
129. Duncan S, Brodie MJ. Sudden unexpected death in epilepsy. Epilepsy Behav 2011;21:344–51.
130. Kotagal P. Neurostimulation: vagus nerve stimulation and beyond. Semin Pediatr Neurol 2011;18:186–94.
131. Englot DJ, Chang EF, Auguste KI. Efficacy of vagus nerve stimulation for epilepsy by patient age, epilepsy duration, and seizure type. Neurosurg Clin N Am 2011;22:443–8.
132. Levy RG, Cooper PN, Giri P. Ketogenic diet and other dietary treatments for epilepsy. Cochrane Database Syst Rev 2012;(3):CD001903.
133. Jarrar RG, Buchhalter JR. Therapeutics in pediatric epilepsy, Part 1: the new antiepileptic drugs and the ketogenic diet. Mayo Clin Proc 2003;78:359–70.
134. Rubenstein JE, Kossoff EH, Pyzik PL, et al. Experience in the use of the ketogenic diet as early therapy. J Child Neurol 2005;20:31–4.
135. Fisher RS. Therapeutic devices for epilepsy. Ann Neurol 2012;71:157–68.
136. Caraballo R, Bartuluchi M, Cersosimo R, et al. Hemispherectomy in pediatric patients with epilepsy: a study of 45 cases with special emphasis on epileptic syndromes. Childs Nerv Syst 2011;27:2131–6.
137. Widjaja E, Li B, Schinkel CD, et al. Cost-effectiveness of pediatric epilepsy surgery compared to medical treatment in children with intractable epilepsy. Epilepsy Res 2011;94:61–8.
138. Nair PP, Kalita J, Misra UK. Status epilepticus: why, what, and how. J Postgrad Med 2011;57:242–52.
139. Verrotti A, Nanni G, Agostinelli S, et al. Benign convulsions associated with mild gastroenteritis: a multicenter clinical study. Epilepsy Res 2011;93:107–14.
140. Tanabe T, Okumura A, Komatsu M, et al. Clinical trial of minimal treatment for clustering seizures in cases of convulsions with mild gastroenteritis. Brain Dev 2011;33:120–4.
141. Khan WA, Dhar U, Salam MA, et al. Central nervous system manifestations of childhood shigellosis: prevalence, risk factors, and outcome. Pediatrics 1999; 103:E18.
142. Shneker BF, Fountain NB. Epilepsy. Dis Mon 2003;49:426–78.
143. Vining EP. Pediatric seizures. Emerg Med Clin North Am 1994;12:973–88.
144. Hancock EC, Osborne JP, Edwards SW. Treatment of infantile spasms. Cochrane Database Syst Rev 2008;(4):CD001770.
145. Trevathan E. Infantile spasms and Lennox-Gastaut syndrome. J Child Neurol 2002;17(Suppl 2):2S9–22.

Diabetic Ketoacidosis in the Pediatric Emergency Department

Laura Olivieri, MD[a], Rose Chasm, MD[b,c,*]

KEYWORDS

- Diabetic ketoacidosis • Cerebral edema • Fluid resuscitation • Insulin

KEY POINTS

- Despite advances in research and treatment, the incidence of pediatric-onset diabetes and diabetic ketoacidosis is increasing.
- Diabetes mellitus is one of the most common chronic pediatric illnesses and, along with diabetic ketoacidosis, is associated with significant cost and morbidity.
- DKA is a complicated metabolic state hallmarked by dehydration and electrolyte disturbances. Treatment involves proper fluid resuscitation with insulin and electrolyte replacement under constant monitoring for cerebral edema, which is the deadliest complication.
- When DKA is recognized and treated immediately, the prognosis is excellent. However, when a patient has prolonged or multiple courses of DKA or if DKA is complicated by cerebral edema, the results can be devastating.

INTRODUCTION

Diabetes mellitus is one of the most common chronic diseases among children and adolescents worldwide. Over the past 20 years, the incidence of type 2 diabetes (formerly known as adult-onset diabetes) has increased among children in the United States.[1] European studies have demonstrated an increased frequency of type 1 diabetes in children and adolescents.

A major complication of diabetes, diabetic ketoacidosis (DKA), is characterized by the metabolic triad of hyperglycemia, anion gap metabolic acidosis, and ketonemia that develops from an absolute or relative insulin deficiency and excess of counter-regulatory hormone. DKA results in dehydration and electrolyte derangements. This

[a] Department of Emergency Medicine, University of Maryland Medical Center, 110 South Paca Street, 6th Floor, Suite 200, Baltimore, MD 21201, USA; [b] Combined Emergency Medicine/Pediatrics Residency, Department of Emergency Medicine, University of Maryland School of Medicine, 110 South Paca Street, 6th Floor, Suite 200, Baltimore, MD 21201, USA; [c] Pediatric Quality Assurance and Risk Management, University of Maryland Emergency Medicine Network, Baltimore, MD, USA
* Corresponding author. 110 South Paca Street, 6th Floor, Suite 200, Baltimore, MD 21201.
E-mail address: rchas001@umaryland.edu

Emerg Med Clin N Am 31 (2013) 755–773
http://dx.doi.org/10.1016/j.emc.2013.05.004
0733-8627/13/$ – see front matter © 2013 Elsevier Inc. All rights reserved.

combination, along with the major complication of cerebral edema, is the most important cause of morbidity and mortality among children with DKA. The mainstay of therapy is rehydration with intravenous (IV) fluids, insulin, and potassium repletion, as needed. Bicarbonate therapy is rarely, if ever, indicated and can lead to complications.

EPIDEMIOLOGY

In 2010, the Centers for Disease Control and Prevention estimated that 215,000 Americans younger than 20 years of age were diabetic.[1] Despite significant advances in diabetes management, the incidence of DKA and diabetes complications remains high, probably as a result of the alarming increase in childhood obesity and its direct link to diabetes. The incidence of DKA at the time diabetes is diagnosed varies by geographic location, ranging from 12% to 80%; approximately one-third of type 1 diabetics have DKA at the time of diagnosis.[2–5] Young children, especially those younger than 5 years of age, are at high risk for DKA. The severity of DKA is also inversely related to age,[6] placing the youngest children at the greatest risk. Other factors that increase the likelihood of DKA at the time of diagnosis of diabetes include ethnic minority status, lack of health insurance, lower body mass index, missed diagnosis at previous health care visits, delayed treatment, and preceding infection.[6] The incidence of DKA among established diabetics is 25%.[7]

Type 2 diabetes is becoming increasingly common among children as a result of obesity.[8] DKA also occurs in type 2 diabetics; 5% to 25% of type 2 diabetics present with DKA at the time of diagnosis.[3,9] In a study of type 1 and type 2 diabetics, the most common cause of DKA was insulin omission, especially in type 1 diabetics. Although less common overall, infection is more often associated with DKA in type 2 diabetics. Although acidosis tends to be more severe in type 1 diabetics, type 2 diabetics require a longer duration of insulin infusion to achieve ketone-free urine, possibly because of underlying insulin resistance.[10]

DKA is associated with significant cost and morbidity.[11] In the United States, the average cost for a hospitalization is $13,000, yielding annual hospital costs exceeding $1 billion.[12] Although the mortality rate associated with DKA is less than 1%, this imbalance accounts for most diabetes-related deaths in children,[13] most of which result from cerebral edema that progresses to brain herniation. Cerebral edema, a rare and devastating complication of DKA, is clinically apparent in 1% to 5% of patients with DKA.[2,14,15] Mortality rates ranging from 20% to 90% have been reported.[15–17] A large proportion of survivors, up to 26%, experience permanent neurologic deficits.[16] Studies have also demonstrated risks of long-term memory dysfunction in children who experienced DKA without cerebral edema.[18]

PATHOPHYSIOLOGY

Insulin is the primary hormone of blood glucose regulation. It is responsible for increasing peripheral glucose uptake and stopping hepatic gluconeogenesis. As blood glucose levels increase, counter-regulatory hormones (glucagon, catecholamines, cortisol, and growth hormone) play reciprocal roles with insulin in attempts to maintain glucose homeostasis. DKA results from an absolute or relative deficiency of insulin and the resulting excess of counter-regulatory hormones. Absolute insulin deficiency occurs in new-onset type 1 diabetes as a result of pancreatic β-cell failure and in established diabetes as a result of insulin omission or insulin pump failure. Relative insulin deficiency can be attributable to insulin resistance or inadequate insulin dosing to balance the increased counter-regulatory hormone levels present during infection, trauma, or other physiologic stressors. Medications such as high-dose glucocorticoids, atypical antipsychotics,[19–21] and immunosuppressive drugs can also trigger DKA.[22,23]

Insulin deficiency leads to impaired glucose uptake and use by tissues. Counter-regulatory hormone excess leads to increased glycogenolysis, gluconeogenesis, proteolysis (which creates more substrates for gluconeogenesis), and lipolysis. Lipolysis generates free fatty acids, which normally undergo β-oxidation to generate acetyl coenzyme A, an entry molecule for the citric acid cycle. In the absence of insulin, the significant lipolysis and fatty acid burden is diverted toward ketogenesis instead. The two main ketones produced are acetoacetate and β-hydroxybutyrate, which dissociate fully at physiologic pH.[24] Acetone is the least abundant product of ketogenesis but does not contribute to acidosis, as it does not dissociate to yield hydrogen ions. It is metabolized through the lung and produces the fruity breath characteristic of DKA. The ratio of β-hydroxybutyrate to acetoacetate, normally 1:1, increases to as high as 10:1 in DKA.[24] Although ketones are weak acids, their severe overproduction overwhelms the buffering capacity of the body, which leads to an anion gap metabolic acidosis. Lactic acidosis and renal dysfunction caused by prerenal azotemia and dehydration may also contribute to acidosis. Respiratory compensation for this acidosis results in the classic shallow rapid breathing (Kussmaul respirations).

Dehydration is a significant consequence of DKA and has several causes. Decreased glucose uptake and increased glucose production via glycogenolysis and gluconeogenesis lead to hyperglycemia, causing extracellular fluid and electrolyte shifts. An osmotic diuresis results when serum glucose levels increase above the renal threshold for glucose reabsorption. This causes free water, glucose, and electrolytes to be lost in urine. Ketone-induced nausea and vomiting, along with the insensible losses associated with Kussmaul respirations, compound fluid losses.

Multiple electrolyte abnormalities occur in the setting of DKA. Sodium, potassium, chloride, phosphorus, calcium, and magnesium are all affected. The most significant and imminently life-threatening electrolyte imbalance is hypokalemia. Potassium shifts out of the cells because of insulin deficiency and the exchange of hydrogen ions to compensate for acidosis. This can cause the serum potassium level to be normal or even increased, despite the total body depletion of potassium that results from osmotic diuresis, gastrointestinal losses, and volume depletion. Under these conditions, the renin-angiotensin-aldosterone system is activated, exacerbating renal potassium excretion via urine.

CLINICAL PRESENTATION

DKA can develop quickly in patients with established diabetes, especially when it is related to insulin omission. However, when DKA acts as the first presentation of diabetes, the symptoms emerge over several days. Typical symptoms are the classic triad of polyuria, polydipsia, and weight loss with or without polyphagia. These symptoms are easy to miss in children who are wearing diapers and being fed by multiple caretakers. Abdominal pain, nausea, and vomiting are also common complaints. Dehydration and electrolyte derangements can lead to muscle pains and cramping. The abdominal pain can mimic an acute abdomen. It can also be an indication of an underlying cause, so further evaluation is warranted if the pain does not resolve with hydration and resolution of ketoacidosis.[12] Persistent candidal infections or new-onset enuresis should raise suspicion for diabetes or DKA. Late findings include changes in mental status, Kussmaul respirations, and fruity, sweet, ketotic breath. Because the presentation of DKA may vary and be subtle in children who may not have an established diagnosis of diabetes or be able to communicate their complaints verbally, a high degree of suspicion is needed to diagnose DKA in the pediatric population.

Complaints of headache or changes in mental status are worrisome as indications of cerebral edema. Focal neurologic deficits can also be seen. Hemodynamic instability and shock are rare in children with DKA, but patients are often dehydrated to varying degrees as a result of fluid shifts, osmotic diuresis, gastrointestinal losses, and insensible losses (see section on assessing dehydration).

DIAGNOSIS

The biochemical criteria for DKA are as follows[12,25–27]:

- Hyperglycemia with blood glucose concentration greater than 200 mg/dL (>11 mmol/L)
- Venous pH less than 7.3 or bicarbonate concentration less than 15 mmol/L
- Ketonuria and ketonemia

The severity of DKA can be categorized as follows[12,25–27]:

- Mild: venous pH less than 7.3, HCO_3 less than 15 mmol/L
- Moderate: venous pH less than 7.2, HCO_3 less than 10 mmol/L
- Severe: venous pH less than 7.1, HCO_3 less than 5 mmol/L

The basic initial diagnostic tests that should be obtained in all patients suspected of having DKA are listed in **Box 1**. Although hypotension is not common in

---

Box 1
Initial diagnostic workup of all patients with DKA

- Vital signs
- Weight
- Capillary blood glucose
- Electrocardiogram
- Serum chemistry
  - Glucose
  - Sodium
  - Potassium
  - Chloride
  - Blood urea nitrogen
  - Creatinine
  - Calcium
  - Magnesium
  - Phosphorus
- Complete blood count
- Venous blood gas
- β-Hydroxybutyrate or urine ketones (see section on ketone testing)

straightforward DKA, tachycardia is. Fever may occur in the setting of infection but is not caused by DKA inherently. Tachypnea is present in later compensatory stages of DKA. It is imperative to weigh all patients so that accurate medication and fluid doses can be calculated.

The measurement of glucose levels in capillary blood samples with bedside meters provides information immediately and is adequate for monitoring changes during treatment. Values should be obtained at least every hour during acute management.

An electrocardiogram must be obtained if potassium measurement is not available immediately, such as via point-of-care testing, as early detection of arrhythmogenic electrolyte imbalances is crucial.[28] U waves are suggestive of hypokalemia, whereas short QT intervals and peaked T waves may progress to prolonged PR intervals, widened QRS complexes, or a sine wave pattern in hyperkalemia.[29]

The complete blood count might show leukocytosis, which is not specific for infection in the setting of DKA[3] and could be related to dehydration. An infectious workup should be initiated if the patient has a history of fever or other suggestive symptoms.

Serum chemistry is obtained for both the individual electrolyte values and to perform the calculations listed in **Box 2**. The serum sodium concentration is corrected to account for the dilutional effect of the degree of hyperglycemia. The anion gap, however, is calculated using the measured serum sodium level rather than a corrected sodium level because glucose is electrically neutral and does not contribute to the anion gap. The anion gap is determined by negatively charged ions and proteins such as albumin. Therefore, in the setting of albumin deficiency, the anion gap should be corrected, assuming a normal serum albumin concentration of 4 g/dL and an expected reduction in the anion gap by 2.5 mEq/L for every 1 g/dL decrease in serum albumin. Albumin levels should be obtained if there is a concern about nephrotic syndrome or severe malnutrition but not necessarily in a previously healthy child.

Venous Blood Gas Analysis

It is well established that venous and arterial pH are well correlated in DKA.[30] Consensus guidelines for management now include venous pH, rather than arterial pH, as part of the biochemical definition of DKA. This eliminates the added risk of pain, hemorrhage, fistula formation, thrombosis, and infection when obtaining a sample for analysis of arterial blood gases.[31] Although arterial blood gases used to be considered essential in the diagnosis of DKA, they have not been found to influence decision making in the emergency department when treating patients with DKA.[32] Based on various studies, the mean difference between arterial and venous pH ranges from 0.015 to 0.05, and venous pH accurately measures the degree of acidosis in adult patients with DKA.[30,32,33] Subtle differences are not likely to be clinically significant. However, it can be difficult to identify mixed acid-base disturbances, thus arterial blood gas analysis may be indicated in certain cases.[30]

Box 2
Calculations using serum chemistry

Corrected sodium = serum sodium + 1.6 × [(serum glucose in mg/dL − 100)/100]

Anion gap = serum sodium − (serum chloride + serum bicarbonate)

Anion gap corrected for albumin = anion gap − 2.5 × (4 − serum albumin in g/dL)

Consensus statements recommend measuring both bicarbonate and pH from venous blood. However, venous blood gas (VBG) analysis is not readily available in all treatment settings, requires extra blood to be drawn, and incurs extra cost. A recent comparison of pH and serum bicarbonate levels in 300 children with diagnosed DKA confirmed excellent correlation between the 2 measures.[34] In addition, the ketoacids present in DKA increase the number of unmeasured anions, resulting in an anion gap metabolic acidosis. Therefore, the anion gap and serum bicarbonate can be used to monitor DKA if VBG analysis is unavailable.

VBG electrolyte testing is a newer aspect of DKA diagnosis and monitoring that may allow the rapid assessment of essential data in a single test. Menchine and colleagues's[35] prospective observational study investigating the diagnostic accuracy of VBG electrolytes in hyperglycemic adults, including sodium, chloride, and bicarbonate, showed 97.8% sensitivity and 100% specificity in diagnosing DKA, suggesting that this method could supplant serum electrolytes in addition to VBG analysis. However, Fu and colleagues[36] showed a difference between VBG potassium and serum potassium levels ranging from 0.9 to 2.9 mmol/L, and 20% of the sample pairs had a difference greater than 0.5 mmol/L, which was the maximum clinically acceptable difference predetermined before the study by surveying 15 physicians. Given the lack of substantial data and the possible inconsistency of the VBG potassium readings, further testing is necessary before VBG can be recommended as an alternative to testing serum for electrolytes.

Ketone Testing

Although β-hydroxybutyrate is the predominant ketone produced in DKA, urine and serum ketone assays typically use the nitroprusside reaction, which detects only acetone and acetoacetate and is semiquantitative using dilutions. During treatment with insulin therapy, β-hydroxybutyrate is oxidized to acetoacetate, causing β-hydroxybutyrate levels to decrease before acetoacetate levels. A ketone assay may give the false impression that the patient is not improving, when, actually, the overall quantity of ketones has decreased. Therefore, when interpreting ketone tests, both the time delay before the development of ketonemia and ketonuria must be considered in diagnosing DKA as well as the earlier clearance of β-hydroxybutyrate rather than urine ketones alone.[24,37] Furthermore, urine ketone testing is affected by hydration status and urine stagnation in the bladder, and false-positive results can be encountered if patients are taking captopril, penicillamine, N-acetylcysteine, mesna, dimercaprol, or isopropyl alcohol.[38] To more precisely measure ketone burden, a quantitative serum β-hydroxybutyrate test should be used.[12,24,27]

The use of β-hydroxybutyrate testing has been proposed as an end point to monitor resolution of ketosis and direct insulin infusion therapy.[27,37,39] Compared with urine ketone testing, serum β-hydroxybutyrate-guided DKA treatment has been associated with shorter intensive care unit (ICU) and hospital stays as well as decreased costs.[39] However, because serum β-hydroxybutyrate assays are not available at all institutions, the anion gap, pH, or bicarbonate can be used to direct DKA treatment.

An additional laboratory study that can benefit inpatient and especially outpatient diabetes management is hemoglobin A1C testing. Although it does not necessarily change emergency department management, it can provide valuable information regarding the chronicity and severity of hyperglycemia in all patients and overall glycemic control in established diabetics if increased, and acuity in well-controlled patients if close to normal limits.

EMERGENCY DEPARTMENT MANAGEMENT

Current practice guidelines are based on both evidence and consensus recommendations. First and foremost, pediatric resuscitation principles should be followed. Airway, breathing, and circulation should be secured. Intravenous access must be obtained. Aspiration precautions should be taken if the patient has an altered level of consciousness. Continuous cardiac monitoring and pulse oximetry are imperative to assess for arrhythmias secondary to hyperkalemia or hypokalemia and to ensure adequate oxygenation. Frequent neurologic monitoring is also warranted. The best outcomes are achieved when children are monitored closely and continuously, with prompt attention to any changes.[40]

Additional hourly monitoring should include vital signs, neurologic checks, blood glucose, and accurate fluid intake and output. Frequent neurologic checks are particularly important in patients at greater risk for cerebral edema, such as those with new-onset diabetes, patients younger than 5 years old, and patients with greater degrees of acidosis, hypocapnia, or azotemia.[14–16] Capillary blood glucose levels should be confirmed with laboratory venous values. Initially, VBGs and chemistries should be checked every 2 hours, but depending on those initial values, may require more frequent monitoring. As previously mentioned, ketone testing should not guide treatment. The serum β-hydroxybutyrate concentration is ideal for monitoring progress; if that reading is not available, anion gap, pH, and bicarbonate can also be used as end points.

Specific aspects of DKA management are as follows[27]:

- Fluid resuscitation to rehydrate and improve tissue perfusion and glomerular filtration rate
- Correction of ketoacidosis and hyperglycemia via inhibition of lipolysis and ketogenesis with insulin
- Restoration of electrolyte balance
- Avoidance of complications, specifically cerebral edema

Fluids

Intravenous fluids are administered for resuscitation and rehydration as well as to decrease the blood glucose level by improving the glomerular filtration rate and, thus, glucose and ketone clearance. Although adults tend to present with large volume deficits requiring aggressive fluid repletion, a more restrictive strategy must be used in the pediatric setting to avoid potential complications. The initial resuscitation of a pediatric patient in DKA calls for administration of an isotonic crystalloid solution as a bolus of 10 to 20 mL/kg over 1 to 2 hours. The dose can be repeated if the patient is hemodynamically unstable.[12,25–27] Children rarely present in hypovolemic shock caused by DKA alone. If a child does not respond to the initial resuscitation bolus, search for other causes of shock. To avoid increasing the risk of cerebral edema and herniation, resuscitation volumes should not exceed 40 to 50 mL/kg during the first 4 hours of treatment, unless the patient is in shock.[12,17,41]

After the initial bolus of IV fluid, the goal of rehydration is to administer the remainder of replacement fluids evenly over 24 to 48 hours with 0.45% to 0.9% saline.[25] Overzealous fluid resuscitation could lead to further complications, particularly cerebral edema,[41,42] although no data have demonstrated increased safety with rehydration over 48 hours. The rate of total fluid administration includes maintenance plus replacement of the fluid deficit based on the patient's estimated degree of dehydration (see section on degree of dehydration) and should not exceed 2 times the maintenance volume. Fluids that were administered before arrival should be accounted for in these calculations, but urinary losses should not.

Weight-based 24-hour maintenance fluid requirements can be calculated as follows[43]:

- 100 mL/kg for the first 10 kg of body weight
- 50 mL/kg for the second 10 kg of body weight
- 20 mL/kg for each kilogram above 20 kg of body weight

Using the 4-2-1 rule, the requirements can be estimated as follows:

- 100 mL/kg/24 h = 4 mL/kg/h for the first 10 kg of body weight
- 50 mL/kg/24 h = 2 mL/kg/h for the second 10 kg of body weight
- 20 mL/kg/24 h = 1 mL/kg/h for each kilogram above 20 kg of body weight

Fluid type

Normal saline (0.9% NaCl) is commonly used as the replacement fluid for patients with DKA and can be switched to half normal saline (0.45% NaCl) once the corrected sodium concentration normalizes (see section on sodium). There is no evidence supporting the use of solutions with tonicity lower than 0.45% NaCl, which can lead to rapid osmolar changes and intracellular movement of fluid,[25] or colloids.

Recent evidence implicates the administration of large volumes of saline in the development of hyperchloremia with a nongap metabolic acidosis,[44,45] which increases with treatment duration and can mask the resolution of DKA if base deficit alone is being monitored as an end point for treatment. The clinical significance of hyperchloremia with acidosis is unclear, but concerns about possible deleterious effects from excessive saline administration have raised controversy with respect to fluid choice. A small blinded, randomized controlled trial failed to show any difference in time to normalization of pH and resolution of DKA between patients resuscitated using normal saline and others who received Ringer's lactate.[46] Recent literature comparing non–calcium-containing balanced crystalloid such as Plasma-Lyte (Plasma-Lyte 148 or Plasma-Lyte A, Baxter Healthcare, Deerfield, IL) with normal saline administration to patients with DKA reported lower serum chloride levels and higher bicarbonate concentrations after resuscitation in the Plasma-Lyte group, consistent with prevention of hyperchloremia and acidosis.[47] The effect of these changes on outcome and mortality rate is unknown. Chua and colleagues[48] attained similar results, that is, faster resolution of acidosis in the first 12 hours of treatment with Plasma-Lyte and stable chloride levels. They reported no difference in the rate of resolution of hyperglycemia, the duration or total dose of IV insulin administration, or length of ICU stay. Further investigation is needed to determine whether the administration of a saline solution to patients with DKA carries any clinically significant risks; there is no evidence of associated morbidity. Currently, the use of saline remains the standard of care.

Rate of rehydration

Because of conflicting theories on the underlying mechanism of cerebral edema in patients with DKA, arguments for both slower and faster rehydration have been put forth. If cerebral edema results from osmotic changes or vasogenic edema associated with a compromised blood-brain barrier, slower rehydration might limit edema. On the other hand, if ischemia and hypoperfusion are the major insults to the brain, then more rapid rehydration could rectify the problem sooner and prevent ischemia when intracellular fluid shifts during treatment with insulin.[15]

Unfortunately, little evidence is available to definitively guide the rapidity of fluid therapy. The large, multicenter Pediatric Emergency Care Applied Research Network (PECARN) trial is investigating the impact of the administration of 0.9% versus 0.45% normal saline at 2 rates on short-term and long-term neurologic outcome,[49] which might clarify the role and implications of fluid resuscitation.

Degree of dehydration

The clinical assessment of dehydration is obfuscated by multiple factors. Although previous studies of nonacidotic children demonstrated the usefulness of multiple physical examination signs, such as reduced skin turgor, increased capillary refill time, dry tongue, and sunken eyes or fontanelle, in assessing degree of dehydration,[50,51] none of these parameters have been found to be accurate predictors of hydration status in DKA because they might not reflect only fluid losses.[50] Acidosis can make a child seem more dehydrated because of the tachypnea of Kussmaul respirations, which results in dry mucous membranes, and vasoconstriction, which leads to cooler extremities.[52,53] The ongoing lipolysis, proteolysis, and weight loss caused by insulin deficiency[50] can also make a child seem clinically more dehydrated. On the other hand, hyperosmolarity tends to preserve intravascular volume (and thus pulses, blood pressure, and urine output) until extreme volume depletion and shock occur.[53,54] Therefore, physical examination findings are often unreliable in estimating dehydration in the setting of DKA.

Historically, children were assumed to be 10% dehydrated at presentation[55] unless they were hemodynamically unstable. Because of concerns about an increased risk of cerebral edema with rapid fluid administration, it has been suggested to assume 5% to 8% dehydration.[56] More recent guidelines advise stratifying the degree of dehydration based on the severity of DKA, estimating 5% to 7% dehydration in moderate DKA and 7% to 10% dehydration in severe DKA.[27]

Multiple prospective studies based on percent loss of body weight (PLBW), calculated by the difference between initial and discharge weight as a percentage of the discharge weight, have shown that the degree of dehydration cannot be predicted clinically.[50,52–54] Using PLBW as a surrogate marker for dehydration, several groups of investigators[50,52,53] have reported median dehydration percentages of 5% to 8%.[50,52,53] Up to 70% of patients were assessed incorrectly; some were overestimated and some underestimated. Ugale and colleagues[53] showed that, although 60% of their study patients presented with severe DKA, their median dehydration was 5.4%. No significant difference was found in the measured degree of dehydration between severity groups, suggesting that patients with severe acidosis are not necessarily more dehydrated than other patients with DKA. Based on the available data, it might be excessive to estimate up to 10% dehydration in patients. Administration of maintenance fluids, based on an assumed 6% deficit, seems more reasonable.

The two-bag system

Because of rapid fluctuations in fluid, electrolyte, and dextrose requirements, patients with DKA require frequent adjustments in fluid and insulin administration. The two-bag system was introduced in the 1990s[57] to facilitate these changes. This system consists of two bags of fluids with identical electrolyte content but different dextrose concentrations (0% and 10%) that are administered simultaneously into the same IV line.

The rate of fluid delivery is determined by the degree of dehydration and individual patient needs, whereas the concentration of dextrose depends on the patient's serum glucose level and its rate of decline during treatment. These factors can be manipulated independently, as different proportions of fluid from each bag are administered.

Initially, no dextrose is given; as hyperglycemia resolves with the infusion of insulin, dextrose is titrated up to control the rate of decrease in blood glucose while continuing the insulin infusion. The IV fluids can therefore be customized to meet the patient's individual glucose, fluid, and insulin needs by creating a fluid dextrose concentration that ranges between 0% and 10% to control the rate of blood glucose decline and prevent hypoglycemia.[58]

Koul[59] described a system of fluids and concentrations to be given based on different serum glucose values:

- If greater than 250 mg/dL (13.8 mmol/L), give normal saline (NS) alone
- If less than 250 mg/dL (13.8 mmol/L), give half of the rate from each bag to make 5% dextrose (D5) NS
- If less than 150 mg/dL (8.33 mmol/L), give 10% dextrose (D10) NS alone at a predetermined rate

Studies have shown multiple advantages to the two-bag system. Rather than changing an individual IV fluid bag each time the dextrose concentration needs to be adjusted during correction of hyperglycemia and acidosis, which can take more than 30 minutes, the two-bag system allows rapid transitioning of fluids when necessary, taking as little as one minute.[58] Based on the billing system in the late 1990s, the two-bag system cost approximately $500 less per DKA admission than the one-bag system, because of the reduction in the number of IV fluid bags required.[57] More recent data have shown a faster rate of bicarbonate and ketone correction with the two-bag system compared with the one-bag system[60]; the significance of this observation requires further study.

The two-bag system is superior to the single-bag system with respect to flexibility, timeliness, and cost-effectiveness. The rate and dextrose concentration of the fluids can be adjusted independently, and the dextrose concentration can be changed quickly in response to updated serum glucose levels without discarding partially used bags of fluids. Studies have not yet demonstrated clinical benefit, but the two-bag system does not increase the risk of complications from DKA[57,58] and could have clinical benefits in addition to its more practical advantages (**Table 1**).

Insulin

Rehydration alone can decrease the blood glucose concentration, but insulin is required to suppress the lipolysis and ketogenesis that drive DKA. Insulin therapy is initiated after volume resuscitation has been started[27,41] and after the serum

Table 1		
Differential rates and dextrose concentrations made possible by the 2-bag system		
Bag A	Bag B	Overall Composition and Rate of Administration
100 mL/h NS +	0 mL/h D10 NS =	NS at 100 mL/h
90 mL/h NS +	10 mL/h D10 NS =	D1 NS at 100 mL/h
80 mL/h NS +	20 mL/h D10 NS =	D2 NS at 100 mL/h
75 mL/h NS +	25 mL/h D10 NS =	D2.5 NS at 100 mL/h
50 mL/h NS +	50 mL/h D10 NS =	D5 NS at 100 mL/h
40 mL/h NS +	40 mL/h D10 NS =	D5 NS at 80 mL/h
20 mL/h NS +	60 mL/h D10 NS =	D7.5 NS at 80 mL/h
0 mL/h NS +	100 mL/h D10 NS =	D10 NS at 100 mL/h

potassium level is known. Low-dose insulin is the standard of care. Start and maintain a low-dose regular insulin IV infusion at 0.1 units/kg/h and continue until the ketoacidosis resolves or until the anion gap closes. Although still a point of contention in the management of adults with DKA, an initial bolus of insulin is not necessary in pediatric patients[61] and may even be harmful by predisposing patients to hypoglycemia and increasing the risk of cerebral edema.[41,62] Theoretically, rapid correction of hyperglycemia may shift osmolarity and lead to cerebral complications, but the rate of glucose correction has not been shown to increase the risk of cerebral edema or brainstem herniation.[15,17]

Hyperglycemia usually resolves before the acidemia, but the insulin infusion must be continued to achieve full resolution of the ketoacidosis (pH >7.3, bicarbonate >15 mmol/L, β-hydroxybutyrate <1 mmol/L, and/or closure of the anion gap). The target serum glucose level during treatment is approximately 200 mg/dL. To avoid hypoglycemia during insulin infusion, dextrose should be added to IV fluids when the blood glucose concentration reaches 250 to 300 mg/dL (14 17 mmol/L)[25] or if the decline in the blood glucose level exceeds 100 mg/dL/h (5.6 mmol/L/h).[27] This practice is facilitated by the two-bag fluid system as described earlier. If hypoglycemia occurs on the maximum dextrose concentration of D10, then lower the insulin drip to no less than 0.05 units/kg/h,[63] as rates less than this can prevent full resolution of the ketoacidosis.

The transition from intravenous to subcutaneous insulin should occur after ketoacidosis resolves. Subcutaneous insulin is given at least 30 minutes before discontinuing the insulin infusion to allow time for absorption and prevent rebound hyperglycemia. The patient must be able to tolerate oral fluids and should begin to eat at that time.

End points used to determine the transition from intravenous to subcutaneous insulin vary, mainly because no evidence-based guidelines have been established. Using a pH of 7.3 as a signal to make the transition might be inadequate, as patients have been found to be ketotic at this pH.[37] Vanelli and colleagues[39] used normalization of the β-hydroxybutyrate concentration as the signal to change the route of administration and reported financial savings and patient benefit stemming from a shorter ICU stay.

Route of administration

Intravenous insulin is indicated for patients with type 1 diabetes and moderate to severe DKA (pH <7.2 and bicarbonate <10 mmol/L). Mild DKA (pH 7.2–7.3 and bicarbonate 10–15 mmol/L) can be treated with either subcutaneous or IV insulin, depending on the clinical situation.[26] If it is not possible to give an IV insulin infusion, insulin therapy can be given as subcutaneous or intramuscular injections of short-acting or rapid-acting insulin analogues, such as lispro or aspart. As with the IV insulin infusion, to maintain a goal blood glucose level of approximately 200 mg/dL, D5 should be added to the IV fluid when the blood glucose concentration decreases to less than 250 mg/dL (14 mmol/L) and the ketoacidosis has not resolved. Several studies have compared different dosages and schedules.[64,65] Although the data thus far seem to support the use of subcutaneous insulin as an alternative mode of DKA treatment that would not require ICU level care, further studies must be done to clarify subcutaneous insulin dosing and schedule.

Sodium

The corrected sodium concentration should be calculated and monitored and should increase with treatment. A failure of the serum sodium level to increase or a decrease in the level despite treatment is associated with an increased risk of cerebral edema.[15,66] In this situation, the sodium content of the fluid being administered may need to be increased.

Potassium

As previously mentioned, despite total body potassium depletion, serum potassium levels might be normal or even increased in response to transcellular shifts resulting from insulin deficiency and acidosis. Potassium levels quickly decrease with insulin therapy; therefore, to prevent fatal arrhythmias secondary to severe hypokalemia, insulin should not be given until an initial potassium level is obtained.[12,25,26,67] If the serum potassium concentration cannot be measured immediately, an electrocardiogram should be obtained to assess for signs of hyperkalemia or hypokalemia.

Potassium needs to be replaced depending on the initial serum concentration. The level must be checked at least hourly. If the initial serum potassium level is increased, give insulin without supplemental potassium until the patient's ability to urinate is ensured. If the initial serum potassium level is normal, give potassium (40 mEq/L) with IV fluids when insulin administration is started. If the initial serum potassium level is low, replete potassium when beginning volume resuscitation and before initiating insulin. Intravenous potassium administration should not exceed a rate of 0.5 mEq/kg/h. If the serum potassium level remains low despite supplementation during insulin infusion, consider adding oral potassium supplementation or slightly decreasing the insulin infusion rate.

Potassium can be given as potassium chloride, potassium phosphate, or potassium acetate. To avoid administering excess chloride and exacerbating hyperchloremia associated with saline administration, potassium can be replenished with half potassium phosphate and half potassium chloride or acetate, as long as serum calcium levels are monitored to avoid hypocalcemia resulting from phosphate administration.[12,27]

Phosphate

Like potassium, phosphate is lost with osmotic diuresis. IV fluids decrease phosphate levels, and insulin exacerbates this change by causing the intracellular movement of phosphate. Symptoms of profound hypophosphatemia emerge with decreasing intracellular concentrations of adenosine triphosphate and 2,3-diphosphoglycerate, that is, when the plasma levels decrease to less than 0.32 mmol/L. Severe hypophosphatemia can occur in the setting of prolonged fasting (>24 hours).[27] No data have demonstrated significant clinical benefits from phosphate repletion,[68] and phosphate administration can result in hypocalcemia. However, if the patient has unexplained severe muscle weakness or decreased cardiac function, phosphate administration should be considered.[27]

Magnesium

Serum magnesium levels can be low in patients with DKA, but they tend to normalize with resolution of the acidosis and with oral intake. There is no evidence supporting repletion of magnesium in the management of DKA.

Bicarbonate

Bicarbonate administration is not recommended or indicated in the management of DKA.[25–27] Historically, the use of bicarbonate in DKA treatment has been controversial. No pediatric studies have investigated the impact of bicarbonate on outcome. Although studies involving small numbers of adult patients have shown transient improvement in biochemical parameters, they have not reported clinical benefits or improved outcomes.[48,69–73] Studies suggest that bicarbonate administration is associated with longer hospital stays for children,[71] paradoxic worsening of ketosis in adults,[69] and hypokalemia.[72] Not only can bicarbonate exacerbate hypokalemia and decrease tissue perfusion by decreasing oxygen delivery but it has also been strongly associated with the development of cerebral edema in children.[15,41]

The mainstay of treatment of acidosis is fluid replacement and insulin. Fluids improve tissue perfusion and increase the glomerular filtration rate, enhancing the excretion of acid, and insulin inhibits the underlying ketone production.

COMPLICATIONS

The most common complications of DKA are hypokalemia and hypoglycemia, which occur in response to treatment, as discussed previously. Thus, blood glucose and electrolyte concentrations must be monitored frequently throughout the course of DKA management. Cerebral edema, the most feared complication, is exclusive to pediatric patients with DKA. Almost no cases have been reported in patients older than 20 years of age.

Cerebral edema is a potentially devastating complication of pediatric DKA. It occurs in up to 1.5% of cases, with a mortality rate as high as 24%.[16] Numerous factors have been implicated in the pathophysiology of DKA-related cerebral edema, but no single mechanism has been definitively proven as causative. Most investigators suspect it is caused by a combination of factors that arise before treatment, which are then exacerbated by therapy. Ischemic and cytotoxic edema secondary to acidosis decrease cerebral perfusion. Vasogenic edema that causes direct damage to cerebral vascular endothelium increases blood-brain permeability.[74] Risk factors for DKA-induced cerebral edema are listed in **Box 3**.

Typically, cerebral edema occurs within 4 to 12 hours after initiation of treatment, but its onset can be delayed up to 24 to 48 hours after initiation of treatment. It has been postulated that cerebral edema could be iatrogenic, related to fluid resuscitation, or the speed with which hyperglycemia is corrected; however, it has been well established that symptomatic cerebral edema can develop in type 1 and type 2 diabetics without aggressive treatment.[14,16,76–79] Death has been described even before initiation of DKA treatment.[79]

Box 3
Risk factors for pediatric DKA-induced cerebral edema

- New-onset diabetes[15]
- Younger age
- Longer duration of DKA symptoms
- Degree of acidosis at presentation (pH <7.1)[17,41]
- Greater hypocapnia (Pco_2 <20 mm Hg)[15,17]
- Greater initial rate of fluid resuscitation for treatment of severe DKA (>50 mL/kg in the first 4 hours)[41]
- Administration of insulin during the first hour of fluid resuscitation[41]
- Higher blood urea nitrogen at presentation[15,75]
- Slower increase in measured serum sodium concentration during treatment of DKA[15,66]
- Bicarbonate treatment[15,73]

Regular neurologic checks along with assessment of vital signs are crucial. Mental status changes, which can range from somnolence to irritability, are worrisome, as are focal neurologic deficits. Age-inappropriate incontinence can be a sign of cerebral edema. Complaints of headache should be considered seriously. The combination of hypertension, bradycardia, and irregular respiration (Cushing triad) is a sign of increased intracranial pressure. Hypoxemia can also result from compression of the brain's respiratory center, leading to impending brain herniation.

Physicians should have a low threshold to diagnose and treat cerebral edema. When it is suspected based on clinical signs and symptoms, treatment should be initiated immediately. Treatment should never be postponed to wait for confirming computed tomography (CT) imaging; changes that indicate cerebral edema that can be seen on CT images occur late in its development. Treatment includes elevation of the head of the bed and reduction of IV fluids by one-third.[27]

Mannitol should be administered at a dose of 0.5 to 1 g/kg IV over 20 minutes. This regimen can be repeated if there is no clinical response within 30 to 120 minutes.[80,81] Mannitol decreases blood viscosity and thus improves cerebral blood flow acutely.[82] Caution with its use is warranted, however, because mannitol can induce diuresis, thereby decreasing intravascular volume and causing hypokalemia. This may result in hypotension and, subsequently, decreased cerebral blood flow.

Alternatively, 3% hypertonic saline can be given at a dosage of 5 to 10 mL/kg over 30 minutes, either instead of or along with mannitol.[83,84] Hypertonic saline lowers intracranial pressure, increases intravascular volume, and increases mean arterial pressure.

Patients might require intubation and mechanical ventilation to manage respiratory depression and avert impending respiratory failure. Patients with intracranial hypertension may be cautiously hyperventilated; however, hyperventilation to a Pco_2 less than 22 mm Hg should be avoided, as one study found poorer neurologic outcomes in intubated patients who were aggressively hyperventilated.[75]

DISPOSITION

Established diabetics with mild DKA who are alert and tolerating oral fluids can be treated in the emergency department and discharged, provided they have close supervision at home, possess the proper medications and supplies, have been educated about insulin administration, have the ability to monitor their blood glucose level, and have access to close follow-up.[27] Patients with new-onset diabetes must be admitted. Patients requiring IV rehydration over an extended period need to be admitted to a unit capable of hourly blood glucose measurement and frequent measurement of vital signs and neurologic checks. Patients with severe DKA should be admitted to the ICU, especially if they have had a long duration of symptoms, any hemodynamic instability, altered mental status, a high risk of cerebral edema (eg, age <5 years), low partial pressure of carbon dioxide (Pco_2), or high BUN.[27]

SUMMARY

Despite advances in research and treatment, the incidence of pediatric-onset diabetes and diabetic ketoacidosis is increasing. Diabetes mellitus is one of the most common chronic pediatric illnesses and, along with diabetic ketoacidosis, is associated with significant cost and morbidity. DKA is a complicated metabolic state hallmarked by dehydration and electrolyte disturbances. Treatment revolves around proper fluid resuscitation with insulin and electrolyte replacement under constant monitoring for cerebral edema, which is the deadliest complication. When DKA is recognized and treated immediately, the prognosis is excellent. However, when a patient has prolonged or multiple courses of DKA or if DKA is complicated by cerebral edema, the results can be devastating.

REFERENCES

1. Centers for Disease Control and Prevention. National diabetes fact sheet: general information and national estimates on diabetes in the United States, 2011. Atlanta (GA): US Department of Health and Human Services; 2011.
2. Klingensmith GJ, Tamborlane WV, Wood J, et al. Diabetic ketoacidosis at diabetes onset: still an all too common threat in youth. J Pediatr 2013;162(2): 330–4.e1.
3. Rewers A, Klingensmith G, Davis C, et al. Presence of diabetic ketoacidosis at diagnosis of diabetes mellitus in youth: the Search for Diabetes in Youth Study. Pediatrics 2008;121:e1258–66.
4. Levy-Marchal C, Patterson CC, Green A, et al. Geographical variation of presentation at diagnosis of type 1 diabetes in children: the EURODIAB study. Diabetologia 2001;44:B75–80.
5. Usher-Smith JA, Thompson M, Ercole A, et al. Variation between countries in the frequency of diabetic ketoacidosis at first presentation of type 1 diabetes in children: a systematic review. Diabetologia 2012;55(11):2878–94.
6. Usher-Smith JA, Thompson MJ, Sharp SJ, et al. Factors associated with the presence of diabetic ketoacidosis at diagnosis of diabetes in children and young adults: a systematic review. BMJ 2011;343:d4092.
7. Rewers A, Chase HP, Mackenzie T, et al. Predictors of acute complications in children with type 1 diabetes. JAMA 2002;287:2511–8.
8. Fagot-Campagna A, Pettitt DJ, Engelgau MM, et al. Type 2 diabetes among North American children and adolescents: an epidemiologic review and a public health perspective. J Pediatr 2000;136(5):664–72.
9. Type 2 diabetes in children and adolescents. American Diabetes Association. Diabetes Care 2000;23:381–9.
10. Newton CA, Raskin P. Diabetic ketoacidosis in type 1 and type 2 diabetes mellitus: clinical and biochemical differences. Arch Intern Med 2004;164: 1925–31.
11. Shrestha SS, Zhang P, Barker L, et al. Medical expenditures associated with diabetes acute complications in privately insured U.S. youth. Diabetes Care 2010; 33:2617–22.
12. Kitabchi AE, Umpierrez GE, Murphy MB, et al, American Diabetes Association. Hyperglycemic crises in diabetes. Diabetes Care 2004;27(Suppl 1):S94–102.
13. Edge JA, Ford-Adams ME, Dunger DB. Causes of death in children with insulin dependent diabetes 1990–96. Arch Dis Child 1999;81:318–96.
14. Lawrence SE, Cummings EA, Gaboury I, et al. Population-based study of incidence and risk factors for cerebral edema in pediatric diabetic ketoacidosis. J Pediatr 2005;146:688–92.
15. Glaser N, Barnett P, McCaslin I, et al. Risk factors for cerebral edema in children with diabetic ketoacidosis. N Engl J Med 2001;344:264–9.
16. Edge JA, Hawkins MM, Winter DL, et al. The risk and outcome of cerebral oedema developing during diabetic ketoacidosis. Arch Dis Child 2001;85(1): 16–22.
17. Mahoney CP, Vleck BW, Del Aguila M. Risk factors for developing brain herniation during diabetic ketoacidosis. Pediatr Neurol 1999;21:721–7.

18. Ghetti S, Lee JK, Sims CE, et al. Diabetic ketoacidosis and memory dysfunction in children with type 1 diabetes. J Pediatr 2010;156(1):109–14.
19. Jin H, Meyer JM, Jeste DV. Phenomenology of and risk factors for new-onset diabetes mellitus and diabetic ketoacidosis associated with atypical antipsychotics: an analysis of 45 published cases. Ann Clin Psychiatry 2002;14:59–64.
20. Wilson DR, D'Souza L, Sarkar N, et al. New-onset diabetes and ketoacidosis with atypical antipsychotics. Schizophr Res 2002;59:1–6.
21. Yood MU, deLorenze G, Quesenberry CP Jr, et al. The incidence of diabetes in atypical antipsychotic users differs according to agent—results from a multisite epidemiologic study. Pharmacoepidemiol Drug Saf 2009;18:791–9.
22. Keshavarz R, Mousavi M, Hassan C. Diabetic ketoacidosis in a child on FK506 immunosuppression after a liver transplant. Pediatr Emerg Care 2002;18:22–4.
23. Ersoy A, Ersoy C, Tekce H, et al. Diabetic ketoacidosis following development of de novo diabetes in renal transplant recipient associated with tacrolimus. Transplant Proc 2004;36:1407–10.
24. Laffel L. Ketone bodies: a review of physiology, pathophysiology and application of monitoring to diabetes. Diabetes Metab Res Rev 1999;15(6):412–26.
25. Dunger DB, Sperling MA, Acerini CL, et al. European Society for Pediatric Endocrinology/Lawson Wilkins Pediatric Endocrine Society consensus statement on diabetic ketoacidosis in children and adolescents. Pediatrics 2004;113: e133–40.
26. Wolfsdorf J, Glaser N, Sperling MA. Diabetic ketoacidosis in infants, children, and adolescents. A consensus statement from the American Diabetes Association. Diabetes Care 2006;29(5):1150–9.
27. Wolfsdorf J, Craig ME, Daneman D, et al. ISPAD Clinical Practice Consensus Guidelines 2009 Compendium. Diabetic ketoacidosis in children and adolescents with diabetes. Pediatr Diabetes 2009;10(Suppl 12):118–33.
28. Malone JI, Brodsky SJ. The value of electrocardiogram monitoring in diabetic ketoacidosis. Diabetes Care 1980;3(4):543–7.
29. Parham WA, Mehdirad AA, Biermann KM, et al. Hyperkalemia revisited. Tex Heart Inst J 2006;33(1):40–7.
30. Brandenburg MA, Dire DJ. Comparison of arterial and venous blood gas values in the initial emergency department evaluation of patients with diabetic ketoacidosis. Ann Emerg Med 1998;31(4):459–65.
31. Kelly AM. The case for venous rather than arterial blood gases in diabetic ketoacidosis. Emerg Med Australas 2006;18:64–7.
32. Ma OJ, Rush MD, Godfrey MM, et al. Arterial blood gas results rarely influence emergency physician management of patients with suspected diabetic ketoacidosis. Acad Emerg Med 2003;10:836–41.
33. Gokel Y, Paydas S, Koseoglu Z, et al. Comparison of blood gas and acid-base measurements in arterial and venous blood samples in patients with uremic acidosis and diabetic ketoacidosis in the emergency room. Am J Nephrol 2000;20:319–23.
34. Nadler OA, Finkelstein MJ, Reid SR. How well does serum bicarbonate concentration predict the venous pH in children being evaluated for diabetic ketoacidosis? Pediatr Emerg Care 2011;27:907–10.
35. Menchine M, Probst MA, Agy C, et al. Diagnostic accuracy of venous blood gas electrolytes for identifying diabetic ketoacidosis in the emergency department. Acad Emerg Med 2011;18(10):1105–8.

36. Fu P, Douros G, Kelly AM. Does potassium concentration measured on blood gas analysis agree with serum potassium in patients with diabetic ketoacidosis? Emerg Med Australas 2004;16:280–3.

37. Noyes KJ, Crofton P, Bath LE, et al. Hydroxybutyrate near-patient testing to evaluate a new end-point for intravenous insulin therapy in the treatment of diabetic ketoacidosis in children. Pediatr Diabetes 2007;8:150–6.

38. Csako G, Elin RJ. Spurious ketonuria due to captopril and other free sulfhydryl drugs. Diabetes Care 1996;19:673–4.

39. Vanelli M, Chiari G, Capuano C. Cost effectiveness of the direct measurement of 3-beta-hydroxybutyrate in the management of diabetic ketoacidosis in children. Diabetes Care 2004;26(3):959.

40. Fiordalisi I, Novotny WE, Holbert D, et al. An 18-yr prospective study of pediatric diabetic ketoacidosis: an approach to minimizing the risk of brain herniation during treatment. Pediatr Diabetes 2007;8(3):142–9.

41. Edge JA, Jakes RW, Roy Y, et al. The UK case–control study of cerebral oedema complicating diabetic ketoacidosis in children. Diabetologia 2006; 49(9):2002–9.

42. Carlotti AP, Bohn D, Halperin ML. Importance of timing of risk factors for cerebral oedema during therapy for diabetic ketoacidosis. Arch Dis Child 2003;88: 170–3.

43. Holliday MA, Segar WE. The maintenance need for water in parenteral fluid therapy. Pediatrics 1957;19:823–32.

44. Skellett S, Mayer A, Durward A, et al. Chasing the base deficit: hyperchloraemic acidosis following 0.9% saline fluid resuscitation. Arch Dis Child 2000;83:514–6.

45. Taylor D, Durward A, Tibby SM, et al. The influence of hyperchloraemia on acid base interpretation in diabetic ketoacidosis. Intensive Care Med 2006;32: 295–301.

46. Van Zyl DG, Rheeder P, Delport E. Fluid management in diabetic-acidosis– Ringer's lactate versus normal saline: a randomized controlled trial. QJM 2012;105:337–43.

47. Mahler SA, Conrad SA, Wang H, et al. Resuscitation with balanced electrolyte solution prevents hyperchloremic metabolic acidosis in patients with diabetic ketoacidosis. Am J Emerg Med 2011;29(6):670–4.

48. Chua HR, Venkatesh B, Stachowski E, et al. Plasma-Lyte 148 vs 0.9% saline for fluid resuscitation in diabetic ketoacidosis. J Crit Care 2012;27(2):138–45.

49. Pediatric Emergency Care Applied Research Network. Current and past research, December 17, 2012. Available at: www.pecarn.org/currentresearch/index.html. Accessed January 16, 2013.

50. Koves IH, Neutze J, Donath S, et al. The accuracy of clinical assessment of dehydration during diabetic ketoacidosis in childhood. Diabetes Care 2004; 27(10):2485–7.

51. Murphy MS. Guidelines for managing acute gastroenteritis based on a systematic review of published research. Arch Dis Child 1998;79:279–84.

52. Fagan MJ, Avner J, Khine H. Initial fluid resuscitation for patients with diabetic ketoacidosis: how dry are they? Clin Pediatr 2008;47:851–5.

53. Ugale J, Mata A, Meert KL. Measured degree of dehydration in children and adolescents with type 1 diabetic ketoacidosis. Pediatr Crit Care Med 2012; 13(2):e103–7.

54. Sottosanti M, Morrison GC, Singh RN, et al. Dehydration in children with diabetic ketoacidosis: a prospective study. Arch Dis Child 2012;97:96–100.

55. Rosenbloom AL. Diabetic ketoacidosis: treatment guidelines. Clin Pediatr (Phila) 1996;35:261–6.
56. Finberg L. Appropriate therapy can prevent cerebral swelling in diabetic ketoacidosis. J Clin Endocrinol Metab 2000;85:507–8.
57. Grimberg A, Cerri RW, Satin-Smith M, et al. The "two bag system" for variable intravenous dextrose and fluid management: benefits in diabetic ketoacidosis management. J Pediatr 1999;134:376–8.
58. Poirier MP, Greer D, Satin-Smith M. A prospective study of the "two-bag system" in diabetic ketoacidosis management. Clin Pediatr (Phila) 2004;43:809–13.
59. Koul PB. Diabetic ketoacidosis: a current appraisal of pathophysiology and management. Clin Pediatr (Phila) 2009;48(2):135–44.
60. So TY, Grunewalder E. Evaluation of the two-bag system for fluid management in pediatric patients with diabetic ketoacidosis. J Pediatr Pharmacol Ther 2009; 14(2):100–5.
61. Lindsay R, Bolte RG. The use of an insulin bolus in low-dose insulin infusion for pediatric diabetic ketoacidosis. Pediatr Emerg Care 1989;5(2):77–9.
62. Hoorn EJ, Carlotti AP, Costa LA, et al. Preventing a drop in effective plasma osmolality to minimize the likelihood of cerebral edema during treatment of children with diabetic ketoacidosis. J Pediatr 2007;150(5):467–73.
63. Klein M, Sathasivam A, Novoa Y, et al. Recent consensus statements in pediatric endocrinology: a selective review. Endocrinol Metab Clin North Am 2009;38(4): 811–25.
64. Umpierrez GE, Jones S, Smiley D, et al. Insulin analogs versus human insulin in the treatment of patients with diabetic ketoacidosis: a randomized controlled trial. Diabetes Care 2009;32(7):1164–9.
65. Della Manna T, Steinmetz L, Campos PR, et al. Subcutaneous use of a fast-acting insulin analog: an alternative treatment for pediatric patients with diabetic ketoacidosis. Diabetes Care 2005;28(8):1856–61.
66. Harris GD, Fiordalisi I, Harris WL, et al. Minimizing the risk of brain herniation during the treatment of diabetic ketoacidemia: a retrospective and prospective study. J Pediatr 1990;117(1 Pt 1):22–31.
67. Arora S, Cheng D, Wyler B, et al. Prevalence of hypokalemia in ED patients with diabetic ketoacidosis. Am J Emerg Med 2012;30:481–4.
68. Becker DJ, Brown DR, Steranka BH. Phosphate replacement during treatment of diabetic ketoacidosis. Am J Dis Child 1983;137:241–6.
69. Hale PJ, Crase J, Nattrass M. Metabolic effects of bicarbonate in the treatment of diabetic ketoacidosis. Br Med J (Clin Res Ed) 1984;289:1035–8.
70. Morris LR, Murphy MB, Kitabchi AE. Bicarbonate therapy in severe diabetic ketoacidosis. Ann Intern Med 1986;105:836–40.
71. Green SM, Rothrock SG, Ho JD, et al. Failure of adjunctive bicarbonate to improve outcome in severe pediatric diabetic ketoacidosis. Ann Emerg Med 1998;31(1):41–8.
72. Viallon A, Zeni F, Lafond P, et al. Does bicarbonate therapy improve the management of severe diabetic ketoacidosis? Crit Care Med 1999;27(12):2690–3.
73. Chua HR, Schneider A, Bellomo R. Bicarbonate in diabetic ketoacidosis: a systematic review. Ann Intensive Care 2011;1:23.
74. Silver SM, Clark EC, Schroeder BM, et al. Pathogenesis of cerebral edema after treatment of diabetic ketoacidosis. Kidney Int 1997;51:1237–44.
75. Marcin JP, Glaser N, Barnett P, et al. Factors associated with adverse outcomes in children with diabetic ketoacidosis-related cerebral edema. J Pediatr 2002; 141:793–7.

76. Glaser N. Cerebral edema in children with diabetic ketoacidosis. Curr Diab Rep 2001;1:41–6.
77. Takaya J, Ohashi R, Harada Y, et al. Cerebral edema in a child with diabetic ketoacidosis before initial treatment. Pediatr Int 2007;49:395–6.
78. Morales AE, Daniels KA. Cerebral edema before onset of therapy in newly diagnosed type 2 diabetes. Pediatr Diabetes 2009;10(2):155–7.
79. Glasgow A. Devastating cerebral edema in diabetic ketoacidosis before therapy. Diabetes Care 1991;14:77–8.
80. Franklin B, Liu J, Ginsberg-Fellner F. Cerebral edema and ophthalmoplegia reversed by mannitol in a new case of insulin-dependent diabetes mellitus. Pediatrics 1982;69:87–90.
81. Shabbir N, Oberfield SE, Corrales R, et al. Recovery from symptomatic brain swelling in diabetic ketoacidosis. Clin Pediatr 1992;31:570–3.
82. Muir A. Cerebral edema in diabetic ketoacidosis: a look beyond rehydration. J Clin Endocrinol Metab 2000;85:509–13.
83. Curtis JR, Bohn D, Daneman D. Use of hypertonic saline in the treatment of cerebral edema in diabetic ketoacidosis (DKA). Pediatr Diabetes 2001;2:191–4.
84. Kamat P, Vats A, Gross M, et al. Use of hypertonic saline for the treatment of altered mental status associated with diabetic ketoacidosis. Pediatr Crit Care Med 2003;4:239–42.

An Update on Common Gastrointestinal Emergencies

Seema Shah, MD

KEYWORDS

- Malrotation • Appendicitis • Pyloric stenosis • Hirschsprung disease
- Intussusception

KEY POINTS

- Infants with pyloric stenosis often present with progressive nonbilious emesis with an intact appetite.
- Although most of the infants with malrotation and volvulus present in the neonatal period maintain a high index of suspicion in any older infant or child presenting with bilious emesis and abdominal pain.
- Intussusception should be considered in an infant presenting with lethargy or altered level of consciousness.
- Laboratory testing is of limited utility in children with appendicitis; careful history and physical examination are more likely to aid in the diagnosis.
- Chronic constipation and malnutrition are common symptoms in delayed presentation of Hirschsprung disease.

IDIOPATHIC HYPERTROPHIC PYLORIC STENOSIS

Background/Epidemiology

Idiopathic hypertrophic pyloric stenosis (IHPS) is a condition where the pyloric muscle abnormally thickens and as a result, there is delayed gastric emptying. This disease affects 2 to 5 in 1000 live births with a male to female predominance of 4:1.[1–3] The exact cause is unknown, despite a multitude of studies that suggest various genetic and environmental associations. Classically, this condition is described as being more common in firstborn males. Recent epidemiologic studies do not suggest a unique position for firstborns, but rather a decline in risk with the increasing birth order.[3] A notable environmental association with IHPS is the sharp decline in incidence after the back to sleep campaign was promoted in Denmark and Sweden.[3] Similarly, the expanded use of erythromycin for pertussis has been associated with

Funding Sources: None.
Division of Emergency Medicine, Rady Children's Hospital, University of California San Diego, 3020 Children's Way, MC 5075, San Diego, CA 92123, USA
E-mail address: sshah@rchsd.org

Emerg Med Clin N Am 31 (2013) 775–793
http://dx.doi.org/10.1016/j.emc.2013.05.002
0733-8627/13/$ – see front matter © 2013 Elsevier Inc. All rights reserved.

emed.theclinics.com

an increased incidence of IHPS. There were 2 studies that identified clusters of increased incidence of pyloric stenosis after the use of erythromycin. Although the increased risk is small, there are data to suggest that infants younger than 2 weeks of are at greatest risk for developing IHPS when exposed to erythromycin.[3,4]

Clinical Features

Infants with IHPS typically are healthy at birth. Symptoms begin with small amounts of emesis with progression to large-volume emesis as the pyloric muscle hypertrophies. The most common age of presentation is between 2 and 5 weeks of life. IHPS is rare after 12 weeks of age. The emesis is frequently projectile and nonbilious. Protracted emesis predisposes to a Mallory-Weiss tear and subsequent hematemesis. Despite persistent emesis, these infants usually have a normal, intact appetite. Early in the course of disease, infants are often well appearing. As the emesis advances, infants begin to show clinical signs of dehydration. Infants with emesis for an extended period of time may show signs of growth failure often appearing cachectic with loss of subcutaneous fat and loose skin.[5] Additional physical examination findings include a visualization of gastric peristalsis and a palpable pyloric mass or "olive," present in 44% to 48% of cases.[6,7] In cases of severe contraction metabolic alkalosis, infants may present with apnea.[8]

Laboratory Analysis

Electrolytes may be normal early in disease. As a result of protracted emesis with dehydration, a hypochloremic metabolic alkalosis may develop. With earlier detection of disease, the incidence of a hypochloremic alkalosis has slowly declined.[7]

Radiographic Studies

Plain radiographs
Plain radiographs of the abdomen most often are nonspecific and may appear normal. Although neither sensitive nor specific, the presence of gastric dilatation with a paucity of distal bowel gas may be suggestive of IHPS. Infrequently, gastric peristalsis may be visualized as the "caterpillar sign" giving the false appearance of a "double bubble" sign (**Fig. 1**).

Pyloric ultrasound
Ultrasound (US) of the pylorus is the preferred diagnostic study with high sensitivity and specificity, which approaches 98% and 100%, respectively.[9,10] Classic sonographic findings include a thickened pylorus with a length greater than 15 mm and diameter greater than 3 mm. An additional US finding is a prolapsed, hypertrophied pyloric mucosa protruding into the gastric antrum, also known as the "antral nipple" sign (**Fig. 2**).[11] The advantages of sonography over an upper gastrointestinal series are that it requires no radiation exposure, may be rapidly obtained, and does not depend up on the transit of gastric materials across the pyloric canal.

Upper gastrointestinal series
An upper gastrointestinal series (UGI) is frequently obtained when differentiating between other causes of neonatal emesis. In IHPS, an UGI series may demonstrate a failure of relaxation of the prepyloric antrum and a string of contrast through the mucosal interstices that outlines the canal called the "string sign."[12] The advantage of an UGI series is that it provides additional information regarding esophageal anatomy and motility, especially when considering additional causes of neonatal emesis such as malrotation, gastroesophageal reflux disease, and other intestinal stenoses and atresias.

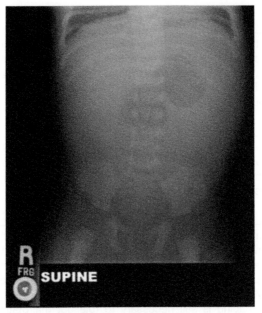

Fig. 1. Pyloric stenosis. Plain abdominal radiograph demonstrates the presence of a caterpillar sign and a paucity of gas distal to the pylorus.

Management

Initial management in patients with IHPS is focused on intravenous hydration with isotonic fluids. Diagnostic workup may include both laboratory testing and radiologic studies as mentioned earlier. Infants are often admitted for intravenous (IV) hydration. Electrolytes abnormalities are corrected before surgical repair to reduce perioperative morbidity. Definitive therapy for IHPS is open or laparoscopic pyloromyotomy. Once surgically repaired, recurrence rarely occurs.

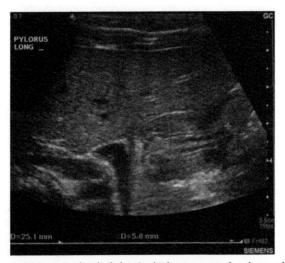

Fig. 2. Pyloric stenosis. Longitudinal abdominal ultrasonography shows thickened muscle and redundant mucosa consistent with the antral nipple sign.

MALROTATION
Background

During normal embryonic development between the 4th and 10th weeks of gestation, a 270° counter-clockwise rotation of the proximal and midgut occurs before settling into the abdomen. Malrotation occurs as a result of incomplete rotation of the bowel with an abnormal fixation of the mesentery of the bowel. It is within this abnormal fixation that a volvulus may occur.

Epidemiology

In the United States, the prevalence of malrotation in infants under the age of 1 year is 3.9 in 10.000 live births.[13] Twenty-five percent of patients with malrotation will present within the 1st month of life and 90% by the 1st year of life. Mortality depends on the degree of bowel ischemia during surgery.[14]

Clinical Features

The classic presentation of malrotation with volvulus is a neonate with sudden onset of bilious emesis. However, there is considerable variability in presentation depending on severity of disease. Bilious emesis indicates any obstruction distal to the ampulla of Vater and is not pathognomonic of malrotation with volvulus. A prospective study identified that 62% of infants with bilious emesis did not have anatomic obstruction; however, further imaging is still necessary to rule out malrotation as a potential cause.[15] Infants frequently present with a normal history or more subtle findings such as feeding problems or gastroesophageal reflux associated with a failure to thrive.[16]

Infants may have a completely normal physical examination. The presence of an acute abdomen, although rare, is a poor prognostic indicator.[16] Approximately 10% to 15% of infants will present with gross hematochezia or guaiac positive stool. The presence of blood is another indicator of poor prognosis due to risk of impending bowel gangrene.[16]

Laboratory Analysis

Laboratory studies are rarely diagnostic; however an elevated white blood cell count, C-reactive protein, lactic acid, and glucose have been associated with bowel ischemia.[17]

Radiographic Studies

Plain radiographs
Plain radiographs of the abdomen often vary from nonspecific findings to a distal bowel obstruction (**Fig. 3**). The presence of a normal bowel gas pattern does not exclude the possibility of malrotation.[14] Plain radiographs and decubitus films of the abdomen are helpful in determining the presence of free intraperitoneal air. The presence of free air requires immediate pediatric surgical consultation and operative intervention.

Upper gastrointestinal series
The preferred imaging modality for determining the presence of malrotation is an UGI series. The diagnostic finding on the UGI series is the abnormal positioning of the duodenal-jejunal junction (**Fig. 4**). Normal positioning of the junction should be located left of the left vertebral pedicle at the level of the inferior margin of the duodenal bulb. In malrotation, the junction is present to the right of the vertebral body.[14] Although the UGI series is the diagnostic imaging of choice, the false-positive rate may be as

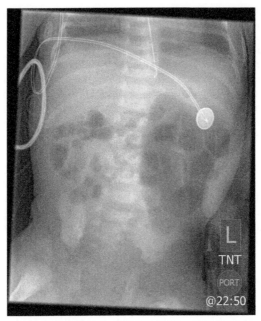

Fig. 3. Malrotation with volvulus. Plain radiographs show the presence of large bowel on the left side of the abdomen.

high as approximately 15% with a false-negative rate of 2% to 3%.[18] Sensitivity of the UGI series for malrotation approaches 93% to 100%.[19] Common reasons for the false positives are usually the result of normal anatomic variation such as a wandering duodenum, duodenum inversum, or mobile duodenum. Additional reasons for the

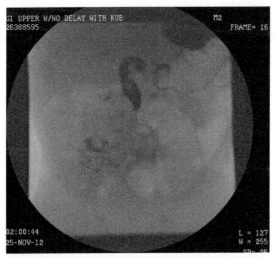

Fig. 4. Malrotation with volvulus. Upper gastrointestinal series demonstrates inferior displacement of the duodenal jejunal junction (DJJ) to the right. DJJ does not pass to the left of the spine and does not rise to the level of the duodenal bulb. Proximal small bowel appears on the right side of the abdomen. Likely corkscrew pattern of duodenum indicating volvulus.

displacement of the junction include a dilated stomach, splenomegaly, renal agenesis, or liver transplantation.[18]

Abdominal ultrasound

US is frequently obtained due to the low risk of radiation exposure and ease of accessibility. Suggestive findings include a reversal of the relationship of the superior mesenteric artery (SMA) to the superior mesenteric vein (SMV). A "whirlpool sign," a swirling, whirlpool-like shape seen when the SMV and mesentery wrap around the SMA in a clockwise direction, may also be visualized on transverse ultrasonography. Several studies have documented variable sensitivity and specificity of this imaging modality.[14]

Management

Once access has been obtained, fluid resuscitation and antibiotics should be initiated, followed by immediate surgical consultation. Unstable patients requiring airway stabilization and aggressive fluid resuscitation will likely require emergent surgical intervention. Further imaging, as described earlier, should be obtained once the patient is adequately resuscitated.

Surgical repair

Originally described by William Ladd in 1930, the Ladd procedure is still performed today with (1) detorsion of the bowel when volvulus is present, (2) lysis of duodenal bands, (3) broadening the mesentery to separate the duodenum and cecum as far away as possible, (4) placement of the small bowel to the right side of the abdomen, and (5) placement of the colon to the left side of the abdomen.[20] The laparoscopic procedure has no difference in complication rates and decrease in length of stay when compared with an open Ladd procedure.[21] Postoperative complications include bowel obstruction from adhesions, volvulus, and incisional hernias.[21,22]

INTUSSUSCEPTION
Background/Epidemiology

Intussusception is the most common cause of pediatric small bowel obstruction and afflicts approximately 56 in 100,000 children annually.[23] The disease involves the telescoping of the bowel into itself, usually including both the large and small bowel. Most intussusceptions are ileocolic and 90% to 95% are presumed to be the result of lymphoid hyperplasia. The remainder is the result of pathologic lead points.[24,25] The typical age of presentation is between 6 months and 2 years, with a peak incidence between 5 and 9 months.[26,27] There have been rare reported cases of infants under 2 months of age with intussusception. Pathologic lead points, such as Meckel diverticulum, benign tumors, or vasculitis from Henoch-Schonlein Purpura, are more common in children older than 2 years of with an incidence of 22% of intussusception cases in this age group.[28]

Clinical Features

The classic presentation of intussusception is a clinical triad of colicky abdominal pain, currant jelly stools, and a palpable abdominal mass. Unfortunately, this triad is present in less than 40% of children.[29–32] Atypical presentations are more common in young infants and older children. In infants younger than 4 months of age, painless intussusception may be present in up to 40%. Other nonspecific neurologic symptoms such as lethargy or altered level of consciousness may also occur.[27,33] Children older than 2 years of age tend to present with more subacute or chronic abdominal pain and few have rectal bleeding.[28]

Laboratory Analysis

Laboratory studies are rarely useful in aiding in the diagnosis of intussusception.

Radiographic Studies

Plain radiographs

In the emergency department, supine and lateral decubitus films are often obtained as screening tools for intussusception. However, the sensitivity and specificity of these studies are very low. Approximately 24% of patients with confirmed intussusception may have normal radiographs.[34] Radiographic findings suggestive of intussusception include the presence of a small bowel obstruction, the appearance of a soft tissue mass in the right upper quadrant, paucity of gas in the right lower quadrant, "target sign," and the "crescent sign." The target sign, seen in approximately 29% of patients with intussusception, is comprised of 2 concentric radiolucencies in the right upper quadrant outlining a soft tissue mass to the right of the spine overlying the kidney.[34] The crescent sign is the presence of a curvilinear mass in the transverse colon beyond the hepatic flexure (**Fig. 5**). The triad of intestinal obstruction, intracolonic mass, and paucity of gas in the right lower quadrant occurs in only 1% of patients.[34] One of the most sensitive indicators of intussusception is the presence of air in the ascending colon visualized on at least 2 of the 3 views of the abdomen reaching a sensitivity of 96% and specificity of 41%.[35]

Abdominal ultrasound

Abdominal US has emerged as the primary diagnostic tool for intussusception with high sensitivity ranging from 98% to 100% and specificity from 88% to 100%.[36–38] Sonographic findings on transverse imaging are a hypoechoic outer rim of homogeneous thickness with a central hyperechoic core designated the "doughnut" or "target" sign (**Fig. 6**).[39] On longitudinal scans, there is an appearance of a

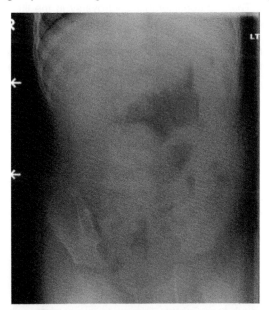

Fig. 5. Intussusception. Plain film demonstration of intracolonic mass. Decubitus plain abdominal radiograph demonstrates soft tissue mass within the colon caused by the head of the intussusception (intussusceptum).

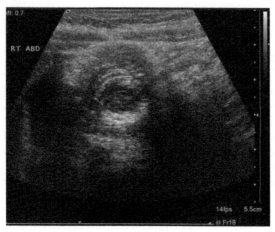

Fig. 6. Intussusception. Abdominal ultrasonography shows an outer hypoechoic region surrounding an echogenic ring also known as the "target sign".

"pseudokidney," a hyperechoic tubular center covered on each side by a hyperechoic rim producing a kidneylike appearance.[26,39]

Management

Initial management should focus on fluid resuscitation. Antibiotics and immediate surgical consultation are required if perforation or peritonitis is suspected. Once a radiographic diagnosis of intussusception is made and perforation is not suspected, nonoperative management is pursued with an air or contrast enema performed by a radiologist (**Fig. 7**). There is considerable controversy in the literature between air and contrast enema with little difference in rates of perforation and recurrence (**Table 1**).

Children at risk for enema reduction failure include infants younger than 3 months, children older than 5 years, duration of symptoms greater than 48 hours, presence of

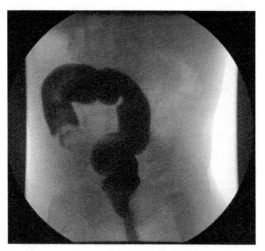

Fig. 7. Intussusception. Contrast enema demonstrating reduction of intussusception.

Table 1
Comparison of air versus contrast enema reduction for intussusception

	Air Enema	Contrast Enema
Success Rate	60%–90%	60%–80%
Rate of Perforation	<3%	<1%
Disadvantage	Tension pneumoperitoneum	Contrast peritonitis
Advantages	Lower radiation dose Better control of intracolonic pressures	Better anatomic definition

hematochezia, significant dehydration, or evidence of small bowel obstruction on plain radiograph.[5] More recent retrospective studies indicate that age may not be a risk factor for failed reduction. These studies demonstrated that a duration of symptoms greater than 24 hours, bloody diarrhea, and lethargy were the most significant risk factors in failed enema reductions.[40,41]

Management after successful enema reduction of intussusception requires observation for recurrent intussusception or bowel perforation. Previous studies recommended admission for 48 hours. This recommendation has not been validated leading to considerable debate on management. The overall recurrence rate for intussusception following enema reduction is 10% with 0% to 5.3% in the first 24 hours.[42] This low early recurrence rate for intussusception demonstrates that few patients would benefit from inpatient observation. More recent studies suggest that, given the low early recurrence rate for enema-reduced intussusception, an emergency department observation for a 6-hour period may be a safe alternative to inpatient management.[43]

APPENDICITIS
Epidemiology

Appendicitis is the most common surgical emergency of childhood afflicting 71,000 children younger than 15 years of age with a male to female ratio of 1.4:1.[44] The incidence is highest in boys aged 10 to 14 years (27.6 per 10,000 population per year) and girls aged 15 to 19 years (20.5 per 10,000 population per year).[45] Children younger than 5 years account for less than 5% of all appendicitis, which poses a diagnostic challenge for clinicians.[46]

Clinical Features

The classic presentation of appendicitis is periumbilical abdominal pain and nausea that migrates to the right lower quadrant followed by emesis and fever.[46,47] Although this sequence of events is present in approximately 50% of adults, it is less common in children.[47] The distinctive physical examination finding of right lower quadrant tenderness is considered to be the single most important diagnostic tool for appendicitis.

Unfortunately, children younger than 5 years are a diagnostic dilemma to clinicians as the result of a lack of communication skills and difficulty in examining these children. Risk factors for missed appendicitis include younger children (5.3 vs 7.9 years), onset of emesis before abdominal pain, constipation, diarrhea, upper respiratory symptoms, lethargy, or irritability.[47] Missed appendicitis not only increases the rate of perforation leading to greater morbidity and mortality but also poses a significant medicolegal risk.[47–50] One study noted that appendicitis was the second most prevalent condition in pediatric malpractice claims from 1985 to 2005 caused by error in diagnosis.[51] Rates of misdiagnosis from initial symptoms vary across age groups.

Most children youger than 3 years old are missed at initial presentation, with some studies noting a missed diagnosis rate approaching 100%.[46,52] In preschool-aged children, the rate of missed appendicitis improves ranging from 19% to 57%. In school-aged children, the rate of missed appendicitis further improves to 12% to 28%.[46,47]

Clinical Prediction Rules

Several clinical predictions rules (CPRs) have been proposed and validated including the Alvarado Score/MANTRELS (Migration, Anorexia, Nausea/vomiting, Tenderness in the right lower quadrant, Rebound pain, Elevation in temperature, Leukocytosis, Shift to the left), Low-Risk Appendicitis Rule, and Pediatric Appendicitis Score (PAS). More recent systematic reviews found the PAS and Alvarado scores to be the most validated CPRs; however, they do not reach the 4-rule performance benchmark of high-performing CPRs.[53] The more recent validation of the Low-Risk Appendicitis Rule yielded a sensitivity of 98%, specificity of 24%, and negative predictive value of 95%when the rule was refined.[54] Components of this refined rule include (1) an absolute neutrophil count of $6.75 \times 10^3/\mu L$ or less and no maximal tenderness in the right lower quadrant or (2) an absolute neutrophil count of $6.75 \times 10^3/\mu L$ or less with maximal tenderness in the right lower quadrant but no abdominal pain with walking/jumping or coughing. Recent commentary on this study noted the low, but not zero, risk for appendicitis; clinicians need to balance the risks of missing appendicitis with the increased risk of negative appendectomies and the potential long-term risks associated with exposure to ionizing radiation.[55]

Laboratory Analysis

Several laboratory studies have been evaluated as potential markers for children with suspected appendicitis. Most data have been equivocal at best.

Complete blood count

A white blood cell (WBC) count and differential is commonly ordered in children, despite limited diagnostic sensitivity and specificity for appendicitis. The WBC count has been studied frequently in the adult population with fewer studies in the pediatric population. Some studies have suggested that neutrophilia may be more sensitive than an elevated WBC count. A more recent study demonstrated that the combination of neutrophilia and increased WBC count results in a higher sensitivity (79%) than either test independently.[56] Neither the WBC count nor the neutrophil count allow for differentiation between perforated from nonperforated appendicitis.[47,57]

C-reactive protein

C-reactive protein (CRP), a nonspecific inflammatory marker, is the most frequently studied biomarker in appendicitis. A meta-analysis performed in the adult population found the WBC count more sensitive than the CRP.[58] Studies in the pediatric population suggest CRP elevations to be more sensitive in children with perforated appendicitis or abscess formation. A study of 209 children with 115 diagnosed with appendicitis established an optimal CRP cutoff value of 3 mg/dL. This CRP cutoff value coincided with a specificity and sensitivity of 65% and 71% respectively. With a CRP value greater than 3 mg/dL and WBC count greater than 12 cells/1000 mm^3, there was a further increase in specificity to 91% and a decrease in sensitivity to 42%.[59] Clinicians should maintain a higher index of suspicion for appendicitis and consider surgical consultation with these elevated values.

Gene expression

Recent advances in the study of gene expression are emerging as diagnostic tools for various disease processes including appendicitis. One study using leukocyte gene expression and cytokine levels identified 80% of the prospective cohorts with appendicitis.[60] Further investigation is warranted.

Radiographic Studies

Plain radiographs

Once thought to be useful in the diagnosis of appendicitis, most recent studies indicate that plain radiographs of the abdomen are often normal or misleading.[46] Previously, a calcified appendicolith identified on plain film was considered diagnostic. More recent studies have demonstrated appendicoliths in only 13% to 22% of cases with appendicitis and 1% to 2% of cases without appendicitis.[46,61,62] As a result of its limited utility, evidenced-based guidelines suggest the use of plain radiographs only when the patient's presentation is concerning for bowel obstruction, free air, mass, or nephrolithiasis.[63]

Abdominal ultrasound

US to evaluate the appendix is the imaging modality of choice in many centers. It is often considered an extension of the physical examination and serves the advantages of being noninvasive, avoiding conscious sedation, and avoiding ionizing radiation exposure.[64,65] The major disadvantages of abdominal US in the evaluation of appendicitis are that it is highly operator dependent and is less accurate than computed tomography (CT).[66] A meta-analysis comparing US to CT in children demonstrated higher pooled sensitivity and specificity for CT at 94% and 95%, respectively, over US, 88% and 94%, respectively.[66] For children with obesity, one study has established that the specificity, sensitivity, and negative predictive value were significantly lower than in nonobese children.[67]

Computed tomography

CT has been the diagnostic imaging of choice, secondary to its widespread availability at most major hospitals and emergency rooms. Compared with US, CT has superior accuracy (**Fig. 8**). An 18-year retrospective institutional review of an adult emergency department found a significant reduction in the negative appendectomy rate following an increase in the proportion of patients who had a preoperative CT.[68] Although CT of the abdomen and pelvis is frequently performed with various methods of contrast, a recent meta-analysis observed that the introduction of high-resolution CT may deter

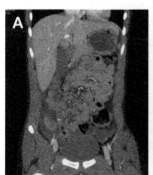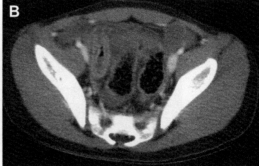

Fig. 8. Appendicitis. Computed tomography. (*A*) Coronal images show appendicolith. (*B*) Images demonstrate dilated and inflammed appendix.

the eventual use of contrast altogether in the adult population.[69] This comprehensive review of 7 studies found the pooled sensitivity and specificity of noncontrast CT to be 93% and 96%, respectively, with a false negative rate of 7.3%. Although well described in the adult literature,[70] there have been few studies in the pediatric population that allow the exclusion of appendicitis from a normal CT scan with a nonvisualized appendix. In one retrospective case control study of pediatric patients, the negative predictive value of a normal CT scan with a nonvisualized appendix was 98.7%.[71]

The widespread availability and fairly good sensitivity of CT is offset by the limitations of equivocal scans, exposure to ionizing radiation, and need for sedation in young children. Unfortunately, the risk of exposure to ionizing radiation is a growing concern. A comprehensive review of the effects of ionizing radiation derived from prediction models by Wakeford[72] validated that low levels of radiation exposure are associated with higher risk of childhood leukemia. Before the review by Wakeford, a Markov-based decision model found that a single abdominal CT in a 5-year-old child has a lifetime risk of radiation-induced cancer of 26.1 per 100,000 in women and 20.4 per 100,000 in men. This study also outlined the utility of US followed by CT if the initial US result was negative. This protocol demonstrated a reduction of CT scans with a concomitant reduction in radiation-induced malignancy by more than 50%.[73]

Magnetic resonance imaging

Magnetic resonance imaging (MRI) is emerging as a promising radiographic study in the diagnosis of appendicitis. MRI of the abdomen was originally studied in pregnant women. Given the reduced risk of ionizing radiation exposure, the concept was applied to the pediatric population. A recent study investigated 208 children after the implementation of a four-sequence expedited noncontrast MRI protocol and found the sensitivity and specificity to be 97% and 97.6%, respectively (**Fig. 9**).[74] The high sensitivity and specificity is partially offset by several limitations: a requirement for sedation in young children, potentially high cost, and lengthy procedural time. With the aforementioned study using a noncontrast expedited MR protocol, the median time from procedure request to final report was 164 minutes. Cost analysis

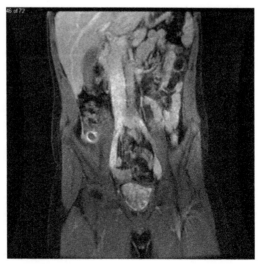

Fig. 9. Appendicitis. MRI of the abdomen and pelvis shows markedly dilated and inflamed appendix.

has been briefly addressed in the European literature,[75] and the most recent pediatric study indicated the cost of a noncontrast MRI to be $104 more than the cost of a CT with IV contrast; however, this is highly institution dependent and warrants further investigation.

Management

Currently, the standard treatment of choice is appendectomy. For nonperforated appendicitis, laparoscopic appendectomy is the preferred surgical approach. Recent advances in surgical techniques have facilitated the single umbilical incision laparoscopy for appendectomy (SILA). A systematic review of 9 studies in the adult population demonstrated no significant difference in operative time, length of stay, pain scores, and conversion or complication rates between SILA and conventional laparoscopic appendectomy.[76] Several pediatric studies have demonstrated similar findings[77]; a prospective study of 415 children using SILA validated its feasibility in the pediatric population.[78]

In cases of perforated appendicitis with abscess formation, the preferred approach is percutaneous drainage of the abscess and IV antibiotics followed by an interval appendectomy.[65] One study comparing early appendectomy to interval appendectomy in cases of perforated appendicitis with abscess formation revealed no differences in length of hospitalization, rate of abscess recurrence, or overall charges.[79]

HIRSCHSPRUNG DISEASE
Background/Epidemiology

Hirschsprung disease (HD), also known as aganglionic megacolon, is the absence of parasympathetic ganglion cells of Auerbach plexus in a variable portion of the distal gut. The most classic form, referred to as "short segment" disease, is limited to the rectosigmoid colon and accounts for 80% of all cases. The incidence is 1 in 5000 with a strong male to female predominance of 4:1.[80] "Long segment" disease extends proximal to the sigmoid colon and can involve the entire large bowel.

Hirschsprung disease may be associated with other congenital cardiac, neurologic, gastrointestinal, or urologic abnormalities. Trisomy 21 is the most common chromosomal abnormality associated in 10% of these infants.[80]

Clinical Features

Eighty percent of infants with Hirschsprung disease present within the neonatal period. The most common presenting symptom in 90% of neonates is the failure to pass meconium in the first 24 hours.[81] Additional symptoms include bilious emesis, infrequent explosive diarrhea, jaundice, and poor feeding. The presenting symptoms in older children vary from the neonatal time period as these patients often have chronic constipation, progressive abdominal distention, and malnutrition.[82] Most of the older children with HD have short segment disease.

Ten percent of children with HD present with fever, abdominal distention, abdominal pain, and sepsis. This is more commonly seen in neonates and infants.[83]

Laboratory Studies

Laboratory studies are of limited utility. WBC count and CRP may be elevated, but these are nonspecific markers.

Radiographic Studies

Plain radiographs are frequently obtained as screening tools.

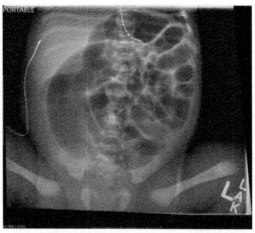

Fig. 10. Hirschsprung Disease. Plain radiograph of the abdomen shows a dilated small bowel and proximal colon with an empty rectum.

Plain radiographs in Hirschsprung disease demonstrate a dilated small bowel and proximal colon with an empty rectum (**Fig. 10**). A contrast enema obtained on an unprepped bowel will reveal a transition zone that reflects the joining of the aganglionic bowel with the dilated ganglionic bowel (**Fig. 11**).[80] Delayed barium evacuation may be noted in plain radiographs taken after the contrast enema is complete (**Fig. 12**).

Management

Fluid resuscitation and antibiotics should be initiated in patients who demonstrate signs of Hirschsprung disease–associated enterocolitis. In stable patients, the

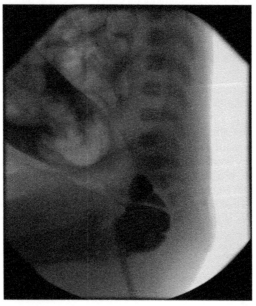

Fig. 11. Hirschsprung Disease. Contrast enema with demonstrating the presence of a transition zone.

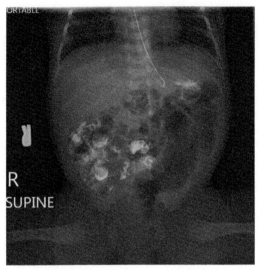

Fig. 12. Hirschsprung Disease. Plain abdominal radiography with delayed barium evacuation after completion of a contrast enema.

diagnosis may be made via a contrast enema or rectal suction biopsy. Discussion with a pediatric surgeon is necessary, but not emergent, for patients presenting without associated enterocolitis.

SUMMARY

Abdominal pain is one of the most common presenting complaints in the emergency department. Early recognition of these conditions requires high indices of suspicion. Despite advances in research and treatment, the diagnosis of pediatric abdominal emergencies remains challenging and can be associated with considerable cost and morbidity. Management often revolves around appropriate fluid resuscitation, electrolyte repletion, obtaining advanced imaging, and prompt surgical consultation.

REFERENCES

1. Applegate MS, Druschel CM. The epidemiology of infantile hypertrophic pyloric stenosis in New York State, 1983 to 1990. Arch Pediatr Adolesc Med 1995; 149(10):1123–9.
2. Mitchell LE, Risch N. The genetics of infantile hypertrophic pyloric stenosis. A reanalysis. Am J Dis Child 1993;147(11):1203–11.
3. MacMahon B. The continuing enigma of pyloric stenosis of infancy: a review. Epidemiology 2006;17(2):195–201.
4. Maheshwai N. Are young infants treated with erythromycin at risk for developing hypertrophic pyloric stenosis? Arch Dis Child 2007;92(3):271–3.
5. Fleisher G, Ludwig S, Henretig FM, editors. Textbook of pediatric emergency medicine. 6th edition. Philadelphia: Lippincott Williams & Wilkins; 2010.
6. Gotley LM, Blanch A, Kimble R, et al. Pyloric stenosis: a retrospective study of an Australian population. Emerg Med Australas 2009;21(5):407–13.
7. Taylor ND, Cass DT, Holland AJ. Infantile hypertrophic pyloric stenosis: has anything changed? J Paediatr Child Health 2013;49(1):33–7.

8. Pappano D. Alkalosis-induced respiratory depression from infantile hypertrophic pyloric stenosis. Pediatr Emerg Care 2011;27(2):124.

9. Niedzielski J, Kobielski A, Sokal J, et al. Accuracy of sonographic criteria in the decision for surgical treatment in infantile hypertrophic pyloric stenosis. Arch Med Sci 2011;7(3):508–11.

10. Hernanz-Schulman M, Sells LL, Ambrosino MM, et al. Hypertrophic pyloric stenosis in the infant without a palpable olive: accuracy of sonographic diagnosis. Radiology 1994;193(3):771–6.

11. Hernanz-Schulman M, Dinauer P, Ambrosino MM, et al. The antral nipple sign of pyloric mucosal prolapse: endoscopic correlation of a new sonographic observation in patients with pyloric stenosis. J Ultrasound Med 1995;14(4):283–7.

12. Hernanz-Schulman M. Pyloric stenosis: role of imaging. Pediatr Radiol 2009; 39(Suppl 2):S134–9.

13. Schulman J, Edmonds LD, McClearn AB, et al. Surveillance for and comparison of birth defect prevalences in two geographic areas–United States, 1983–88. MMWR CDC Surveill Summ 1993;42(1):1–7.

14. Applegate KE. Evidence-based diagnosis of malrotation and volvulus. Pediatr Radiol 2009;39(Suppl 2):S161–3.

15. Godbole P, Stringer MD. Bilious vomiting in the newborn: how often is it pathologic? J Pediatr Surg 2002;37(6):909–11.

16. Bonadio WA, Clarkson T, Naus J. The clinical features of children with malrotation of the intestine. Pediatr Emerg Care 1991;7(6):348–9.

17. Lin YP, Lee J, Chao HC, et al. Risk factors for intestinal gangrene in children with small-bowel volvulus. J Pediatr Gastroenterol Nutr 2011;53(4):417–22.

18. Applegate KE, Anderson JM, Klatte EC. Intestinal malrotation in children: a problem-solving approach to the upper gastrointestinal series. Radiographics 2006;26(5):1485–500.

19. Sizemore AW, Rabbani KZ, Ladd A, et al. Diagnostic performance of the upper gastrointestinal series in the evaluation of children with clinically suspected malrotation. Pediatr Radiol 2008;38(5):518–28.

20. Shew SB. Surgical concerns in malrotation and midgut volvulus. Pediatr Radiol 2009;39(Suppl 2):S167–71.

21. Stanfill AB, Pearl RH, Kalvakuri K, et al. Laparoscopic Ladd's procedure: treatment of choice for midgutmalrotation in infants and children. J Laparoendosc Adv Surg Tech A 2010;20(4):369–72.

22. El-Gohary Y, Alagtal M, Gillick J. Long-term complications following operative intervention for intestinal malrotation: a 10-year review. Pediatr Surg Int 2010; 26(2):203–6.

23. Parashar UD, Holman RC, Cummings KC, et al. Trends in intussusception-associated hospitalizations and deaths among US infants. Pediatrics 2000; 106:1413–21.

24. Bajaj L, Roback MG. Postreduction management of intussusception in a children's hospital emergency department. Pediatrics 2003;112(6 Pt 1):1302–7.

25. Ein SH. Leading points in childhood intussusception. J Pediatr Surg 1976;11: 209–11.

26. Waseem M, Rosenberg HK. Intussusception. Pediatr Emerg Care 2008;24(11): 793–800.

27. Newman J, Schuh S. Intussusception in babies under 4 months of age. CMAJ 1987;136:266–9.

28. Turner D, Rickwood AM, Brereton RJ. Intussusception in older children. Arch Dis Child 1980;55:544–6.

29. Reijnen JA, Festen C, Joosten HJ, et al. Atypical characteristics of a group of children with intussusception. Acta Paediatr Scand 1990;79:675–9.
30. Sato M, Ishida H, Konno K, et al. Long-standing painless intussuscep- tion in adults. Eur Radiol 2000;10:811–3.
31. Klein EJ, Kapoor D, Shugerman RP. The diagnosis of intussusception. Clin Pediatr (Phila) 2004;43(4):343–7.
32. Kuppermann N, O'Dea T, Pinckney L, et al. Predictors of intussusception in young children. Arch Pediatr Adolesc Med 2000;154:250–5.
33. Kleizen KJ, Hunck A, Wijnen MH, et al. Neurological symptoms in children with intussusception. Acta Paediatr 2009;98(11):1822–4.
34. Hernandez JA, Swischuk LE, Angel CA. Validity of plain films in intussusception. Emerg Radiol 2004;10(6):323–6.
35. Roskind CG, Kamdar G, Ruzal-Shapiro CB, et al. Accuracy of plain radiographs to exclude the diagnosis of intussusception. Pediatr Emerg Care 2012;28(9): 855–8.
36. Henderson AA, Anupindi SA, Servaes S, et al. Comparison of 2-view abdominal radiographs with ultrasound in children with suspected intussusception. Pediatr Emerg Care 2013;29(2):145–50.
37. Bhisitkul DM, Listernick R, Shkolnik A, et al. Clinical application of ultrasonography in the diagnosis of intussusception. J Pediatr 1992;121(2):182–6.
38. Hryhorczuk AL, Strouse PJ. Validation of US as a first-line diagnostic test for assessment of pediatric ileocolic intussusception. Pediatr Radiol 2009;39(10): 1075–9.
39. Swischuk LE, Hayden CK, Boulden T. Intussusception: indications for ultrasonography and an explanation of the doughnut and pseudokidney signs. Pediatr Radiol 1985;15(6):388–91.
40. Fike FB, Mortellaro VE, Holcomb GW 3rd, et al. Predictors of failed enema reduction in childhood intussusception. J Pediatr Surg 2012;47(5):925–7.
41. Kaiser AD, Applegate KE, Ladd AP. Current success in the treatment of intussusception in children. Surgery 2007;142(4):469–75 [discussion: 475–7].
42. Gilmore AW, Reed M, Tenenbein M. Management of childhood intussusception after reduction by enema. Am J Emerg Med 2011;29(9):1136–40.
43. Chien M, Willyerd FA, Mandeville K, et al. Management of the child after enema-reduced intussusception: hospital or home? J Emerg Med 2013; 44(1):53–7.
44. Hall MJ, DeFrances CJ, Williams SN, et al. National Hospital Discharge Survey: 2007 summary. Natl Health Stat Report 2010;(29):1–20, 24. PubMed PMID: 21086860.
45. Addiss DG, Shaffer N, Fowler BS, et al. The epidemiology of appendicitis and appendectomy in the United States. Am J Epidemiol 1990;132(5): 910–25.
46. Rothrock SG, Pagane J. Acute appendicitis in children: emergency department diagnosis and management. Ann Emerg Med 2000;36(1):39–51.
47. Rothrock SG, Skeoch G, Rush JJ, et al. Clinical features of misdiagnosed appendicitis in children. Ann Emerg Med 1991;20(1):45–50.
48. Bansal S, Banever GT, Karrer FM, et al. Appendicitis in children less than 5 years old: influence of age on presentation and outcome. Am J Surg 2012;204(6): 1031–5.
49. Trautlein JJ, Lambert R, Miller J. Malpractice in the emergency room: a critical review of undiagnosed appendicitis cases and legal actions. Qual Assur Util Rev 1987;2(2):54–6.

50. Körner H, Söndenaa K, Söreide JA, et al. Incidence of acute nonperforated and perforated appendicitis: age-specific and sex-specific analysis. World J Surg 1997;21(3):313–7.
51. McAbee GN, Donn SM, Mendelson RA, et al. Medical diagnoses commonly associated with pediatric malpractice lawsuits in the United States. Pediatrics 2008;122(6):e1282–6.
52. Barker AP, Davey RB. Appendicitis in the first three years of life. Aust N Z J Surg 1988;58(6):491–4.
53. Kulik DM, Uleryk EM, Maguire JL. Does this child have appendicitis? A systematic review of clinical prediction rules for children with acute abdominal pain. J Clin Epidemiol 2013;66(1):95–104.
54. Kharbanda AB, Dudley NC, Bajaj L, et al, Pediatric Emergency Medicine Collaborative Research Committee of the American Academy of Pediatrics. Validation and refinement of a prediction rule to identify children at low risk for acute appendicitis. Arch Pediatr Adolesc Med 2012;166(8):738–44.
55. Bundy DG. Clinical prediction rule identifies children at low risk for appendicitis. J Pediatr 2013;162(3):654–5.
56. Wang LT, Prentiss KA, Simon JZ, et al. The use of white blood cell count and left shift in the diagnosis of appendicitis in children. Pediatr Emerg Care 2007;23(2):69–76.
57. Nance ML, Adamson WT, Hedrick HL. Appendicitis in the young child: a continuing diagnostic challenge. Pediatr Emerg Care 2000;16(3):160–2.
58. Hallan S, Asberg A. The accuracy of C-reactive protein in diagnosing acute appendicitis–a meta-analysis. Scand J Clin Lab Invest 1997;57(5):373–80.
59. Kwan KY, Nager AL. Diagnosing pediatric appendicitis: usefulness of laboratory markers. Am J Emerg Med 2010;28(9):1009–15. http://dx.doi.org/10.1016/j.ajem.2009.06.004.
60. Muenzer JT, Jaffe DM, Schwulst SJ, et al. Evidence for a novel blood RNA diagnostic for pediatric appendicitis: the riboleukogram. Pediatr Emerg Care 2010;26(5):333–8.
61. Olutola PS. Plain film radiographic diagnosis of acute appendicitis: an evaluation of the signs. Can Assoc Radiol J 1988;39(4):254–6.
62. Rothrock SG, Green SM, Hummel CB. Plain abdominal radiography in the detection of major disease in children: a prospective analysis. Ann Emerg Med 1992;21(12):1423–9.
63. Warner BW, Kulick RM, Stoops MM, et al. An evidenced-based clinical pathway for acute appendicitis decreases hospital duration and cost. J Pediatr Surg 1998;33(9):1371–5.
64. Strouse PJ. Pediatric appendicitis: an argument for US. Radiology 2010;255(1):8–13.
65. Hennelly KE, Bachur R. Appendicitis update. Curr Opin Pediatr 2011;23(3):281–5.
66. Doria AS, Moineddin R, Kellenberger CJ, et al. US or CT for diagnosis of appendicitis in children and adults? A meta-analysis. Radiology 2006;241(1):83–94.
67. Kutasy B, Hunziker M, Laxamanadass G, et al. Increased incidence of negative appendectomy in childhood obesity. Pediatr Surg Int 2010;26(10):959–62.
68. Raja AS, Wright C, Sodickson AD, et al. Negative appendectomy rate in the era of CT: an 18-year perspective. Radiology 2010;256(2):460–5.
69. Hlibczuk V, Dattaro JA, Jin Z, et al. Diagnostic accuracy of noncontrast computed tomography for appendicitis in adults: a systematic review. Ann Emerg Med 2010;55(1):51–9.

70. Ganguli S, Raptopoulos V, Komlos F, et al. Right lower quadrant pain: value of the nonvisualized appendix in patients at multidetector CT. Radiology 2006; 241(1):175–80.
71. Garcia K, Hernanz-Schulman M, Bennett DL, et al. Suspected appendicitis in children: diagnostic importance of normal abdominopelvic CT findings with non-visualized appendix. Radiology 2009;250(2):531–7.
72. Wakeford R. The risk of childhood leukaemia following exposure to ionising radiation-a review. J Radiol Prot 2013;33(1):1–25.
73. Wan MJ, Krahn M, Ungar WJ, et al. Acute appendicitis in young children: cost-effectiveness of US versus CT in diagnosis-a Markov decision analytic model. Radiology 2009;250(2):378–86.
74. Moore MM, Gustas CN, Choudhary AK, et al. MRI for clinically suspected pediatric appendicitis: an implemented program. Pediatr Radiol 2012;42(9): 1056–63.
75. Cobben L, Groot I, Kingma L, et al. A simple MRI protocol in patients with clinically suspected appendicitis: results in 138 patients and effect on outcome of appendectomy. Eur Radiol 2009;19(5):1175–83.
76. Gill RS, Shi X, Al-Adra DP, et al. Single-incision appendectomy is comparable to conventional laparoscopic appendectomy: a systematic review and pooled analysis. Surg Laparosc Endosc Percutan Tech 2012;22(4):319–27.
77. Garey CL, Laituri CA, Ostlie DJ, et al. Single-incision laparoscopic surgery in children: initial single-center experience. J Pediatr Surg 2011;46(5):904–7.
78. Lacher M, Muensterer OJ, Yannam GR, et al. Feasibility of single-incision pediatric endosurgery for treatment of appendicitis in 415 children. J Laparoendosc Adv Surg Tech A 2012;22(6):604–8.
79. St Peter SD, Aguayo P, Fraser JD, et al. Initial laparoscopic appendectomy versus initial nonoperative management and interval appendectomy for perforated appendicitis with abscess: a prospective, randomized trial. J Pediatr Surg 2010;45(1):236–40.
80. Amiel J, Lyonnet S. Hirschsprung disease, associated syndromes, and genetics: a review. J Med Genet 2001;38(11):729–39.
81. Holschneider AM, Puri P. Hirschsprung's disease and allied disorders. 2nd edition. Amsterdam: Harwood Academic Publishers; 2000.
82. Khan AR, Vujanic GM, Huddart S. The constipated child: how likely is Hirschsprung's disease? Pediatr Surg Int 2003;19:439–42.
83. Pini Prato A, Rossi V, Avanzini S, et al. Hirschsprung's disease: what about mortality? Pediatr Surg Int 2011;27(5):473–8.

Pediatric ENT Emergencies

Michael J. Stoner, MD[a,b,]*, Marlie Dulaurier, MD[a,b]

KEYWORDS

- Foreign bodies • Trauma • Peritonsillar abscess • Mastoiditis
- Retropharyngeal abscess • Tonsillectomy • Epistaxis

KEY POINTS

- Importance should be paid to the airway in children who present with ENT complaints.
- Most nasal and ear foreign bodies can be removed in the emergency department.
- Risks of retained nasal foreign bodies include infection, nasal septum perforation, and aspiration.
- Lodged disk battery and magnets always require emergent removal.
- Complications of posterior pharyngeal trauma are rare but include deep pharyngeal infection, mediastinitis, and deep neck vessel trauma.
- The most common postoperative adverse effects of tonsillectomy include inadequate pain control with poor intake and wound bleeding.
- Posttonsillectomy bleeding occurs at two times, early within the first 24 hours, and later at postoperative days 5 to 8.

FOREIGN BODIES

Young children are constantly exploring their surroundings and are more apt to place objects in locations that can pose a threat to well-being. This includes the nasal passages, the external ear canals, and the mouth. Although foreign bodies in the ears and nose are not usually an emergency, there are instances when it can be an emergency situation. Foreign bodies in the throat or airway can pose a complete airway obstruction immediately and is a true emergency (**Table 1**).

Nasal Foreign Bodies

Nasal foreign bodies are most common in children between the ages of 2 and 5 years, and include any object small enough to fit up the nostril, such as food, buttons, toys, and erasers. Although nasal foreign bodies only make up about 0.1% of emergency department (ED) visits, most of these can and should be removed in the ED.[1] Nasal

[a] Section of Emergency Medicine, Nationwide Children's Hospital, 700 Children's Drive, Columbus, OH 43205, USA; [b] Department of Pediatrics, OSU College of Medicine, Columbus, OH, USA
* Corresponding author.
E-mail address: Michael.Stoner@nationwidechildrens.org

Emerg Med Clin N Am 31 (2013) 795–808
http://dx.doi.org/10.1016/j.emc.2013.04.005
0733-8627/13/$ – see front matter © 2013 Elsevier Inc. All rights reserved.

Location	Common Foreign Bodies	Removal Technique	Indications for Referral
Table 1 Common pediatric ears, nose, and pharynx foreign body management			
Ear	Beads, paper, toys, pebbles	Irrigation with water Grasping foreign body with forceps, cerumen loop, right-angle ball hook, or suction catheter Acetone to dissolve Styrofoam foreign body	Need for sedation Canal or tympanic membrane trauma Foreign body is nongraspable, tightly wedged, or touching tympanic membrane Sharp foreign body Removal attempts unsuccessful
Nasal	Beads, buttons, toy parts, pebbles, candle wax, food, paper, cloth, button batteries	Patient "blows nose" with opposite nostril obstructed Grasping with forceps, curved hook, cerumen loop, or suction catheter Thin, lubricated, balloon-tip catheter[3] Parent's kiss; positive pressure may also be delivered by bag mask[5]	Bleeding disorder Removal attempts unsuccessful Septum or bone destruction, granulation tissue from chronic foreign body or button battery
Pharynx	Plastic, balloons, pins, seeds, nuts, bones, coins	Magills if able to see, such as a balloon, but often need to be removed endoscopically, requiring sedation and, thus, referral	Inadequate visualization Need for sedation Signs of airway compromise

Data from Heim SW, Maughan KL. Foreign bodies in the ear, nose, and throat. Am Fam Physician 2007;76(8):1185–9.

foreign bodies usually present with the complaint of "my child put something in his/her nose," but can also present with pain or discomfort, foul smelling nasal discharge, recurrent epistaxis, or rhinorrhea/congestion alone; a key historical piece of information is unilateral drainage. The most concerning object that children can insert into their nares is a button battery. The availability of these has soared in the past few years. Button batteries are now found in many toys, flashlights, handheld games, watches, remote controls, and talking or musical greeting cards. In the case of alkaline batteries, they can corrode and release caustic material, which leads to damage of the nasal tissue, necrosis, and subsequent nasal septal perforation. Nasal septal perforation has been reported to occur in as little as 7 hours.[2] Another common nasal foreign body that has a high rate of complications is magnets. If there is a magnet in each nare, or a magnet on one side and a ferrous object on the other, these can cause pressure, leading to mucosal breakdown and ultimately a septal perforation if not removed. Other more common complications of nasal foreign bodies include local irritation, pain, ulceration, infection, and epistaxis.

Removal of nasal foreign bodies is divided into two categories: positive pressure and mechanical extraction.[3] Positive pressure refers to using pressure to "blow" the object out. The simplest strategy for this is to have the child blow the object out while obstructing the opposite nostril. This can take a lot of coaxing and is often futile in the younger population, but worth trying. It may be more successful to pinch off both nares, instructing the child to blow as hard as he or she can, then letting pressure off the affected nostril. Making it a game or a challenge for the child may get them more involved, thereby increasing success at removal. Make sure the child inhales through their mouth before blowing, so as not to suck the foreign body further back into their nasal passage. Another pearl that may aid in removal is the instillation of a vasoconstrictor before any attempts at removal. This can include a nasal deconges-tant drop or spray, such as phenylephrine or oxymetazoline hydrochloride, or nebu-lized epinephrine.[4] A point of caution: although this may make removal a bit easier by drying up secretions, reducing mucosal swelling, and decreasing traumatic epistaxis, it also may increase the risk for the foreign body to be displaced further into the nasal cavity and possibly aspirated.[3] If the blowing technique is not fruitful, there is still the option of using positive pressure. A common technique for this is termed the "parent's kiss." This is a technique whereby the patient's parent is instructed to blow into the child's mouth, while occluding the unaffected nostril, thereby increasing pressure and in essence blowing the child's nose for them (**Fig. 1**). The use of the child's parent is to allow the child to relax and anticipate a "kiss" from them. It is important to instruct the parent on technique, including a good seal before attempting. One concern that has been noted is the concern for barotrauma, although pressure is low, around 60 mm Hg, which is comparable with a sneeze.[5] Two other positive pressure techniques that are similar include using air from a mechanical device, either an Ambu bag or air or oxygen from the wall at 10 to 15 L/min and instilling it into the unaffected nare using a tight-fitting tube or cath-eter.[3] Finally, the same can be done using a bulb syringe and sterile saline to flush out the foreign body. This method, although effective, can be a little harder to tolerate. All of these positive pressure techniques include the risk of aspiration, so it is best to

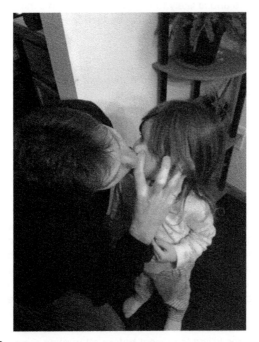

Fig. 1. Parent's kiss.

reserve these techniques for nasal foreign bodies that can be visualized and are not too far posterior.

Mechanical extraction includes a wide range of techniques. For most of these, proper preparation is necessary. Preparation of the nose includes proper visualization, possibly the use of a local decongestant if there is not a high risk of it moving further posterior, and analgesia. Some authors recommend using topical 1% lidocaine, up to 0.3 mL/kg, 10 minutes before attempting removal. One way to do this is with a nasal atomizer; however, the clinician must be careful to ensure that the patient does not sniff the foreign body further into the nasal cavity. Lidocaine can be uncomfortable initially to the nasal mucosa, so risk and benefits must first be considered. Restraints in the form of extra holders, a sheet, papoose or, in certain situations, procedural sedation may be necessary. Common tools for mechanical extraction include straight or alligator forceps. These work well for objects that have a surface on which to grab. That being said, they are a poor option for round objects, such as beads, often pushing them in further while trying to grab the object. Catheters with a balloon on the end, such as a small urinary or vascular catheter, can be used. This is inserted into the nasal passage past the object. The balloon is then inflated and the catheter, along with the object, is expelled. This method works well for objects that are further posterior. There have been reports of foreign body removal using cyanoacrylate glue. A small amount is put onto a stick, such as the back of a throat swab, and held to the foreign body until the glue dries. As the swab is carefully removed, the object comes with it. This only works on dry and usually anterior foreign bodies. Care must be taken not to push it back further while waiting for the glue to dry.[3] Magnets are good tools to use when presented with a metallic foreign body that is anteriorly located. Finally, objects can be removed with rigid instruments. A bead with a hole in the middle can be grabbed with a small surgical hook or bent paperclip. A rigid metal ear curette works very well to scoop an object out of the nose. A typical disposable plastic one bends and is likely to be unsuccessful. This method, although effective, can be a bit traumatic to the nasal mucosa if done aggressively, or if the child is fighting back.

Ear Foreign Bodies

Foreign bodies in the ear canal are also a frequent presentation to the ED. Reports have shown the median age to be 7 years, with most children younger than 8 years of age. Beads are common offenders, with other common objects including pebbles, toys, and paper. Insects are also quite common, mostly in patients older than 10 years of age, and are not placed but rather crawled into the ear canal.[6,7] Although there is no risk of aspiration as with nasal foreign bodies, foreign bodies in the ear can be quite uncomfortable, and certain objects, such as a button battery, can be damaging. When attempting removal of foreign bodies in the ear canal, proper preparation is a must. The ear canal can be very sensitive, so proper analgesia or a topical anesthetic is optimal, as is proper positioning and control. Tools for removal include magnets, hooks, or forceps. Finally, irrigation has great success with removing objects from the external ear canal. There are many irrigation devices on the market, but one can be made easily using a syringe and 18- to 20-gauge angiocatheter. This method should be avoided if there is concern for perforation of the tympanic membrane. Irrigation should be used cautiously if the foreign body is organic (ie, corn, bean, and so forth) in nature, because these objects are likely to swell in the presence of water, making it very difficult to remove. Occasionally, patients may present with the sensation of intense pain and movement in their ear canal as a result of an insect in the external ear canal. Removal requires killing the insect before attempting removal. One of the best ways to euthanize the insect is to instill alcohol, mineral oil, or lidocaine into the ear canal. This should be avoided if there is a perforation in the tympanic membrane.[8] Ear, nose, and throat (ENT) consultation or referral should be considered for objects that have been in the canal for greater than 24 hours, objects that are laying on the tympanic membrane, or certain types of objects. These include objects that are spherical or sharp-edged shape, disk batteries, and vegetable matter, because these are most likely to be difficult to remove and necessitate otomicroscopy-guided foreign body removal. The disk battery necessitates ENT consultation in the ED, and should not be left for removal at a later time.[6]

Airway Foreign Bodies

Pharyngeal foreign bodies are a true emergency because they can cause complete obstruction of the airway. Common objects include food, balloons, plastic bags, or toys. Patients may present with increased work of breathing, stridor, or respiratory failure. In a patient with complete obstruction, immediate airway maneuvers must be initiated. This includes the Heimlich maneuver, jaw thrust, and nasal or oral airways. If these techniques do not improve respiratory status, direct laryngoscopy may be necessary with removal of the foreign body using a Magill forceps or passing an endotracheal tube past the obstruction. If these attempts fail, emergent cricothyrotomy or tracheostomy is necessary.

Partial obstructions are much more common. Partially obstructing objects including toys, seeds, nuts, bones, food, and coins usually present with a cough or gag, or may present with stridor and mimic croup.[8] The key history from parents is that symptoms developed acutely with no preceding illness, often while the child was playing or eating. However, at times the inciting event may not have been witnessed and may not have occurred acutely; these patients may present with persistent wheezing unresponsive to usual treatments or recurrent stridor, this scenario requires a high index of suspicion to diagnose. If the object is radiopaque, it can be visualized with radiography. If it is not, one must have a high clinical suspicion to pursue the work-up. If the patient is able to maintain his or her own airway, offer oxygen and look into the mouth making sure not to agitate the patient. If an object is visible and able to be grasped, remove it; otherwise, keep the child in a position of comfort and have them taken to the operating room for further evaluation with direct visualization.

TRAUMA
Oral Injuries

Traumatic injuries to the mouth or posterior pharynx may present as decreased oral intake, drooling, or bloody emesis. A common scenario is a child running with an object, such as a pencil or toothbrush in their mouth, falling or hitting something, and forcing it into the posterior pharynx.[8] Although quite uncommon, there are reports of children being brought to the ED with a foreign body (pencil, toothbrush, and fence posts) still lodged in the posterior pharynx. This is a true airway emergency, and the patient must be kept as calm as possible to avoid further trauma and airway compromise. ENT should be consulted immediately and preparations made to have emergency airway equipment available at the bedside to secure an airway if necessary. For injuries that involve posterior pharyngeal trauma without an immediate airway compromise, the most concerning injury is trauma involving the lateral soft palate and tonsil pillars because of the location of the internal carotid artery (**Fig. 2**).

In a series of 335 patients looking at posterior pharyngeal penetrating injuries, the authors found two (0.6%) with injury to the internal carotid artery and none with

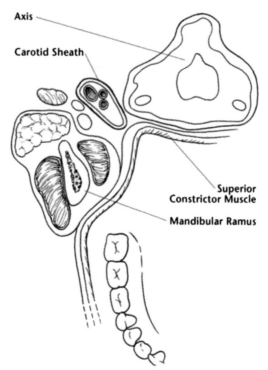

Axis

Carotid Sheath

Superior
Constrictor Muscle

Mandibular Ramus

Fig. 2. Proximity of carotid sheath to posterior pharynx. (*From* Randall DA, Kang DR. Current management of penetrating injuries of the soft palate. Otolaryngol Head Neck Surg 2006;135(3):356–60; with permission.)

neurologic sequelae.[9] In another review, Randall and Kang[10] describe concerns and management of these injuries. The authors recommend that lacerations be left to heal without closure unless there is concern for a foreign body or there is a large laceration or hanging flap. With the abundance of oral flora, many clinicians have become concerned about the development of infection leading to the practice of prescribing prophylactic antibiotics. Although there is no great evidence for or against this practice, it is recommended to consider prophylactic antibiotics aimed at oral flora for lacerations greater than 1 to 2 cm. The management of lateral injuries over the internal carotid artery has evolved. With the concern for an intimal tear leading to a thrombus and ultimately stroke, management in the past has included imaging, anticoagulation, and in-hospital observation. In the review by Randall and Kang,[10] they found report of only 32 cases of carotid thrombus with neurologic impairment, making this exceedingly rare. A total of 244 patients were identified using retrospective data that sustained an "at risk" injury to the lateral palate. Of these, there were no patients that developed neurologic complications. They therefore concluded that the risk of this injury is less than 1%, and recommend instead close observation with further work-up for any neurologic changes. The reported lucid period is thought to last 48 to 60 hours, which had led to the recommendation of a 3-day in-hospital observation. With the frequency of this injury and the reported rarity of any sequelae, unless there are social or other issues that may preclude this, observation can be done at home.

Nasal Injuries

The nose is an area of frequent blunt trauma. Families are frequently worried about a nasal fracture, which rarely requires emergent evaluation or management. However, a hematoma of the nasal septum may cause significant consequences if not recognized and managed appropriately. The definition is a blood collection between the nasal septal cartilage and its surrounding perichondrium. The proposed mechanism is rupture of the small blood vessels supplying the nasal septum resulting from trauma causing a hematoma to form, thus separating the septal perichondrium from cartilage. Cartilage destruction may follow as a result of ischemia and pressure necrosis with resultant septal perforation and saddle-nose deformity, if it is not detected and managed. Diagnostically, one looks for a boggy, bluish mass bulging from the septum. The septum may be gently palpated with a blunt instrument or cotton swab. Topical anesthetics can aid with this examination. Treatment includes incision and drainage with packing, which is best performed under anesthesia or sedation, usually by ENT.[11] Antibiotics should also be initiated to cover nasopharyngeal flora. The most common complication of septal hematomas is abscess formation, which if not recognized may lead to such problems as intracranial extension, orbital cellulitis, meningitis, or sinus thrombus.

Epistaxis

Nosebleeds are a common presenting complaint to the ED. The nose is especially vulnerable to bleeding because of its rich blood supply. Most episodes are minor in nature and easily treated at home. However, epistaxis can be profuse and life-threatening. The most common cause of nosebleeds is the result of digital trauma, blunt trauma, or mucosal irritation from upper respiratory infections. Epistaxis can be classified as either anterior or posterior according to the location of bleeding. Anterior bleeding accounts for most epistaxis episodes and usually arises from Kieselbach plexus in the anterior nasal septum. Posterior bleeds originate from the sphenopalatine artery in the posterior nasal cavity and nasopharynx and tend to bleed more profusely. Posterior bleeds can result in airway compromise, hemodynamic instability, and aspiration.

The initial evaluation of the patient with epistaxis involves the assessment of the airway, breathing, and circulation. It is important to quickly identify patients with hemodynamic instability and to stabilize. Physical examination should be geared toward identifying the location of the bleed to allow proper management. This can be accomplished with suctioning, topical vasoconstrictors, and a nasal speculum with good light source. Treatment of mild epistaxis that is anterior usually involves supportive care, limiting digital trauma or blowing, nasal saline, moisturizing ointments, and reducing mucosal irritation. If actively bleeding, patients or parents should be instructed to apply direct pressure for 5 to 15 minutes without interruption with head bent forward to prevent aspiration. If direct pressure does not resolve the bleeding, one should consider topical vasoconstrictors and limited cautery with silver nitrate. If an anterior bleed cannot be resolved with these measures, then nasal packing should be the next line of treatment. Packing can be removed within the next 30 minutes and the site reexamined. Posterior bleeds are more difficult to control and usually do not respond to the same measures of treatment as anterior bleeds. Posterior nasal packing or a balloon may be necessary to tamponade the bleeding. Otolaryngology should be involved in the care of patients with posterior bleeds for emergent and definitive management. In addition, children with a posterior nasal packing or epistaxis balloon should be treated with a course of antibiotics that provides staphylococcal and streptococcal coverage to decrease the incidence of sinusitis or toxic shock syndrome.

INFECTION

ED visits for acute infections, such as otitis media, sinusitis, or pharyngitis, although quite common are rarely an emergency. It is the less common infections that can be a true ENT emergency and are the focus of this next section.

Mastoiditis

Otitis media is a common pediatric ailment, but left untreated it can progress to mastoiditis in a small percentage of cases. Mastoiditis was the most common complication of acute otitis media in the preantibiotic era. The mastoid sinuses are air cells in the mastoid process of the temporal bone. Relatively small at birth, the complete sinus does not fully develop until age 3, which is why mastoiditis is rare, although not impossible, before 3 years of age. The diagnosis is typically clinical; physical examination reveals a downward and outward protrusion of the auricle with erythema and swelling over the mastoid process. Treatment involves admission and treatment with broad-spectrum antibiotics. If treatment is delayed, the patient will likely require surgery to decrease secondary complications, such as hearing loss, labrynthitis with associated dizziness, or cranial nerve VII involvement with facial nerve paralysis. Mastoiditis can also spread to the brain leading to meningitis or cerebral sinovenous thrombosis.[12] Cerebral sinovenous thrombosis secondary to mastoiditis predominantly affects the transverse sinus. Diagnosis takes a high degree of suspicion, but associated symptoms include headache, papilledema, vomiting, and cranial nerve VI paralysis. Treatment revolves around treating the infection and anticoagulation therapy to restore blood flow and prevent further sequelae. A study by Vieira and colleagues[13] found that even though recanalization is the goal with anticoagulation therapy, a large portion did not recanalize and that recanalization did not correlate with a better prognosis in the long term. Transverse sinus thrombosis from mastoiditis frequently recovers without sequelae regardless of whether or not there was recanalization.

Orbital (Septal) Cellulitis

Orbital (septal) cellulitis is an infection of the soft tissues of the orbit behind the orbital septum. In contrast, preseptal cellulitis is an infection of the eyelids and periocular region anterior to orbital septum. Treatment of periorbital cellulitis usually only requires antibiotics and rarely progresses into septal cellulitis unless the thin septum is incomplete (**Fig. 3**).[14,15] Orbital cellulitis is usually secondary to extension of infection from a sinusitis, with the exception of penetrating trauma or hematogenous spread. That said, an odontogenic abscess can extend into the maxillary sinus and continue to penetrate superiorly into the orbit, just as infection from a nasal foreign body can extend into the orbit. Anatomically, the orbit has the frontal sinus above, the maxillary sinus below, and the ethmoids medial to it, with ethmoiditis being the most common cause for extension, only having the lamina papyracea between them. Because orbital cellulitis is usually secondary to sinusitis, the causative bacteria are typically respiratory and presentation commonly occurs in older children. In contrast, periorbital cellulitis is typically seen in younger children. Clinically, orbital cellulitis presents with unilateral swelling, tenderness, and erythema. The patient may also have fever and be ill appearing. These patients may also have signs of increased intraocular pressure, including visual changes, pain on extraocular movements, decreased range of motion,

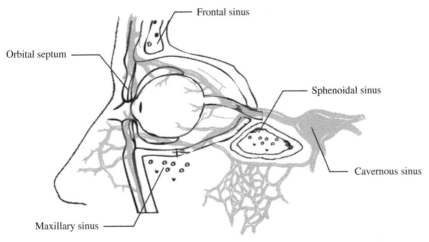

Fig. 3. Orbital and periorbital anatomy. (*From* Hauser A, Fogarasi S. Periorbital and orbital cellulitis. Pediatr Rev 2010;31:242–9; with permission.)

chemosis, afferent pupillary defect, and proptosis. Orbital cellulitis does not extend above the brow, as can periorbital cellulitis.[15,16] Contrast-enhanced computed tomography (CT) scan of the sinuses and orbits with axial and coronal thin cuts is the diagnostic test of choice to confirm and further delineate the degree of involvement (**Fig. 4**). If there is concern for cavernous sinus thrombosis or further soft tissue details are necessary, magnetic resonance imaging is the next imaging technique of choice.[16] Treatment includes admission and intravenous antibiotics targeted at *Staphylococcus aureus, Streptococcus pyogenes,* and typical respiratory pathogens. Indications for surgery include presence of a large abscess or clinical signs of increased pressure, such as decreased range of motion or significant visual acuity loss (20/60). Surgery is also indicated for failure to improve after 48 hours despite aggressive medical

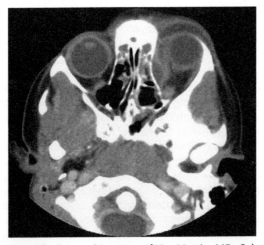

Fig. 4. Orbital cellulitis with abscess. (*Courtesy of* Lisa Martin, MD, Columbus, OH.)

management.[16] Complications of orbital cellulitis include osteomyelitis, cavernous sinus thrombosis, proptosis, and ophthalmoplegia. Late findings include loss of vision, subdural empyema, extradural or intracerebral abscesses, and meningitis.

Retropharyngeal Abscesses

Retropharyngeal abscesses are a collection of fluid in the retropharyngeal space. These usually start as an upper-respiratory infection or pharyngitis, leading to inflammation of the retropharyngeal lymph nodes and eventually suppuration. Although most common in children up to 5 to 6 years of age, it can also occur in older children. This is thought to be caused by the presence of a paramedian chain of lymph nodes that run in the retropharyngeal space that usually spontaneously regress after 5 years of age.[17] Clinically, children usually present with fever, neck pain, sore throat, or difficulty swallowing. In the younger nonverbal child, fever and decreased oral intake may be the only clues to the diagnosis. As the disease progresses, patients may develop torticollis, drooling, and respiratory distress including stridor. In the ED, the first step after a thorough history and physical examination is a lateral soft tissue neck radiograph.[17] If the child is in significant distress immediate consultation with an otolaryngologist should be obtained and consideration given to a portable lateral soft tissue neck scan. Although the lateral neck radiograph has been considered a good screening tool, there is evidence to suggest that it may miss some cases, and with the availability of CT scanners, a CT should be considered in children with a high degree of clinical suspicion.[18,19] After the diagnosis has been made, ENT consultation is in order. If the child is having any airway or secondary complications, urgent surgical drainage is needed. Depending on the results of the CT, many treatment options include a period of intravenous antibiotics, followed by surgical drainage if not improving in 24 to 48 hours.[18,20]

In a study by Hoffmann and colleagues[18] the authors gave more concise guidelines, starting with surgical intervention for any abscess that was greater than 20 mm versus intravenous antibiotics for those smaller than 20 mm, with a 48-hour recheck. If not clinically better, they were then either taken back to the CT scanner or to the operating room. Complications of missed or delayed diagnosis and treatment include airway obstruction and progression of the illness causing cervical necrotizing fasciitis or mediastinitis, with the latter being the most common. Other complications include aspiration pneumonia, jugular venous thrombosis, or aneurysm of the carotid artery. As one would imagine, these are more common in the younger population where presentation and diagnosis may be delayed.[21]

Peritonsillar Abscess

Peritonsillar abscess (PTA) is another deep infection of the head and neck. It is the most common deep infection of the neck, affecting all age groups, although more prominent in the teenage to young adult years. In a study out of Calgary, Millar and colleagues[22] looked at 229 pediatric patients suspected of having a PTA. They found the highest occurrence in the 14 to 17 years of age range with a rate of 40 per 100,000 child-years at risk. The youngest child affected in their sample was 21 months of age. The abscess forms when the oral flora invades the peritonsillar space, forming an abscess between the palatine tonsil and its capsule.[23] Clinically, the patient complains of sore throat, fever, and may be drooling and have an altered "muffled" voice. On examination, the patient has pharyngeal erythema, asymmetric peritonsillar swelling, bulging soft palate, and deviation of the uvula away from the side of infection. The addition of trismus or uvular deviation is more consistent with abscess than only cellulitis or phlegmon. True diagnosis of a PTA requires the demonstration of a collection of fluid in the peritonsillar space. This can be done either with needle aspiration, ultrasound, or a CT scan. The choice of diagnostic method is based on practitioner's local practices, comfort, and ENT consultation and CT availability. If there is no abscess (phlegmon) or after the fluid has been drained, treatment consists of hydration, pain control, and antibiotics. If the patient is nontoxic, able to tolerate oral intake, and has adequate pain control they can be treated as an outpatient with close ENT follow-up and antibiotics; otherwise they should be admitted.[22,23]

There has been controversy over the use of steroids. Although steroids have been shown to decrease pain in adults with pharyngitis, their use in PTA is unclear. A study of adult patients found the number of days to recovery to be reduced with one dose of intravenous steroids. A similar study in the pediatric population was unable to find a significant improvement with steroids when used for PTA.[22,24]

Complications of PTA include airway obstruction and aspiration. Infection in the peritonsillar space can erode into the carotid sheath and cause sepsis or hemorrhage.[23] Another complication that occurs when infection spreads past the tonsil is Lemierre syndrome, which occurs when infection disrupts the mucosa of the oropharynx, leading to deeper tissue infection with involvement of the internal jugular vein. This in turn causes septic thrombophlebitis of the vein and ultimately metastatic infection, usually into the lungs. The classic causal bacterium is *Fusobacterium necrophorum*, but others have also been implicated. Many times the pulmonary symptoms and sepsis arise after the pharyngeal infection has resolved, so good history and high index of suspicion are needed. Patients have a history of recent pharyngitis and present with neck pain, fever, or rigors. Other presenting signs and symptoms are usually related to site of septic emboli. Treatment of Lemierre syndrome focuses on treatment of sepsis and multiorgan dysfunction including antibiotics to cover for polymicrobial infection, including anaerobes. If no improvement is seen, thrombectomy or ligation of the internal jugular vein may be necessary.[25]

POSTPROCEDURAL COMPLICATIONS
Posttonsillectomy Hemorrhage

Tonsillectomy is the second most common procedure performed in children in the United States. Often it is done on an ambulatory basis with approximately 3% being done in an inpatient setting.[26] The procedure is done at two peaks in childhood, first from 5 to 8 years of age, then from 17 to 21 years of age. Primary reasons for tonsillectomy include recurrent tonsillar infections and sleep-related disorders, such as obstructive sleep apnea. With the increase in the number of tonsillectomies that occur and because they are primarily done as an outpatient, if a postprocedure complication does arise, it likely finds its way into an ED. Hemorrhage is a common complication after tonsillectomy, and occurs at two points: primary bleeding within the first 24 hours, and secondary when the eschar comes off at approximately 5 to 8 days postprocedure with rates up to 2.2% and 3%, respectively (**Fig. 5**).[26,27] Treatment consist of stopping the bleeding and fluid or blood resuscitation as needed. The bleeding can be stopped with direct pressure or by applying epinephrine or thrombin. If this does not work, return to the operating room may be necessary. Consultation with the ENT surgeon earlier rather than later is advised.

Posttonsillectomy Pain

Another common adverse event from tonsillectomy is pain, often leading to dehydration from inadequate oral intake. Pain is expected for the first 3 to 5 days postsurgery, and it is recommended to use pain controllers aggressively to keep pain under control.

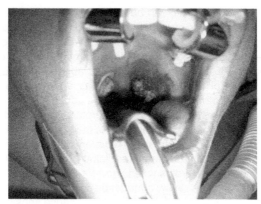

Fig. 5. Posttonsillectomy bleeding. (*Courtesy of* Charles Elmaraghy, MD, Columbus, OH.)

Historically, ENT surgeons have avoided nonsteroidal anti-inflammatory drugs (NSAIDs) with the concern that they may increase the tendency to bleed. Instead, they have used acetaminophen or acetaminophen with codeine. In a review of trials looking at NSAID use, the authors found NSAIDs did not significantly alter the number of perioperative bleeding events requiring surgical intervention or those not requiring surgical intervention. They also found the rate of nausea and vomiting to be lower in the NSAID group.[28] With this in mind, there are also data looking at the analgesic that is commonly prescribed for posttonsillectomy pain, acetaminophen with codeine. In the summer of 2012, the Food and Drug Administration released a warning about three children who had died from codeine. They refer to a small (1%–7%) number of the population that metabolizes codeine into its active drug, morphine, at an ultra-rapid rate, thereby exposing the child to increased doses. These children not only get exceptional pain control, they are exposed to increased side effects, such as respiratory depression. This, in the face of an already swollen posterior pharynx, can lead to upper airway obstruction, respiratory depression, and death.[29]

SUMMARY

When dealing with pediatric cases in the ED, ENT cases are frequent occurrences. Whether it is from trauma, a foreign body, infection, or a complication of a previous procedure, the emergency physician needs to have an understanding of the various conditions and how to manage them. That, and the availability of a good local otolaryngologist, ensures that the emergency physician is well prepared.

REFERENCES

1. Mackle T, Conlon B. Foreign bodies of the nose and ears in children: should these be managed in the accident and emergency setting? Int J Pediatr Otorhinolaryngol 2006;70:425–8.
2. Loh WS, Leong JL, Tan HK. Hazardous foreign bodies: complications and management of button batteries in nose. Ann Otol Rhinol Laryngol 2003;112(4):379–83.
3. Kiger JR, Brenkert TE, Losek JD. Nasal foreign body removal in children. Pediatr Emerg Care 2008;24(11):785–92 [quiz: 790–2].

4. Douglas AR. Use of nebulized adrenaline to aid expulsion of intra-nasal foreign bodies in children. J Laryngol Otol 1996;110(6):559–60.
5. Purohit N, Ray S, Wilson T, et al. The parent's kiss: an effective way to remove paediatric nasal foreign bodies. Ann R Coll Surg Engl 2008;90(5):420–2.
6. Schulze S, Kerschner J, Beste D. Pediatric external auditory canal foreign bodies: a review of 698 cases. Otolaryngol Head Neck Surg 2002;127:73.
7. Ansley JF, Cunningham MJ. Treatment of aural foreign bodies in children. Pediatrics 1998;101(4):638–41.
8. Heim SW, Maughan KL. Foreign bodies in the ear, nose, and throat. Am Fam Physician 2007;76(8):1185–9.
9. Soose RJ, Simon JP, Mandell DL. Evaluation and management of pediatric oropharyngeal trauma. Arch Otolaryngol Head Neck Surg 2006;132:446–51.
10. Randall DA, Kang DR. Current management of penetrating injuries of the soft palate. Otolaryngol Head Neck Surg 2006;135(3):356–60.
11. Canty PA, Berkowitz RG. Hematoma and abscess of the nasal septum in children. Arch Otolaryngol Head Neck Surg 1996;122:1373–6.
12. Wang NE, Burg JM. Mastoiditis: a case-based review. Pediatr Emerg Care 1998; 14(4):290–2.
13. Vieira JP, Luis C, Monteiro JP, et al. Cerebral sinovenous thrombosis in children: clinical presentation and extension, localization and recanalization of thrombosis. Eur J Paediatr Neurol 2010;14(1):80–5.
14. Givner L. Periorbital versus orbital cellulitis. Pediatr Infect Dis J 2002;21(12): 1157–8.
15. Hauser A, Fogarasi S. Periorbital and orbital cellulitis. Pediatr Rev 2010;31:242–9.
16. Sethuraman U, Kamat DM. Eye infection: cures for a common ailment, Part 2. Consultant For Pediatricians 2012;11(12):405–9.
17. Grisaru-Soen G, Komisar O, Aizenstein O, et al. Retropharyngeal and para-pharyngeal abscess in children: epidemiology, clinical features and treatment. Int J Pediatr Otorhinolaryngol 2010;74(9):1016–20.
18. Hoffmann C, Pierrot S, Contencin P, et al. Retropharyngeal infections in children. Treatment strategies and outcomes. Int J Pediatr Otorhinolaryngol 2011;75: 1099–103.
19. Uzomefuna V, Glynn F, Mackle T, et al. Atypical locations of retropharyngeal abscess: beware of the normal lateral soft tissue neck X-ray. Int J Pediatr Otorhinolaryngol 2010;74(12):1445–8.
20. Page NC, Bauer EM, Lieu JE. Clinical features and treatment of retropharyngeal abscess in children. Otolaryngol Head Neck Surg 2008;138:300–6.
21. Baldassari CM, Howell R, Amorn M, et al. Complications in pediatric deep neck space abscesses. Otolaryngol Head Neck Surg 2011;144(4):592–5.
22. Millar KR, Johnson DW, Drummond D, et al. Suspected peritonsillar abscess in children. Pediatr Emerg Care 2007;23(7):431–8.
23. Galioto N. Peritonsillar abscess. Am Fam Physician 2008;77(2):199–202.
24. Ozbek C, Aygenc E, Tuna EU, et al. Use of steroids in the treatment of peritonsillar abscess. J Laryngol Otol 2004;118(6):439–42.
25. Davies O, Than M. Lemierre's syndrome: diagnosis in the emergency department. Emerg Med Australas 2012;24:673–6.
26. Subramanyam R, Varughese A, Willging JP, et al. Future of pediatric tonsillectomy and perioperative outcomes. Int J Pediatr Otorhinolaryngol 2012. http://dx.doi.org/10.1016/j.ijporl.2012.10.016.
27. Windfuhr JP, Chen YS. Hemorrhage following pediatric tonsillectomy before puberty. Int J Pediatr Otorhinolaryngol 2001;58:197–204.

28. Cardwell ME, Siviter G, Smith AF. Nonsteroidal anti-inflammatory drugs and perioperative bleeding in paediatric tonsillectomy. Cochrane Database of Systematic Reviews 2005;(2):CD003591.
29. FDA Drug Safety Communication. Codeine use in certain children after tonsillectomy and/or adenoidectomy may lead to rare, but life-threatening adverse events or death. Silver Spring (MD): United States Food and Drug Administration; 2012.

Pediatric Ultrasound
Applications in the Emergency Department

Kimberly Leeson, MD, RDMS*, Ben Leeson, MD, RDMS

KEYWORDS

- Bedside ultrasound • Pediatrics • Emergency department

KEY POINTS

- Bedside ultrasound is an important diagnostic and therapeutic tool for the pediatric emergency practitioner.
- Ultrasound may be a diagnostic alternative to imaging modalities that expose children to ionizing radiation.
- Bedside ultrasound can reduce time, number of attempts and complications associated with pediatric emergency procedures.
- The scope of pediatric emergency bedside ultrasound continues to grow and physicians are discovering how valuable US is to their practice.

 Videos of ultrasound accompany this article at http://www.emed.theclinics.com/

PEDIATRIC EMERGENCY ULTRASOUND: A REVIEW
Introduction

Bedside emergency ultrasound (EUS) was introduced to the emergency department (ED) over 20 years ago. Although initially used to evaluate adult trauma patients, many new applications of EUS have evolved to aid the emergency physician in diagnostic, procedural, and therapeutic interventions and the scope of bedside ultrasound (US) continues to grow. Advancing technology has also helped spur this growth in the ED and led to improving US portability, resolution, cost, and accessibility. As more physicians embrace the use of US, they are demanding that US machines be available in their patient care environments. Furthermore, US is becoming a sophisticated diagnostic tool that is accessible to rural and less developed regions of the world.

US is an ideal imaging modality for children. Ease of use, portability, lack of radiation exposure, and adequate image resolution because of children's smaller body habitus make US appealing in pediatrics. Many US scanning techniques easily translate from

Texas A&M – Christus Spohn Emergency Medicine Residency, 2606 Hospital Boulevard, 5 West, Corpus Christi, TX 78405, USA
* Corresponding author.
E-mail address: Kimberly.Leeson@christushealth.org

Emerg Med Clin N Am 31 (2013) 809–829
http://dx.doi.org/10.1016/j.emc.2013.05.005   emed.theclinics.com
0733-8627/13/$ – see front matter © 2013 Elsevier Inc. All rights reserved.

adult applications to the pediatric population and EUS has been adopted by many pediatric practitioners. The use of bedside US often translates into shorter ED length of stays and better patient satisfaction.[1,2] As more concerns mount regarding risks from ionizing radiation, safer imaging methods for children are being explored.

Special Considerations for Pediatric Patients

"Children are not just small adults" and pediatric patients have special treatment considerations. First, there are many diseases and conditions that are specific to childhood, such as congenital heart disease, necrotizing enterocolitis, and pyloric stenosis. Fortunately, children are often spared many of the diseases that are common in adulthood, like diabetes and coronary artery disease. Childhood anatomy differs significantly from adults. Children are not only smaller than adults but they also display differences in physiology, such as faster respiratory rates, lower blood pressure, and bones containing more cartilage and growth plates. Their heads are proportionally larger than those of adults, predisposing them to more head trauma. Body habitus can affect image acquisition and diagnostic accuracy of EUS. Children tend to be smaller than adults and US images are often easier to obtain and display better resolution. Yet, challenges develop when adult-sized US probes are used to image tiny infants. One size does not fit all. Pediatric patients may require different US equipment designed to image smaller bodies.

Unfortunately, obesity is rising among all age groups and complications from childhood obesity are cropping up at an alarming rate. The incidence of obesity in children has increased from less than 5% to 20% in the United States over the past 30 years.[3] Pediatricians are seeing more cases of Type II diabetes, renal stones, and liver and gallbladder disease previously encountered largely in the adult population because of this trend. The epidemiology of these weight-related illnesses will undoubtedly affect physician decisions about imaging choices for pediatric patients of the future and prompt physicians to order US tests that historically were reserved for the adult patient.

The use of computed tomography (CT) has dramatically increased (approximately 8-fold) since 1980.[4] Some estimate that more than 7 million CTs are performed annually on children in the United States.[5] Concern regarding the dangers of radiation exposure from increased use of CT scanning has developed in recent years. Radiation exposure is especially concerning for children for several reasons. Children are more sensitive to radiation because they have rapidly dividing cells, have longer life expectancies and a larger window of opportunity for expressing radiation damage, and may receive a higher dose of radiation if settings are not adjusted for their smaller sizes.[4] The concept of ALARA or "as low as reasonably achievable" attempts to balance the need for efficient and reliable imaging with reducing the amount of radiation exposure. Educating physicians about the risks of radiation exposure can help limit the indiscriminate use of CT imaging on children.[6] Physicians are encouraged to limit the use of CTs and consider alternate forms of imaging such as MRI and US whenever possible.

Traditional Emergency US Applications

Trauma
The use of US to evaluate patients with blunt abdominal trauma (BAT) was the first and most widely used EUS application. Traumatic injuries remain the leading cause of death and hospitalization in pediatric patients after infancy.[7] As in adults, pediatric trauma patients are initially evaluated for free fluid in the pericardium, peritoneum, and thoracic cavity using US. Advantages to the use of US in this setting include

avoidance of ionizing radiation, and the noninvasive, quick, repeatable nature of this examination. In addition, the patient does not need to leave the ED setting and the images are interpreted in real-time with no other specialty involvement.

A focused assessment with sonography in trauma (FAST) examination consists of obtaining images in the right upper quadrant (Morrison's pouch), left upper quadrant (splenorenal junction) (**Fig. 1A, B**), subxiphoid (cardiac) (see **Fig. 1C**), and the pelvis (**Fig. 2**). The right and left upper quadrant views should include the diaphragm to evaluate for hemothorax. A FAST examination is considered positive if free fluid is visualized. Although a positive FAST examination in the pediatric patient with associated BAT suggests hemoperitoneum and abdominal injury, a negative FAST does not exclude injury. Fox and colleagues[8] found that FAST has a low sensitivity for clinically important free fluid, lower than in the adult population, but has a high specificity.

CT remains the imaging modality of choice for blunt abdominal trauma in children who are hemodynamically stable whereby solid organ injury is suspected. Fenton and colleagues[9] showed that only 2% of pediatric patients undergoing CT scan were taken to the operating room for exploratory laparotomy. This minority of patients may be due to the more conservative nonoperative management of many pediatric intraperitoneal injuries, such as liver and splenic lacerations.

Pediatric patients undergoing a trauma evaluation for BAT should receive a CT scan if (1) hemodynamically stable with a positive FAST examination, (2) a physical examination suggests abdominal injury, (3) hematoma or contusion to the torso, or

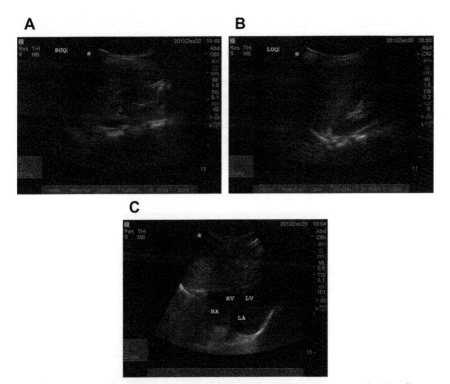

Fig. 1. (A) Fast exam images of the right upper quadrant (Morrison's pouch). (B) Left upper quadrant. (C) Cardiac (subxiphoid) view. LA, left atrium; LV, left ventricle; RA, right atrium; RV, right ventricle.

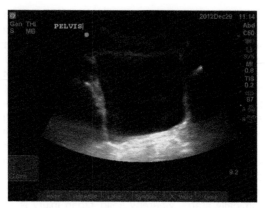

Fig. 2. Negative FAST examination image of the pelvis with full urinary bladder.

(4) neurologic impairment. Hemodynamically unstable patients with a positive FAST examination should go to the operating room for exploratory laparotomy. Hemodynamically stable patients with a negative FAST should undergo serial examinations and possibly serial FAST examinations to rule out evolving injuries whereby free fluid may not be immediately seen.[10–12]

The extended FAST (eFAST) is used to evaluate the thoracic cavity for pneumothorax and hemothorax further. In addition to the right upper quadrant, left upper quadrant, subxiphoid, and pelvic views, images are also obtained over the anterior chest. US has been shown to have superior sensitivity than supine chest radiograph for the detection of pneumothoraces.[13,14] The patient is examined in the supine position by placing a high-frequency probe over the anterior chest wall in a longitudinal plane. Normally, the pleura can be visualized sliding back and forth with respirations (**Fig. 3** and Videos 1 and 2). If the sliding lung sign is absent, a pneumothorax should be suspected. Be aware that if the patient is not ventilating well, as may happen with pain or right mainstem intubation, the sliding lung sign may be diminished or absent and may result in a false positive examination.

Some meta-analyses assessing the value of the FAST examination in the pediatric population report poor sensitivities, and the use of the FAST examination as a screening examination in trauma has been questioned.[15,16] Some investigators

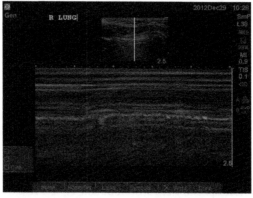

Fig. 3. Pleura can be visualized sliding back and forth with respirations.

recommend abandoning the use of the FAST examination as a screening tool for pediatric trauma patients and using it in cases of traumatic hemodynamic instability to search for causes of bleeding instead. Further investigation is required to determine definitively when and how best to incorporate bedside US into the management of the injured child.

Abdomen

Appendicitis The use of bedside US to diagnose appendicitis has gained considerable support in recent years. This condition, the most common childhood surgical emergency, has a variable presentation that makes diagnosis challenging. Imaging studies such as CT and US are being used with greater frequency and have reduced the number of negative appendectomies performed. Nevertheless, which imaging modality is best for children with suspected appendicitis remains a debate. US is not as sensitive as CT, but CT scan exposes children to ionizing radiation.[17] A large retrospective review found considerable variation in the use of CT and US with appendicitis. This study found institutions that had increased US use or combined US and CT had lower negative appendectomy rates. Overall, there was a trend toward decreased use of CT in children.[18] Some advocate a staged US and CT pathway when evaluating for appendicitis in children with US being the first imaging modality. With this approach, CT is reserved only for children with inconclusive US studies, thereby decreasing the number of unnecessary CTs performed.[19,20]

US findings of appendicitis include an appendiceal diameter greater than 6 mm, echogenic periappendiceal inflammatory fat changes, noncompressible lumen, an appendicolith, or periappendiceal free fluid (**Fig. 4** and Videos 3 and 4). A meta-analysis examining the use of CT and US found pooled sensitivity and specificity for diagnosis of appendicitis in children were 88% (95% confidence interval [CI]: 86%, 90%) and 94% (95% CI: 92%, 95%), respectively, for US studies and 94% (95% CI: 92%, 97%) and 95% (95% CI: 94%, 97%) for CT studies.[21] Positive predictive values and negative predictive values of 98% have been described for US use in evaluating appendicitis.[22] Although some experienced emergency physicians are beginning to incorporate EUS for appendicitis evaluation into their practice, this continues to remain a study that largely takes place in the radiology suite.

Cholecystitis Cholecystitis is relatively uncommon in children, yet the incidence of biliary tract disease has been climbing in this age group since the 1970s.[23] Tsung

A   **B**

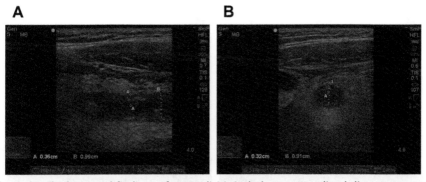

Fig. 4. (A, B) Ultrasound findings of appendicitis include an appendiceal diameter greater than 6 mm, echogenic periappendiceal inflammatory fat changes, noncompressible lumen, an appendicolith, or periappendiceal free fluid.

and colleagues[24] present a small case series of pediatric patients diagnosed with cholecystitis using bedside US. Normal sonographic findings include gallbladder wall thickness less than or equal to 3 mm in children up to age 16 and normal common bile duct diameter of 3 mm or less (measured inner to inner wall) in children up to age 13.[25,26] Measurements outside these parameters were considered abnormal, in addition to the sonographic presence of gallstones, pericholecystic fluid, and a sonographic Murphy sign, whereby pain is elicited by applying direct pressure with the US probe over the gallbladder. The use of bedside US as a screening test in children presenting to the ED with epigastric or right upper quadrant abdominal pain may reduce the likelihood of misdiagnosis and delayed diagnosis in this condition.[24]

Hypertrophic pyloric stenosis Hypertrophic pyloric stenosis is an acute abdominal condition in infants who present to the ED. It is the most common cause of intestinal obstruction in this age group and US is the imaging modality of choice. A small case series by Malcom and colleagues[27] suggests that emergency physicians can be trained to use bedside US to diagnose this condition. The pylorus can be imaged in the short axis in the right upper quadrant between the gallbladder and stomach.[28] Sonographic features of hypertrophic pyloric stenosis include a muscle wall thickness of greater than 3.5 to 4 mm and a pyloric channel length of 15 mm or longer (**Fig. 5**).[29]

Intussusception Intussusception, the leading cause of bowel obstruction in the young child, is another condition that is often diagnosed by US.[30] US has gained favor over traditional contrast enema studies for suspected intussusception because it is risk-free, noninvasive, inexpensive, fast, and painless.[31] Mendez and colleagues[32] found that US was as specific for diagnosing intussusception as the combination of highly suggestive radiographs with several clinical features (abdominal pain, lethargy, and vomiting). There have been no formal studies examining the use of EUS, but 2 case reports describe using bedside US in the ED to identify this condition.[31,33] The sonographic findings of intussusception include a soft tissue mass in the right mid abdomen with the classic "target" or "donut" sign, "crescent" sign, and "pseudokidney" signs (**Fig. 6** and Video 5).[33]

Other abdominal conditions diagnosed by EUS reported in case reports and small studies of pediatric patients include omental infarction, intestinal *Ascaris lumbricoides*, acute mesenteric lymphadenitis, and congenital colon abnormalities.[34–37] One case report identified a congenital diaphragmatic hernia in a young infant

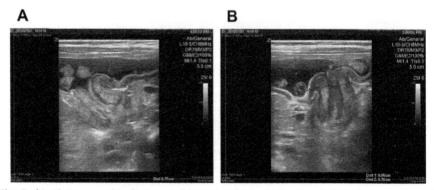

Fig. 5. (*A, B*) Sonographic features of hypertrophic pyloric stenosis include a muscle wall thickness of greater than 3.5 to 4 mm and a pyloric channel length of 15 mm or longer.

A   B

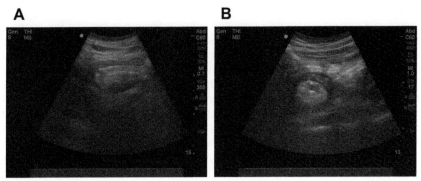

Fig. 6. Sonographic findings of intussusception include a soft tissue mass in the right mid abdomen with the classic "target" or "donut" sign, "crescent" sign, and "pseudokidney" signs.

presenting with respiratory distress and upper respiratory infection symptoms.[38] In this report, US demonstrated liver tissue located at the fourth intercostal space, an unexpectedly high position.

Renal/bladder

EUS can be useful to determine the amount of urine present before urine specimen collection. If insufficient volume is present, the clinician can postpone collecting a sample by catheterization or superpubic aspiration and either wait or hydrate the patient until enough urine is present.[39] Baumann and colleagues[40] found a significant increase in successful first attempt catheterization of children younger than 3 years of age with volumetric bladder US performed by trained nurses. One disadvantage in this study was that the use of US resulted in more than double the time to urine collection.

Urolithiasis is an uncommon condition in the pediatric population, but when present may present in atypical ways. The incidence of pediatric nephrolithias has increased over the last decade with a 7-fold increased incidence.[41] A small study of children with symptoms of urolithiasis that compared CT to US found US failed to detect renal calculi in 41% compared with 5% with CT. The authors recommended foregoing US in favor of CT when considering renal calculi as a diagnosis in children.[42] On the other hand, DiSandro recommends approaching the pediatric patient with possible urolithiasis like adults with similar complaints with the exception of imaging studies. He advocates the use of renal and bladder sonography with plain radiographs of the kidneys, ureter, and bladder to limit radiation exposure. Although conventional US accuracy to locate urinary tract stones is low (50%–70%), other features such as hydronephrosis and color Doppler US twinkling can increase accuracy.[43–45] "Twinkling artifact is a color phenomenon visible behind a strongly reflecting interface such as urinary tract stones, parenchymal calcification or bones during color Doppler examination. It manifests itself as a color signal but without real flow behind the structures. It imitates turbulent flow."[46] Although EUS is frequently used to evaluate for hydronephrosis in adult patients who present to the ED with symptoms of renal colic in the ED, currently there is very limited literature examining this practice in children.

Other urological conditions encountered in pediatrics that may be diagnosed by US include posterior urethral valves and hemolytic uremic syndrome.[47,48] Sonographically, HUS is characterized by increased renal cortical echogenicity.[49] The use of EUS to detect these conditions is not widely used, however.

Cardiac

Although performing a complete pediatric echocardiogram is beyond the scope of practice for most pediatric emergency medical physicians, being able to determine gross abnormalities quickly can help guide management in acute life-threatening situations. Cardiac US is an integral part of the FAST examination. It is also a useful diagnostic tool when evaluating patients with unexplained hypotension and patients presenting to the ED with pulseless electrical activity. Indications for cardiac EUS include chest trauma, chest pain, dyspnea, tachycardia, hypotension/shock, and cardiac arrest. The emergency sonologist should not get bogged down in learning all of the complexities of echocardiography, but should instead focus on recognizing normal cardiac EUS and a few key findings, such as pericardial effusions and their size, cardiac standstill, overall assessment of cardiac function, signs of right heart strain, and volume assessment.[50] Emergency physicians are encouraged to quantify global cardiac function as either normal, hypokinetic, or hyperdynamic (**Fig. 7**, Video 6). Longjohn and colleagues[51] found substantial agreement between emergency physicians and formal cardiology ECHO sonologists in assessing left ventricular ejection fraction. Determining global cardiac function rapidly is a skill the emergency physician can develop with little training that can help facilitate prompt consultation or appropriate transfer.

Procedures

Intravenous access

Children who present to the ED often require intravenous (IV) access. Obtaining IV access in the pediatric patient can be challenging and requires considerable expertise. Medical conditions such as dehydration can complicate this procedure.[52] US-guided peripheral IV placement has been shown to decrease the need for central lines in adult intensive care unit patients and this technique is being used regularly in pediatric EDs.[53] Oakley and colleagues[54] found that although US-guided peripheral IVs took longer to place, there was a higher success rate and better performance of the IV. A randomized trial evaluating the use of EUS for IV placement in pediatric ED patients found the use of US resulted in less time, fewer attempts, and fewer needle redirections than traditional line approaches (**Fig. 8**).[52]

US has also been shown to decrease the number of needle sticks, time, and complications associated with obtaining central venous access. The pediatric population has smaller vessels than adults and direct vessel visualization through US improves

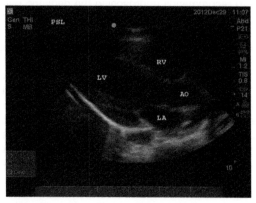

Fig. 7. Global cardiac function is described as either normal, hypokinetic or hyperdynamic. AO, aorta; LA, left atrium; LV, left ventricle; RV, right ventricle.

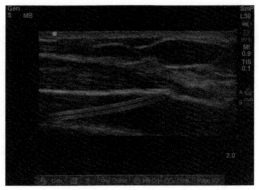

Fig. 8. Longitudinal view of a peripheral vein with an IV catheter seen within the vessel lumen.

accuracy and success rates compared with traditional landmark methods of vessel cannulation. One study looking at US-guided central line placement in infants found US use resulted in increased success with a relatively low complication rate of 22%.[55] Reports on real-time US use for central line placement in children is limited to a several cases series and a few randomized trials and most studies were not conducted in the ED.[56–58] Although anesthesiologists have reported improved success using US for arterial cannulation over blind needle sticks, there are no reports of adopting this practice in the pediatric emergency medicine literature.[59]

Soft tissue infection

US is useful for evaluating and treating soft tissue conditions. It is important to differentiate between cutaneous abscess and cellulitis in children presenting to the ED because the treatments are significantly different. Although some abscesses may be quite evident, others can be challenging to distinguish from cellulitis, which requires a different management approach. In addition, the location of the best site for abscess incision and drainage, with the largest accessible cavity of purulent material, may not be easily discerned from a visual inspection of the skin, and it is impossible to avoid deeper structures such as blood vessels and nerves without looking beneath the skin surface.

Normal soft tissue has a characteristic appearance. The dermis and epidermis appear bright or hyperechoic in relation to the deep subcutaneous fat globules that are present without much separation between each globule (**Fig. 9**A). Cellulitis classically appears as "cobblestoning," with the appearance of dark, hypoechoic fluid separating the fat globules (see **Fig. 9**B). Abscesses have a variable appearance, but most often are identified as an anechoic or hypoechoic (dark or black) elliptical-shaped collection of fluid (see **Fig. 9**C). Gentle compression of the abscess with the US probe can elicit fluid movement, sometimes referred to as the squish sign further supporting the diagnosis.[60,61]

EUS is an important tool in abscess identification and safe incision and drainage. One study demonstrated that pediatric emergency physicians could learn the technique to perform and interpret EUS examinations for soft tissue infections with excellent agreement with an expert emergency sonologist after a brief training program.[62] Another study emphasized the importance of this examination in demonstrating that the use of EUS to examine soft tissue infections changed emergency physician management approximately one-half the time.[63] A similar study in the pediatric population found the use of US changed management 22% of the time.[64]

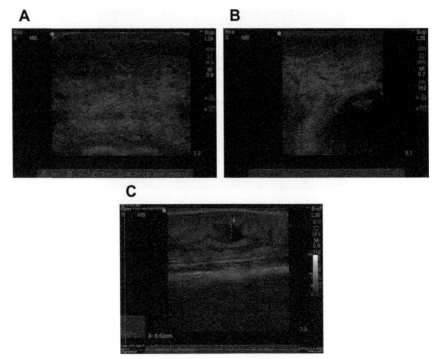

Fig. 9. (*A*) Dermis and epidermis appear bright or hyperechoic in relation to the deep sub-cutaneous fat globules that are present without much separation between each globule. (*B*) Cellulitis appears as "cobblestoning," with the appearance of dark, hypoechoic fluid separating the fat globules. (*C*) Abscesses most often are identified as an anechoic or hypoechoic (*dark or black*) elliptical-shaped collection of fluid.

Peritonsillar abscess

Peritonsillar abscess (PTA) can be difficult to distinguish from peritonsillar cellulitis. The clinical findings for both conditions overlap with trismus, erythema, and edema. Studies have found that blind needle aspiration of PTAs can have failure rates as high as 10% to 24%. Intraoral US can easily localize a peritonsillar fluid collection and guide drainage (**Fig. 10**). By using a high-frequency intracavitary probe and probe

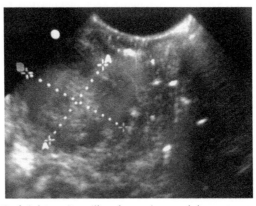

Fig. 10. Intraoral US of right peritonsillar abscess in an adolescent man.

cover, the examiner can image the posterior pharynx in 2 planes. Lyon and Blaivas report a case series of adult patients suspected of having PTA who underwent EUS. Eighty-one percent were found to have PTAs; all of those patients underwent US-guided aspiration and were discharged home. There were no complications and no return visits to the ED.[65]

Necrotizing fasciitis

Necrotizing fasciitis is a rare, rapidly progressing soft tissue infection that requires early diagnosis and intervention. It is important to distinguish this condition from cellulitis, which often is more benign and can appear similarly, especially early in the disease course. US can demonstrate the features of necrotizing fasciitis that include fascial thickening, fluid accumulation along fascial planes, and subcutaneous soft tissue edema and gas.[66,67] Prompt recognition of this dangerous condition can lead to early antibiotic and surgical debridement, the mainstays of therapy with necrotizing fasciitis.

Pelvic/Obstetrics

Abdominal and pelvic pain in the adolescent girl are common complaints evaluated in the ED. Bedside US can be a valuable tool in this patient population to rule in intrauterine pregnancy, which essentially excludes ectopic pregnancy in girls without risk factors for heterotopic pregnancy. One prospective study demonstrated 100% sensitivity and 95% specificity for pelvic EUS diagnosing intrauterine pregnancy by emergency physicians.[68] In addition, identifying intraperitoneal or pelvic free fluid quickly at the bedside in an adolescent woman with a positive pregnancy test may indicate a ruptured ectopic pregnancy and decreased time to definitive obstetrics/gynecologic management. Several studies indicate that pelvic EUS in the ED can be accurately performed by emergency physicians and may significantly decrease the amount of time to diagnosis and treatment of ectopic pregnancy when compared with US performed in the radiology suite.[69–72] Shih found that pelvic sonography performed by emergency physicians can be sensitive, specific, and safe and can shorten ED length of stays.[73]

The role of EUS for evaluating the nonpregnant female patient with abdominal pain is less clear. Sonographic identification of conditions such as ovarian torsion, ovarian cyst, and tubo-ovarian abscess requires advanced sonographic training and experience. Further studies are indicated to determine if broadening the scope of pelvic EUS in the ED is warranted.

Musculoskeletal

US is useful when managing musculoskeletal injuries or conditions in the pediatric population. It may be used quickly and repeatedly at the bedside with no concerns for exposure to ionizing radiation. Pediatric bony anatomy is more complex than adults, with growth plates complicating radiographic image interpretations. Fortunately, US has the advantage of being able to visualize the cartilaginous regions of pediatric joints that can make fracture detection challenging with traditional radiographic imaging. US findings in fractures include subperiosteal hematomas, bending or plastic deformity, cortical disruption, and reverberating echoes.[74]

Although sensitivity of point of care US in detecting fractures in children and young adults was only 73% in one study, US has been found to be helpful, especially in diagnosing mid shaft fractures and in settings where access to diagnostic imaging is limited.[74] Several studies describe using US to diagnose clavicle fractures as well as wrist fractures with adequate sensitivities.[75–78] One study found US to have an overall accuracy of 94% for detecting nonangulated distal forearm fractures and patients reported less pain with US than with radiographs.[79] One review suggests that more evidence is needed to determine if US is an acceptable alternative to radiography in pediatric forearm fractures.[78] US has been used successfully to diagnose and localize rib fractures in the adult population, but whether this application is as useful in nonverbal pediatric patients who cannot express localized chest wall pain continues to be an area for investigation.[80] A single case report describes the use of US to diagnose rib fractures secondary to nonaccidental trauma in a 9 month old. The infant was found to have chest wall crepitus but negative oblique rib films and skeletal surveys.[81]

In addition to aiding with fracture diagnosis, US has been used during fracture anesthesia and reduction. EUS can facilitate hematoma block placement and help the clinician assess fracture reduction adequacy, particularly with forearm fractures. Advantages to EUS for fracture reduction include real-time evaluation of the reduction and limiting ionizing radiation exposure from serial radiographs and fluoroscopy.[82,83]

US may be used for subcutaneous foreign body (FB) detection and localization in children. Some benefits to using US include real-time visualization of the FB and improved sensitivity to detect radiolucent FBs such as wood and plastic.[84] In the pediatric population, Friedman and colleagues[85] reported equal sensitivity and improved specificity than radiography in a small case series. Combining US with patient perception resulted in the highest sensitivity for FB detection.

New Applications in Pediatric Emergency US

Skull fractures

Pediatric closed head trauma is commonly evaluated in the ED. Children's heads are proportionally larger than those of adults, making them more prone to injury. Among neurologically normal children, the incidence of intracranial injury ranges from 5% to 25%.[86,87] Skull fractures are the most common abnormal finding, which increases the likelihood of underlying intracranial injury (**Fig. 11** and Video 7).[88] Clinicians are reluctant to expose children to brain CT scanning, the best diagnostic test, when the suspicion for intracranial injury is low. US can be a useful tool to determine if a skull fracture is present or not and can prompt more targeted use of CT scans in the pediatric patients. Several studies suggest that US may be used to identify skull fractures in a cost-effective, safe, noninvasive manner.[74,88,89]

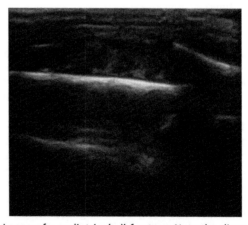

Fig. 11. Ultrasound image of a pediatric skull fracture. Note the disrupted cortical surface.

Transfontanellar US

Transfontanellar ultrasound (TFUS) to identify intracranial injuries may be a viable alternative to CT for minor head trauma in the infant patient. Trenchs and colleagues[90] evaluated infants up to 1 year of age with TFUS as the first neuroimaging test to rule out intracranial injuries. CT was performed if TFUS was inconclusive or difficult to perform, due to a small fontanelle. Two patients had nonoperative small epidural hemorrhages. The authors concluded that TFUS is a reliable alternative to CT in infants who sustain minor head trauma. Although subarachnoid hemorrhage is demonstrated well with TFUS, extra-axial blood such as epidural and subdural may be missed. Some sources suggest that the use of Doppler US can improve sensitivity. This US application is not widely used in EDs to date and CT and MRI remain the best diagnostic tests for intracranial traumatic injury in children.

Much attention has been given to the use of orbital US to identify increased intracranial pressure noninvasively by measurement of the optic sheath diameter. This noninvasive US measurement is well described in the adult literature.[91,92] A small study by Le and colleagues[93] determined that bedside sonographic measurement of the optic sheath was not a good predictor of increased intracranial pressure in children. Further research is required to determine the usefulness of this US application.

Lung US

Historically, lung US has been performed as an extension of the FAST examination to evaluate for hemothorax and pneumothorax in trauma patients. Limited studies demonstrate that lung US may also be useful in diagnosing pulmonary thromboembolism, pneumonia, and pulmonary contusion in children.[94–96] Identifying pleural effusions and other sonographic features such as A and B lines can help the clinician narrow the differential for children presenting with respiratory complaints. A recent study by Shah and colleagues suggests that ED physicians are capable of diagnosing pneumonia with US in the pediatric population with high specificity.[97]

Arthrocentesis

US is a useful tool for evaluating children who present to the ED with hip pain, painful limp, or refusal to bear weight. Septic arthritis is a dangerous part of the differential diagnosis with these complaints. Bedside US can identify whether a hip effusion is present and aid in performing hip arthrocentesis. Smith reports a case whereby EUS was used to diagnose and drain a hip effusion after failed blind attempts and Tsung and Blaivas report a small case series of hip effusion diagnosis and drainage by emergency physicians.[98,99]

Volume assessment and unexplained hypotension

US has been used in the adult population to search for causes of hypotension. Several case reports of EUS in pediatric patients presenting with shock are described.[100–102]

Fluid responsiveness by sonographic evaluation of inferior vena cava diameter has been described in adults. Currently, the data are inconclusive.[103] Several studies describe a method of using sonographic inferior vena cava/aortic diameter indices to evaluate pediatric fluid volume status successfully.[104–106] There continues to be a need for prospective trials examining this US application in children.

Lumbar puncture

Lumbar punctures (LP) are routinely performed in the pediatric ED. LPs can be challenging because of physician inexperience and children's smaller anatomy. US can be very helpful for identifying the ideal needle insertion site for LPs, especially in obese patients where this procedure can be more technically difficult. One study in children found that the LP needle angle should be more acute in younger patients than in older children.[107] Other studies used US to determine the best position to increase the interspinous space size in children. One found the sitting flexed-hip position for LP to be best and the flexed-hip lateral recumbent position is acceptable as well. Neck flexion did not influence interspace site.[108] Cadigan and colleagues[109] recommend a tight, lateral flexed position to maximize interspinous space size for LP. Further research is needed to determine if US use during LP results in more procedural success in children.

Male Genitourinary

Acute scrotal pain comprises 0.5% of complaints to the ED.[110] Common diagnoses include testicular torsion and epididymitis. Timely diagnosis and treatment of torsion are essential to preserve fertility and avoid orchiectomy and US is the test of choice. Delays for imaging can occur, especially in EDs without nighttime in-house sonographers. Emergency physicians can learn to perform testicular US successfully and reduce the amount of time to diagnosis. Traditional 2-dimensional US combined with power and spectral Doppler to assess for flow is essential.[111] Studies on emergency physician use of testicular ultrasonography have been limited to several case reports and retrospective studies comparing accuracy to other diagnostic methods such as surgery and US performed in the radiology department.[112–114] Other scrotal conditions such as orchitis, testicular rupture and hernias, and testicular masses can be diagnosed with EUS.[114,115]

Endotracheal tube placement

Endotracheal tube positioning is usually confirmed with plain radiographs. Efforts to reduce radiation exposure prompted the use of US to confirm appropriate tube placement. Uya and colleagues[116] found that pediatric emergency medicine fellows with no formal airway US training could accurately determine endotracheal tube position in adult cadaveric models after a short teaching module.[117]

Nerve blocks

Recently, emergency physicians have explored alternate methods of pain control for painful conditions and procedures. Regional nerve blocks are a safe alternative to conscious sedation for some patients. Emergency physicians are becoming more acquainted with regional anesthesia using US-guided nerve blocks.[118] To date, study data are limited and only a few case reports of emergency physician–performed US-guided nerve blocks are found in the pediatric literature.[119]

SUMMARY

The field of emergency US is evolving rapidly. New applications for the use of US at the bedside crop up at a remarkable pace. Nevertheless, there remains considerable room for scientific investigation regarding the use of bedside US in the pediatric patient population, not only in the traditional EUS applications but in newer applications as well.

Pediatric emergency training programs lag behind emergency medicine residencies in the amount of US training provided and many pediatric EDs lack bedside US equipment. The Accreditation Council for Graduate Medical Education requires emergency medicine training programs to demonstrate competency in EUS for its graduates but does not have pediatric-specific guidelines.[120] A recent survey of pediatric emergency medicine fellowship directors found that 95% reported some EUS use and 79% offered structured EUS rotations for fellows.[121] One survey of pediatric emergency medicine fellowship programs found that although most programs had access to EUS equipment, only 16% had US curriculums tailored for the pediatric emergency physician.[122] Currently no standard training requirement for pediatric emergency bedside US exists. Physician educators are developing an understanding of the current capabilities of pediatric EUS, as well as an awareness of its limitations and uncertainties that are ripe for future investigation. Pediatric EM educators identify a need for a pediatric emergency US national curriculum so more training programs can incorporate EUS in fellowship training.[122] As bedside US continues to mature, more pediatric emergency physicians will incorporate this valuable technology into their practices.

ACKNOWLEDGMENTS

The authors thank Jeremy Johnson, DO for ultrasound images and videos.

SUPPLEMENTARY DATA

Supplementary data related to this article can be found at http://dx.doi.org/10.1016/j.emc.2013.05.005.

REFERENCES

1. Blaivas M, Harwood RA, Lambert MJ. Decreasing length of stay with emergency ultrasound examination of the gallbladder. Acad Emerg Med 1999;6(10): 1020–3.
2. Blaivas M, Sierzenski P, Plecque D, et al. Do emergency physicians save time when locating a live intrauterine pregnancy with bedside ultrasonography? Acad Emerg Med 2000;7(9):988–93.
3. Ogden CL, Carroll MD, Curtin LR, et al. Prevalence of high body mass index in US children and adolescents, 2007-2008. JAMA 2010;303(3):242–9.
4. Radiation risks and pediatric computed tomography (CT): a guide for healthcare providers.
5. Brenner DJ, Hall EJ. Computed tomography–an increasing source of radiation exposure. N Engl J Med 2007;357(22):2277–84.
6. Shah NB, Platt SL. ALARA: is there a cause for alarm? Reducing radiation risks from computed tomography scanning in children. Curr Opin Pediatr 2008;20(3): 243–7.
7. Dowd MD, Keenan HT, Bratton SL. Epidemiology and prevention of childhood injuries. Crit Care Med 2002;30(Suppl 11):S385–92.
8. Fox JC, Boysen M, Gharahbaghian L, et al. Test characteristics of focused assessment of sonography for trauma for clinically significant abdominal free fluid in pediatric blunt abdominal trauma. Acad Emerg Med 2011;18(5):477–82.
9. Fenton SJ, Hansen KW, Meyers RL, et al. CT scan and the pediatric trauma patient–are we overdoing it? J Pediatr Surg 2004;39(12):1877–81.
10. Retzlaff T, Hirsch W, Till H, et al. Is sonography reliable for the diagnosis of pediatric blunt abdominal trauma? J Pediatr Surg 2010;45(5):912–5.
11. Henderson SO, Sung J, Mandavia D. Serial abdominal ultrasound in the setting of trauma. J Emerg Med 2000;18(1):79–81.
12. Blackbourne LH, Soffer D, McKenney M, et al. Secondary ultrasound examination increases the sensitivity of the FAST exam in blunt trauma. J Trauma 2004; 57(5):934–8.

13. Kirkpatrick AW, Sirois M, Laupland KB, et al. Hand-held thoracic sonography for detecting post-traumatic pneumothoraces: the Extended Focused Assessment with Sonography for Trauma (EFAST). J Trauma 2004;57(2):288–95.

14. Blaivas M, Lyon M, Duggal S. A prospective comparison of supine chest radiography and bedside ultrasound for the diagnosis of traumatic pneumothorax. Acad Emerg Med 2005;12(9):844–9.

15. Stengel D, Bauwens K, Sehouli J, et al. Emergency ultrasound-based algorithms for diagnosing blunt abdominal trauma. Cochrane Database Syst Rev 2005;(2): CD004446.

16. Holmes JF, Gladman A, Chang CH. Performance of abdominal ultrasonography in pediatric blunt trauma patients: a meta-analysis. J Pediatr Surg 2007;42(9): 1588–94.

17. Bundy DG, Byerley JS, Liles EA, et al. Does this child have appendicitis? JAMA 2007;298(4):438–51.

18. Bachur RG, Hennelly K, Callahan MJ, et al. Advanced radiologic imaging for pediatric appendicitis, 2005-2009: trends and outcomes. J Pediatr 2012;160(6): 1034–8.

19. Ramarajan N, Krishnamoorthi R, Barth R, et al. An interdisciplinary initiative to reduce radiation exposure: evaluation of appendicitis in a pediatric emergency department with clinical assessment supported by a staged ultrasound and computed tomography pathway. Acad Emerg Med 2009;16(11): 1258–65.

20. Krishnamoorthi R, Ramarajan N, Wang NE, et al. Effectiveness of a staged US and CT protocol for the diagnosis of pediatric appendicitis: reducing radiation exposure in the age of ALARA. Radiology 2011;259(1):231–9.

21. Doria AS, Moineddin R, Kellenberger CJ, et al. US or CT for diagnosis of appendicitis in children and adults? A meta-analysis. Radiology 2006;241(1):83–94.

22. Kessler N, Cyteval C, Gallix B, et al. Appendicitis: evaluation of sensitivity, specificity, and predictive values of US, Doppler US, and laboratory findings. Radiology 2004;230(2):472–8.

23. Bailey PV, Connors RH, Tracy TF Jr, et al. Changing spectrum of cholelithiasis and cholecystitis in infants and children. Am J Surg 1989;158(6):585–8.

24. Tsung JW, Raio CC, Ramirez-Schrempp D, et al. Point-of-care ultrasound diagnosis of pediatric cholecystitis in the ED. Am J Emerg Med 2010;28(3):338–42.

25. McGahan JP, Phillips HE, Cox KL. Sonography of the normal pediatric gallbladder and biliary tract. Radiology 1982;144(4):873–5.

26. Hernanz-Schulman M, Ambrosino MM, Freeman PC, et al. Common bile duct in children: sonographic dimensions. Radiology 1995;195(1):193–5.

27. Malcom GE 3rd, Raio CC, Del Rios M, et al. Feasibility of emergency physician diagnosis of hypertrophic pyloric stenosis using point-of-care ultrasound: a multi-center case series. J Emerg Med 2009;37(3):283–6.

28. Hayden CK, Swischuk LE, Lobe TE, et al. Ultrasound: the definitive imaging modality in pyloric stenosis. Radiographics 1984;4:517–30.

29. Hernanz-Schulman M. Infantile hypertrophic pyloric stenosis. Radiology 2003; 227(2):319–31.

30. Cochran AA, Higgins GL 3rd, Strout TD. Intussusception in traditional pediatric, nontraditional pediatric, and adult patients. Am J Emerg Med 2011;29(5): 523–7.

31. Halm BM, Boychuk RB, Franke AA. Diagnosis of intussusception using point-of-care ultrasound in the pediatric ED: a case report. Am J Emerg Med 2011;29(3): 354.e1–3.

32. Mendez D, Caviness AC, Ma L, et al. The diagnostic accuracy of an abdominal radiograph with signs and symptoms of intussusception. Am J Emerg Med 2012;30(3):426–31.

33. Kairam N, Kaiafis C, Shih R. Diagnosis of pediatric intussusception by an emergency physician-performed bedside ultrasound: a case report. Pediatr Emerg Care 2009;25(3):177–80.

34. Rimon A, Daneman A, Gerstle JT, et al. Omental infarction in children. J Pediatr 2009;155(3):427–31.e1.

35. Kessler DO, Gurwitz A, Tsung JW. Point-of-care sonographic detection of intestinal ascaris lumbricoides in the pediatric emergency department. Pediatr Emerg Care 2010;26(8):586–7.

36. Toorenvliet B, Vellekoop A, Bakker R, et al. Clinical differentiation between acute appendicitis and acute mesenteric lymphadenitis in children. Eur J Pediatr Surg 2011;21(2):120–3.

37. Rodesch G, Dargent JL, Haller A, et al. An unusual presentation of a cystic duplication of the sigmoid colon entirely lined with squamous epithelium. J Pediatr Surg 2009;44(9):1831–4.

38. Soto F, Soltero R, Rovira H. Complicated bronchiolitis: another use for your bedside ultrasound in the emergency department. Bol Asoc Med P R 2009; 101(3):51–3.

39. Baumann BM, Welsh BE, Rogers CJ, et al. Nurses using volumetric bladder ultrasound in the pediatric ED. Am J Nurs 2008;108(4):73–6.

40. Baumann BM, McCans K, Stahmer SA, et al. Volumetric bladder ultrasound performed by trained nurses increases catheterization success in pediatric patients. Am J Emerg Med 2008;26(1):18–23.

41. Schissel BL, Johnson BK. Renal stones: evolving epidemiology and management. Pediatr Emerg Care 2011;27(7):676–81.

42. Palmer JS, Donaher ER, O'Riordan MA, et al. Diagnosis of pediatric urolithiasis: role of ultrasound and computerized tomography. J Urol 2005;174(4 Pt 1):1413–6.

43. DiSandro M. Pediatric urolithiasis: children as little adults. J Urol 2010;184(5): 1833–4.

44. Ulusan S, Koc Z, Tokmak N. Accuracy of sonography for detecting renal stone: comparison with CT. J Clin Ultrasound 2007;35(5):256–61.

45. Mitterberger M, Aigner F, Pallwein L, et al. Sonographic detection of renal and ureteral stones. Value of the twinkling sign. Int Braz J Urol 2009;35(5):532–9 [discussion: 540–1].

46. Grochal, FJ, P. Twinkling artifact. Available at: http://www.sonoworld.com/fetus/page.aspx?id=1969.

47. Schecter J, Chao JH. Posterior urethral valves diagnosed by bedside ultrasound in the ED. Am J Emerg Med 2012;30(4):633.e1–2.

48. Glatstein M, Miller E, Garcia-Bournissen F, et al. Timing and utility of ultrasound in diarrhea-associated hemolytic uremic syndrome: 7-year experience of a large tertiary care hospital. Clin Pediatr (Phila) 2010;49(5):418–21.

49. Kenney PJ, Brinsko RE, Patel DV, et al. Sonography of the kidneys in hemolytic uremic syndrome. Invest Radiol 1986;21(7):547–50.

50. Labovitz AJ, Noble VE, Bierig M, et al. Focused cardiac ultrasound in the emergent setting: a consensus statement of the American Society of Echocardiography and American College of Emergency Physicians. J Am Soc Echocardiogr 2010;23(12):1225–30.

51. Longjohn M, Wan J, Joshi V, et al. Point-of-care echocardiography by pediatric emergency physicians. Pediatr Emerg Care 2011;27(8):693–6.

52. Doniger SJ, Ishimine P, Fox JC, et al. Randomized controlled trial of ultrasound-guided peripheral intravenous catheter placement versus traditional techniques in difficult-access pediatric patients. Pediatr Emerg Care 2009;25(3):154–9.
53. Gregg SC, Murthi SB, Sisley AC, et al. Ultrasound-guided peripheral intravenous access in the intensive care unit. J Crit Care 2010;25(3):514–9.
54. Oakley E, Wong AM. Ultrasound-assisted peripheral vascular access in a paediatric ED. Emerg Med Australas 2010;22(2):166–70.
55. Di Nardo M, Tomasello C, Pittiruti M, et al. Ultrasound-guided central venous cannulation in infants weighing less than 5 kilograms. J Vasc Access 2011; 12(4):321–4.
56. Alderson PJ, Burrows FA, Stemp LI, et al. Use of ultrasound to evaluate internal jugular vein anatomy and to facilitate central venous cannulation in paediatric patients. Br J Anaesth 1993;70(2):145–8.
57. Verghese ST, McGill WA, Patel RI, et al. Ultrasound-guided internal jugular venous cannulation in infants: a prospective comparison with the traditional palpation method. Anesthesiology 1999;91(1):71–7.
58. Froehlich CD, Rigby MR, Rosenberg ES, et al. Ultrasound-guided central venous catheter placement decreases complications and decreases placement attempts compared with the landmark technique in patients in a pediatric intensive care unit. Crit Care Med 2009;37(3):1090–6.
59. Brzezinski M, Luisetti T, London MJ. Radial artery cannulation: a comprehensive review of recent anatomic and physiologic investigations. Anesth Analg 2009; 109(6):1763–81.
60. Robben SG. Ultrasonography of musculoskeletal infections in children. Eur Radiol 2004;14(Suppl 4):L65–77.
61. Dewitz AF, B. Emergency ultrasound. In: Ma OJ, editor. Soft tissue applications. 2nd edition. New York: McGraw-Hill; 2008.
62. Marin JR, Alpern ER, Panebianco NL, et al. Assessment of a training curriculum for emergency ultrasound for pediatric soft tissue infections. Acad Emerg Med 2011;18(2):174–82.
63. Tayal VS, Hasan N, Norton HJ, et al. The effect of soft-tissue ultrasound on the management of cellulitis in the emergency department. Acad Emerg Med 2006; 13(4):384–8.
64. Sivitz AB, Lam SH, Ramirez-Schrempp D, et al. Effect of bedside ultrasound on management of pediatric soft-tissue infection. J Emerg Med 2010;39(5):637–43.
65. Lyon M, Blaivas M. Intraoral ultrasound in the diagnosis and treatment of suspected peritonsillar abscess in the emergency department. Acad Emerg Med 2005;12(1):85–8.
66. Tsai CC, Lai CS, Yu ML, et al. Early diagnosis of necrotizing fasciitis by utilization of ultrasonography. Kaohsiung J Med Sci 1996;12(4):235–40.
67. Chao HC, Kong MS, Lin TY. Diagnosis of necrotizing fasciitis in children. J Ultrasound Med 1999;18(4):277–81.
68. Mateer JR, Aiman EJ, Brown MH, et al. Ultrasonographic examination by emergency physicians of patients at risk for ectopic pregnancy. Acad Emerg Med 1995;2(10):867–73.
69. Burgher SW, Tandy TK, Dawdy MR. Transvaginal ultrasonography by emergency physicians decreases patient time in the emergency department. Acad Emerg Med 1998;5(8):802–7.
70. Durston WE, Carl ML, Guerra W, et al. Ultrasound availability in the evaluation of ectopic pregnancy in the ED: comparison of quality and cost-effectiveness with different approaches. Am J Emerg Med 2000;18(4):408–17.

71. Kaplan BC, Dart RG, Moskos M, et al. Ectopic pregnancy: prospective study with improved diagnostic accuracy. Ann Emerg Med 1996;28(1):10–7.
72. Rodgerson JD, Heegaard WG, Plummer D, et al. Emergency department right upper quadrant ultrasound is associated with a reduced time to diagnosis and treatment of ruptured ectopic pregnancies. Acad Emerg Med 2001;8(4):331–6.
73. Shih CH. Effect of emergency physician-performed pelvic sonography on length of stay in the emergency department. Ann Emerg Med 1997;29(3):348–51 [discussion: 352].
74. Eksioglu F, Altinok D, Uslu MM, et al. Ultrasonographic findings in pediatric fractures. Turk J Pediatr 2003;45(2):136–40.
75. Cross KP, Warkentine FH, Kim IK, et al. Bedside ultrasound diagnosis of clavicle fractures in the pediatric emergency department. Acad Emerg Med 2010;17(7): 687–93.
76. Chien M, Bulloch B, Garcia-Filion P, et al. Bedside ultrasound in the diagnosis of pediatric clavicle fractures. Pediatr Emerg Care 2011;27(11):1038–41.
77. Willis H, Medicine STE. Towards evidence based emergency medicine: best BETs from the Manchester Royal Infirmary. BET 2: can ultrasound be used to diagnose clavicle fractures in children? Emerg Med J 2012;29(7):599–600.
78. May G, Grayson A. Towards evidence based emergency medicine: best BETs from the Manchester Royal Infirmary. Bet 4: the use of ultrasound in the diagnosis of paediatric wrist fractures. Emerg Med J 2009;26(11):822–5.
79. Chaar-Alvarez FM, Warkentine F, Cross K, et al. Bedside ultrasound diagnosis of nonangulated distal forearm fractures in the pediatric emergency department. Pediatr Emerg Care 2011;27(11):1027–32.
80. Chan SS. Emergency bedside ultrasound for the diagnosis of rib fractures. Am J Emerg Med 2009;27(5):617–20.
81. Kelloff J, Hulett R, Spivey M. Acute rib fracture diagnosis in an infant by US: a matter of child protection. Pediatr Radiol 2009;39(1):70–2.
82. Durston W, Swartzentruber R. Ultrasound guided reduction of pediatric forearm fractures in the ED. Am J Emerg Med 2000;18(1):72–7.
83. Chen L, Kim Y, Moore CL. Diagnosis and guided reduction of forearm fractures in children using bedside ultrasound. Pediatr Emerg Care 2007;23(8):528–31.
84. Manthey DE, Storrow AB, Milbourn JM, et al. Ultrasound versus radiography in the detection of soft-tissue foreign bodies. Ann Emerg Med 1996;28(1):7–9.
85. Friedman DI, Forti RJ, Wall SP, et al. The utility of bedside ultrasound and patient perception in detecting soft tissue foreign bodies in children. Pediatr Emerg Care 2005;21(8):487–92.
86. Klassen TP, Reed MH, Stiell IG, et al. Variation in utilization of computed tomography scanning for the investigation of minor head trauma in children: a Canadian experience. Acad Emerg Med 2000;7(7):739–44.
87. Schunk JE, Rodgerson JD, Woodward GA. The utility of head computed tomographic scanning in pediatric patients with normal neurologic examination in the emergency department. Pediatr Emerg Care 1996;12(3):160–5.
88. Riera A, Chen L. Ultrasound evaluation of skull fractures in children: a feasibility study. Pediatr Emerg Care 2012;28(5):420–5.
89. Ramirez-Schrempp D, Vinci RJ, Liteplo AS. Bedside ultrasound in the diagnosis of skull fractures in the pediatric emergency department. Pediatr Emerg Care 2011;27(4):312–4.
90. Trenchs V, Curcoy AI, Castillo M, et al. Minor head trauma and linear skull fracture in infants: cranial ultrasound or computed tomography? Eur J Emerg Med 2009;16(3):150–2.

91. Amini A, Kariman H, Arhami Dolatabadi A, et al. Use of the sonographic diameter of optic nerve sheath to estimate intracranial pressure. Am J Emerg Med 2013;31(1):236–9.

92. Hightower S, Chin EJ, Heiner JD. Detection of increased intracranial pressure by ultrasound. J Spec Oper Med 2012;12(3):19–22.

93. Le A, Hoehn ME, Smith ME, et al. Bedside sonographic measurement of optic nerve sheath diameter as a predictor of increased intracranial pressure in children. Ann Emerg Med 2009;53(6):785–91.

94. Kosiak M, Korbus-Kosiak A, Kosiak W, et al. Is chest sonography a breakthrough in diagnosis of pulmonary thromboembolism in children? Pediatr Pulmonol 2008;43(12):1183–7.

95. Copetti R, Cattarossi L. Ultrasound diagnosis of pneumonia in children. Radiol Med 2008;113(2):190–8.

96. Stone MB, Secko MA. Bedside ultrasound diagnosis of pulmonary contusion. Pediatr Emerg Care 2009;25(12):854–5.

97. Shah VP, Tunik MG, Tsung JW. Prospective evaluation of point-of-care ultrasonography for the diagnosis of pneumonia in children and young adults. Arch Pediatr Adolesc Med 2012;1–7.

98. Smith SW. Emergency physician-performed ultrasonography-guided hip arthrocentesis. Acad Emerg Med 1999;6(1):84–6.

99. Tsung JW, Blaivas M. Emergency department diagnosis of pediatric hip effusion and guided arthrocentesis using point-of-care ultrasound. J Emerg Med 2008; 35(4):393–9.

100. Pershad J. A 10-year-old girl with shock: role of emergency bedside ultrasound in early diagnosis. Pediatr Emerg Care 2002;18(3):182–4.

101. Pershad J, Chin T. Early detection of cardiac disease masquerading as acute bronchospasm: the role of bedside limited echocardiography by the emergency physician. Pediatr Emerg Care 2003;19(2):E1–3.

102. Gilmore B, Noe HN, Chin T, et al. Posterior urethral valves presenting as abdominal distension and undifferentiated shock in a neonate: the role of screening emergency physician-directed bedside ultrasound. J Emerg Med 2004;27(3):265–9.

103. Bodson L, Vieillard-Baron A. Respiratory variation in inferior vena cava diameter: surrogate of central venous pressure or parameter of fluid responsiveness? Let the physiology reply. Crit Care 2012;16(6):181.

104. Kosiak W, Swieton D, Piskunowicz M. Sonographic inferior vena cava/aorta diameter index, a new approach to the body fluid status assessment in children and young adults in emergency ultrasound–preliminary study. Am J Emerg Med 2008;26(3):320–5.

105. Levine AC, Shah SP, Umulisa I, et al. Ultrasound assessment of severe dehydration in children with diarrhea and vomiting. Acad Emerg Med 2010;17(10): 1035–41.

106. Chen L, Hsiao A, Langhan M, et al. Use of bedside ultrasound to assess degree of dehydration in children with gastroenteritis. Acad Emerg Med 2010;17(10): 1042–7.

107. Bruccoleri RE, Chen L. Needle-entry angle for lumbar puncture in children as determined by using ultrasonography. Pediatrics 2011;127(4):e921–6.

108. Abo A, Chen L, Johnston P, et al. Positioning for lumbar puncture in children evaluated by bedside ultrasound. Pediatrics 2010;125(5):e1149–53.

109. Cadigan BA, Cydulka RK, Werner SL, et al. Evaluating infant positioning for lumbar puncture using sonographic measurements. Acad Emerg Med 2011;18(2):215–8.

110. Lewis AG, Bukowski TP, Jarvis PD, et al. Evaluation of acute scrotum in the emergency department. J Pediatr Surg 1995;30(2):277–81 [discussion: 281–2].
111. Blaivas M, Brannam L. Testicular ultrasound. Emerg Med Clin North Am 2004; 22(3):723–48, ix.
112. Blaivas M, Sierzenski P. Emergency ultrasonography in the evaluation of the acute scrotum. Acad Emerg Med 2001;8(1):85–9.
113. Blaivas M, Batts M, Lambert M. Ultrasonographic diagnosis of testicular torsion by emergency physicians. Am J Emerg Med 2000;18(2):198–200.
114. Blaivas M, Sierzenski P, Lambert M. Emergency evaluation of patients presenting with acute scrotum using bedside ultrasonography. Acad Emerg Med 2001; 8(1):90–3.
115. Pogorelic Z, Juric I, Biocic M, et al. Management of testicular rupture after blunt trauma in children. Pediatr Surg Int 2011;27(8):885–9.
116. Uya A, Spear D, Patel K, et al. Can novice sonographers accurately locate an endotracheal tube with a saline-filled cuff in a cadaver model? A pilot study. Acad Emerg Med 2012;19(3):361–4.
117. Dennington D, Vali P, Finer NN, et al. Ultrasound confirmation of endotracheal tube position in neonates. Neonatology 2012;102(3):185–9.
118. Barnett P. Alternatives to sedation for painful procedures. Pediatr Emerg Care 2009;25(6):415–9 [quiz: 420–2].
119. Frenkel O, Mansour K, Fischer JW. Ultrasound-guided femoral nerve block for pain control in an infant with a femur fracture due to nonaccidental trauma. Pediatr Emerg Care 2012;28(2):183–4.
120. Education, A.C.f.G.M. emergency medicine guidelines. 12/29/12. Available at: http://www.acgme.org/acgmeweb/tabid/292/ProgramandInstitutionalGuidelines/Hospital-BasedAccreditation/EmergencyMedicine/EmergencyMedicineGuidelines.aspx. Accessed December 29, 2012.
121. Marin JR, Zuckerbraun NS, Kahn JM. Use of emergency ultrasound in United States pediatric emergency medicine fellowship programs in 2011. J Ultrasound Med 2012;31(9):1357–63.
122. Cohen JS, Teach SJ, Chapman JI. Bedside ultrasound education in pediatric emergency medicine fellowship programs in the United States. Pediatr Emerg Care 2012;28(9):845–50.

Pediatric Procedural Sedation and Analgesia

Garrett S. Pacheco, MD, Angelique Ferayorni, DO*

KEYWORDS

- Sedation • Analgesia • Pediatrics • Procedures

KEY POINTS

- Analgesia and sedation are often underused in pediatrics.
- Review of available treatment agents for pain and sedation.
- Understand that a child's developmental level can affect pain assessment.
- Review of adverse reactions to commonly used sedation and analgesia.

Sedation and analgesia have historically been criticized for being poorly delivered in the pediatric population. In 2001, the American Academy of Pediatrics Task Force on Pain in Infants, Children, and Adolescents identified barriers in the treatment of pain including the myth that children do not feel pain the way adults do, the lack of pain assessment in pediatrics, and lack of knowledge of pain treatment.[1] Since its release, there have been encouraging improvements in the recognition and treatment of pain. For example, a recent clinical report has identified several studies that have shown an increase in opiate use in children with fractures as an example of the trend to address pediatric pain adequately.[2]

The practice of pediatric sedation and pain control has significantly evolved with new pharmacologic agents, painless interventions, improved continuous monitoring, and safety protocols. Despite such advances, clinicians can still be reluctant to use sedation and analgesia with pediatric patients.[3] The emergency physician should have a firm understanding of the available modalities for treating pain and must be able to provide sedation for painful or anxiety-provoking procedures in the emergency department. This article focuses on various delivery methods for procedural sedation and analgesia (PSA) as well as future trends in the field.

Disclosures: None.
Department of Pediatrics and Emergency Medicine, University of Arizona, 1501 North Campbell Avenue, Tucson, AZ 85724-5057, USA
* Corresponding author.
E-mail address: aferayorni@gmail.com

Emerg Med Clin N Am 31 (2013) 831–852
http://dx.doi.org/10.1016/j.emc.2013.04.002
0733-8627/13/$ – see front matter © 2013 Elsevier Inc. All rights reserved.

SEDATION CONTINUUM

Although a patient who is conscious but cooperative is ideal, physicians often need a deeply sedated patient who is immobile to achieve procedural success. In 1992, the Committee on Drugs of the American Academy of Pediatrics (AAP) released its original *Guidelines for Monitoring and Management of Pediatric Patient During and After Sedation for Diagnostic and Therapeutic Procedures.* These guidelines define conscious sedation as a stage of sedation that allows an appropriate response by the patient to physical stimulation or verbal command.[4] The intention of the Committee was for conscious sedation to be viewed as a minimal state of sedation; however, this concept was ambiguous. In 2002, an addendum was made and the terms were adopted by The Joint Commission.

Conscious sedation was redefined as being moderate sedation and analgesia. At this stage of sedation the patient should have a depressed level of consciousness during which the patient responds purposefully to verbal commands, either alone or accompanied by light tactile stimulation. At the same time, a lesser stage of sedation was acknowledged, termed minimal sedation anxiolysis.[5] A patient who approaches deep sedation may have suppressed or lost protective airway reflexes or ventilatory compromise. They are not easily aroused. General anesthesia occurs when the patient is often unarousable, has often lost protective airway reflexes, and may have impaired ventilation and cardiovascular function. Dissociative sedation does not fit in one of these categories. The patient experiences amnesia, analgesia, and sedation. Patients are minimally responsive to tactile stimulation, but able to protect their airways. The depth of sedation should vary depending on each clinical situation. These levels of sedation represent a continuum (**Fig. 1**). The physician should be comfortable supporting or reversing the patient should they go beyond the intended sedation level.

UNDERSTANDING A CHILD'S DEVELOPMENTAL LEVEL

To reduce the incidence of pain and anxiety that accompanies a diagnostic or therapeutic procedure, nonpharmacologic interventions should be pursued. Nonpharmacologic measures include cognitive and behavioral approaches. When sedation is desired and a nonpharmacologic tool is selected, it is important to keep in mind the developmental and cognitive ability of the patient. Reasoning is rarely useful for children between the ages of 2 and 7 years. However, verbal preparation that is developmentally appropriate can start at the age of 3 years old to help reduce anxiety. Children 8 years old and older benefit from an explanation for the required procedure. Preparation and distraction are important aspects of the preprocedural checklist. Child life

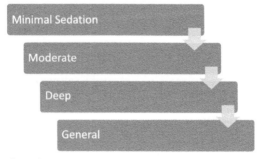

Fig. 1. Sedation level continuum.

has shown an increasing role in this portion of the preparation.[6] Child life specialists aid in the planning and rehearsing of coping mechanisms for the child and establish therapeutic relationships with children and parents to support family involvement in each child's care before a procedure. Play therapy can facilitate understanding and distraction. Music, video, and imagery are tools to aid in preparation and distraction. Distraction tools include movies, toy robots, dolls, virtual reality goggles, music, bubbles, short stories, games, and iPads or digital tablets. Medical supplies, such as playing with syringes, can also be used to prepare the patient and reduce the fear and anxiety of unfamiliar objects. Medical dolls have also been used to prepare patients for procedures. Preparing adolescents for painful procedures is as important as preparing younger children. Adolescents, as well as patients of all ages have the potential to regress during procedures. Much attention is spent on the patient, and the practitioner should also keep in mind that the parents can escalate and add anxiety to a situation or be a source of calm and control for the child.

The primary modality of the child life program incorporates play. Play is reassuring for children and familiar, which reduces the discomfort and intimidation of the health care experience.[6] Child life provides praise during a procedure and positive reinforcement.

EMERGENCY DEPARTMENT PREPARATION AND PRESEDATION

Presedation, intrasedation, and postsedation assessment are paramount to a successful sedation. Presedation includes a detailed history and physical examination to aid in the approach for adequate sedation. The clinician must determine whether analgesia, anxiolysis, or sedation is required or whether a combination will facilitate success. Clinicians should ask specifically about previous medical history, surgeries with prior anesthesia, medication allergies, family history, and current use of medications. The physical examination should focus on the airway, respiratory systems, and cardiovascular systems. Loss of an adequate airway is a serious complication. A primary focus should be on physical constraints that may interfere with endotracheal intubation to avoid this complication.

The clinician must ask about obstructive airway concerns such as signs of snoring, stridor, symptomatic asthma, history of heart disease, gastroesophageal reflux, or swallowing issues. A common approach to obtain important information in emergent situations is to use the AMPLE approach to obtain a focused history, which is an acronym for asking specifically about patient allergies, medication use, past medical history, the patient's last meal consumed, and the event or incident that led to the presentation requiring the procedure.

Evidence specific for children regarding identification and management of the difficult airway is limited, but much has been extrapolated from experience with adults, including the Mallampati classification (**Fig. 2**). The Mallampati grading system is used to assess for potential difficult airway. Mallampati scores that are high may also predict difficult bag-mask ventilation and airway obstruction once muscle-relaxing sedative agents are administered. Mallampati I is when the examiner can visualize the tonsillar pillars. Class II is when the uvula alone is visualized. Class III is when the soft palate is seen, and class IV is when solely the hard palate is visualized. Emergency physicians should be cautious with patients who may have airway challenges such as Pierre Robin syndrome with micrognathia and trisomy 21 because of the patients' large tongues and cervical spine instability. In addition to an appropriate history and physical examination, patients should be classified according to the American Society of Anesthesiologists (ASA) Physical Status Classification (**Table 1**).[7] Children who are in ASA category III or higher may not be candidates for elective procedural

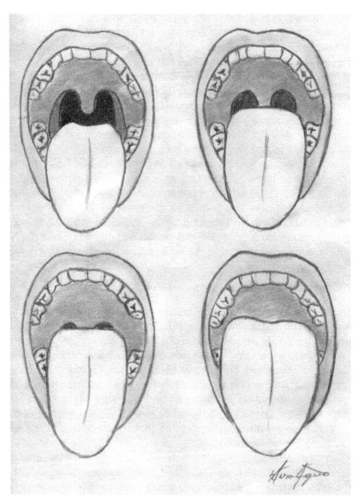

Fig. 2. Mallampati grading system. Class I (*upper left*), the examiner can visualize the tonsillar pillars. Class II (*upper right*), the uvula alone is visualized. Class III (*lower left*), the soft palate is seen. Class IV (*lower right*), solely the hard palate is visualized.

Table 1	
ASA classification: does anesthesia contribute to operative mortality?	
ASA I	Healthy patient without systemic disease
ASA II	Patient with mild systemic disease
ASA III	Patient with severe systemic disease
ASA IV	Patient with severe systemic disease posing a threat to life
ASA V	Moribund patient who cannot survive without surgery

Data from Cohen M, Duncan P, Tate R. Does anesthesia contribute to operative mortality? JAMA 1988;260(19):2859–63.

sedation in the emergency department. Alternative means to providing safe analgesia and anesthesia should be explored, but it is common for ASA III patients to have a procedure performed in the emergency department if necessary. The risks and benefits of performing the procedure in the emergency department must be assessed ahead of time.

Preparation, preparation, preparation is a mantra in emergency medicine. It is often an afterthought in the chaotic environment of the emergency department. However, procedural sedation is often planned and the practitioner is able to have all needed equipment at the bedside. The mnemonic SOAP ME is useful to remind the practitioner of what may be needed at the bedside: suction, oxygen, and bag-mask apparatus for positive pressure ventilation that is age fitting; appropriately sized airway equipment (including airway adjuncts such as oropharyngeal/nasopharyngeal airway, endotracheal tubes, laryngoscope, and blade with functioning light source); pharmaceuticals not only for the procedure, but reversal agents; and monitoring equipment as well as emergency cart with code medications and defibrillator.

The next consideration should be the child's risk of aspiration (**Table 2**). In the emergency setting this may be a luxury not afforded to the physician, but it still must be considered. Most patients who undergo sedation and analgesia are sufficiently conscious to protect their airways, but the potential to progress to a deeper state of sedation exists and raises the risk for aspiration. Therefore, it is recommended that the patient ingest nothing by mouth before any procedure requiring sedation.[8] Often there are institution-specific guidelines with similar restrictions seen and clinicians should seek out their own institution's guidelines.

Some investigators have argued there to be no correlation between fasting status and the incidence of aspiration. A large-scale report from The Pediatric Sedation Research Consortium documented only a single aspiration in 30,037 pediatric sedations outside the operating room. Emesis was only reported in 1 of 200 patients, which typically was in the recovery phase of the sedation.[9] There is weak evidence to support fasting requirements before procedural sedation in the emergent setting; however, The Joint Commission has regarded trivializing nothing-by-mouth status before PSA to be poor medical practice.

Preferably, 1 physician should be responsible for the sedation while another physician performs the procedure. However, in the community hospital setting this may not be practical. Monitoring may be performed by an emergency nurse while a single physician safely and effectively performs the procedure and sedation.[10] The emergency physician should understand and be competent in sedation drug pharmacology,

Table 2
Practice guidelines for preoperative fasting and the use of pharmacologic agents to reduce the risk of pulmonary aspiration

Ingested Material	Minimum Fasting Period
Clear liquids	Stop 2 h before procedure
Human milk	Stop 4 h before procedure
Infant formula or nonhuman milk	Stop 6 h before procedure
Light meal (eg, toast and clear liquid)	Stop 6 h before procedure

Adapted from American Society of Anesthesiologists Committee. Practice guidelines for preoperative fasting and the use of pharmacologic agents to reduce the risk of pulmonary aspiration: application to healthy patients undergoing elective procedures: an updated report by the American Society of Anesthesiologists Committee on Standards and Practice Parameters. Anesthesiology 2011;114(3):495–511.

anticipate possible complications, and be prepared for necessary resuscitation and recovery of care.

INTRASEDATION

Once the patient has had appropriate presedation evaluation, additional preparation includes setting up your intrasedation continuous monitoring, which is necessary for a successful sedation. The degree to which a child's respiratory or cardiovascular status is continuously monitored is scenario specific. Children who receive simple/minimal anxiolysis generally do not require any ongoing monitoring beyond initial, and possibly repeated, vital signs. When continuous monitoring is desired, it should include pulse oximetry, cardiac, blood pressure, and capnography. Monitoring is appropriate and recommended for patients who are ASA class II to III and is mandatory for patients in class IV and V.

Capnography is an adjunct that is an important portion of continuous monitoring. Arterial hypoxia identified with pulse oximetry appears after hypoventilation. Increased end-tidal carbon dioxide levels have been reported with children receiving respiratory depressant sedative agents.[11] When hypoventilation occurs, capnography provides an early indication and is an additional tool to assess for potential ventilatory failure.[12] Often practitioners place the patient on nasal cannula oxygen, and hypoxia is not appreciated. Capnography in this setting leads to early detection of apnea because of the absence of the end-tidal waveform being the earliest sign of airway obstruction. Continuous capnometry should be considered in patients who are sensitive to both carbon dioxide tension as well as oxygen saturation, including those with increased intracranial pressure or certain cardiac lesions.[13]

SELECTING AN AGENT FOR PSA

When selecting an agent for PSA it is important for the emergency practitioner to understand the pharmacology of the agent used and to define the goals of the procedure. Procedures are often done that are anxiety provoking, but painless. An example is the anxiety produced by diagnostic imaging. Some procedures are painful and solely require analgesia. An example is the nondisplaced fracture that needs to be splinted and requires little to no manipulation. Then there are procedures that cause both anxiety and pain and manipulation is required, such as the face laceration repair, the reduction of a distal radius fracture, or incision and drainage of an abscess. Here the physician desires an agent that treats pain and anxiety, but may also want an agent that achieves amnesia. By knowing the pharmacology of each agent, the emergency practitioner can choose a particular agent with the desired effect, and is able to avoid particular side effects (**Fig. 3**). Choosing an agent correctly can help avoid dreaded complications such as cardiovascular depression and hypotension.

ANALGESIA

Analgesia is best defined as the alleviation of pain without intentionally producing a sedated state. A change in mental status may be achieved incidentally when analgesic medications are used. Pain is often undertreated in pediatrics, which is thought to be secondary to problems quantifying pain in young children.[3] There are a variety of agents that can be helpful to the emergency physician when trying to achieve analgesia with or without an element of sedation.

Infants have physiologic and behavioral responses to pain (ie, increased blood pressure, respiratory rate, and heart rate; crying; flushing; diaphoresis; facial expression;

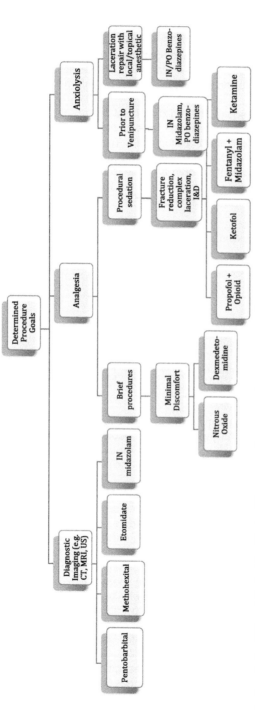

Fig. 3. Agents for PSA and their side effects. CT, computed tomography; IN, intranasal; MRI, magnetic resonance imaging; I&D, incision and drainage; PO, by mouth; US, ultrasound.

and body movements). However, it is often difficult to quantify pain in infants. For this reason, researchers have attempted to develop tools for pediatric pain assessment. In the neonatal intensive care unit there are assessment tools such as the Neonatal Pain Agitation and Sedation Scale (N-PASS) and the Neonatal Infant Pain Scale (NIPS) that attempt to identify pain and allow the practitioner to adequately address it in this special population.[14] Preschoolers (3–4 years old) can use the OUCHER scale. This scale combines both numeric and face scales for young children to point to when describing their pain.[15]

The FACES scale requires the child to point to the face that best describes the pain.[16] The FACES scale is reserved for patients 3 to 12 years old. Older children can be assessed using a visual analog scale. This method has a child 8 to 11 years old rate the intensity of their pain on a horizontal or numeric scale from 0 to 10. School-aged or adolescent children are able to perform self-reported numeric pain rating scales. In this case, pain is rated from 1 to 10. Self-reporting is the ideal measure to assess pediatric pain when appropriate.[17]

Wong-Baker FACES® Pain Rating Scale

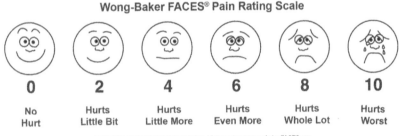

0	2	4	6	8	10
No Hurt	Hurts Little Bit	Hurts Little More	Hurts Even More	Hurts Whole Lot	Hurts Worst

©1983 Wong-Baker FACES® Foundation. Visit us at www.wongbakerFACES.org. Used with permission. Originally published in Whaley & Wong's Nursing Care of Infants and Children. ©Elsevier Inc.

It is important to keep in mind the desired effect and the age of the patient when selecting an agent for analgesia. Nonpharmacologic interventions should always be considered when approaching a child who requires analgesia, or for the completion of diagnostic or therapeutic procedure, but the practitioner must always ensure that pain is adequately addressed.

Topical agents including a eutectic mixture of lidocaine and prilocaine (EMLA), lipodermal lidocaine 4% (LMX), and lidocaine/epinephrine/tetracaine (LET) are excellent options for infants receiving a painful procedure. Also, nonnutritive sucking and high-concentration sucrose solutions have been efficacious. Approximately 1 to 2 mL of 24% to 50% sucrose can be used, typically placed in the cheek with a syringe or pacifier.[18] The onset is within 2 minutes. This option is useful up to 6 months of age and can be effective in term or preterm (<1 month) neonates.[19] The mechanism of action is thought to be release of endogenous endorphins.[17] A variety of commercially available products are available or it can be made up without difficulty.

Topical agents can also be used in older children to pretreat and lessen the pain of venipuncture, laceration repair, or even for lumbar puncture. The agents that are commonly used include LET (lidocaine 4%, epinephrine 0.1%, and tetracaine 0.5%).[20] LET is most appropriate for small lacerations less than 5 cm to avoid intoxication and excess administration. This agent has been shown to be more effective for scalp and facial lacerations than for truncal and extremity lacerations. Resch and colleagues[21] showed 85% complete anesthesia when repairing uncomplicated face and scalp lacerations with primary closure. LET is available as an aqueous solution or gel.

From 1 to 3 mL are applied to an open wound. The onset of action is within 20 to 30 minutes. LET can be toxic to the cardiovascular system and central nervous system (CNS). A concerning side effect is methemoglobinemia, and LET should be used with caution on mucous membranes.[22] Distal anatomic areas such as the tip of the phalange, nose, or penis may be contraindicated because of LET's epinephrine component.

LMX-4 is another topical agent available for use. The onset of action is within 30 minutes and the effect can last up to 1 hour. EMLA is another common agent used in the emergency department. The product contains a eutectic mixture of local anesthetics (2.5% lidocaine and 2.5% prilocaine) in a cream base. EMLA and LMX-4 can be used on intact skin and used to prepare for venous or arterial puncture, placement of an intravenous (IV) catheter and lumbar puncture. EMLA is applied topically in a dose of 1 g for patients less than 5 kg to 2 g for patients more than 5 kg applied over 10 cm. EMLA takes approximately 1 hour to achieve peak effect, which can last up to 2 hours even after the cream is removed and has been argued to be the disadvantage of EMLA in the emergency department. EMLA has similar side effects to those present in other topical agents, including methemoglobinemia.[22]

Another option to painlessly obtain IV access is needle-free injection of lidocaine using the J-tip. This system is needle free and is limited to a single use. The device uses highly pressurized carbon dioxide to push lidocaine through skin and 5 to 8 mm of subcutaneous tissue. The onset of action is 1 to 3 minutes. The needleless administration of lidocaine into the epidermis is associated with minimal discomfort. There is not much literature to support its use in preterm infants or neonates. Ferayorni and colleagues[23] showed that needle-free injection of lidocaine administered before lumbar puncture in infants can offer analgesia.

Other options for noninvasive intervention include intranasal midazolam and fentanyl. Nasal therapy is an effective option because of avoidance of first-pass hepatic metabolism. There is a fast onset and increased bioavailability with either option. The mode of delivery is through an atomizer (**Fig. 4**) added to the end of a syringe. One study showed that the intranasal route showed faster sedation onset, greater proportion of patients achieving adequate sedation, and higher rate of satisfied parents. The same study showed that pediatric sedation with buccal or nasal midazolam aerosol is effective, but not clearly superior to the oral route.[24] Even in the best of these groups, only one-fourth of the children were inadequately sedated. The intranasal route showed faster sedation onset and a greater proportion of patients receiving adequate sedation. Intranasal midazolam dripped into the nares had not been well tolerated because of its acidity and the resulting pain of administration. Intranasal midazolam is dosed 0.2 to 0.3 mg/kg and has an onset of 10 minutes.[25,26] The dose cannot be lowered because of association of failed sedation and potential for paradoxic effect.

Other medications that can be administered intranasally include fentanyl and ketamine. Intranasal fentanyl can be given at a dose of 1 to 2 μg/kg and the onset of effect is at 10 minutes. Intranasal fentanyl is an effective and a safe alternative to IV or intramuscular (IM) morphine for managing acute pain in children presenting to the emergency department. Intranasal fentanyl can decrease IV placement for analgesia by 60% and it reduces the time to analgesia administration by about half.[27] Intranasal ketamine was shown to edge midazolam with success rates approaching 89%. Combining midazolam did not improve the level of sedation.[28]

Fentanyl administered via nebulizer is another quick and effective option to achieve analgesia when vascular access is not available, and is another option to add to the so-called ouchless emergency department. In a randomized clinical trial by Miner and colleagues,[29] 41 patients either received IV fentanyl citrate 1.5 μg/kg or nebulized

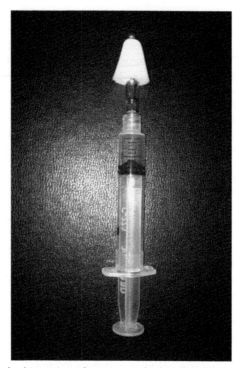

Fig. 4. Atomizer attached to syringe for intranasal administration.

fentanyl 3 μg/kg. The nebulized fentanyl group had similar visual analog scores to the IV route and appeared to be a feasible and safe alternative (**Table 3**).

Ibuprofen is a nonsteroidal antiinflammatory medication that is available for use against mild to moderate pain. Ibuprofen is available for use in children 6 months old and older. The mechanism of action includes prostaglandin inhibition. The agent is metabolized by the liver and it is subsequently excreted in the urine. The dose for pain reduction is 10 mg/kg every 6 to 8 hours with a maximum daily dose of 40 mg/kg.[30]

The most commonly used agent for pain management in children is acetaminophen. It is a safe choice for the treatment of pediatric pain. The dose is 15 mg/kg every 4 hours with a maximum dose of 90 mg/kg/d for children.[30]

Ketorolac is a potent nonsteroidal antiinflammatory agent that is available in both IV, IM, and oral form. Its effects are most comparable and compatible with ibuprofen. The medication is strictly contraindicated in renal failure, peptic ulcer disease, allergy to nonsteroidal antiinflammatory drugs (NSAIDs), bleeding disorder, and platelet dysfunction. Recommended dosing for children is age dependent. Per the manufacturer recommendations, children between 2 and 16 years old are dosed 0.5 mg/kg IV with a maximum dose of 15 mg. This group can receive up to 1 mg/kg intramuscularly and a maximum dose of 30 mg. Children older than 16 years or more than 50 kg can receive 30 mg IV every 6 hours and intramuscularly receive 60 mg for 1 dose. Both routes have a maximum allowance of 120 mg/d.[30]

Morphine sulfate is a commonly used opiate medication that has a rapid onset of 4 to 6 minutes. The duration of effect is 2 to 3 hours when given intravenously. The appropriate dosing is 0.1 to 0.2 mg/kg IV, IM, or subcutaneously.[30]

Table 3
Profile of analgesia agents

Analgesics	Dose (mg/kg)	Route	Maximum Unit Dose (mg/kg)	Duration	Precautions	Comments
Morphine	0.1–0.2	IM/IV/SQ	10	3–4 h	Histamine release/respiratory depression	Better absorbed SQ than IM
Fentanyl	0.001–0.005	IM/IV/IN	0.05	0.5–1 h	Rigid chest	Decrease dose in infants
Remifentanil	0.001–0.003	IV	0.05	3–4 min	Rigid chest	—
Hydromorphone	0.015	IM/IV	—	2.5 h	—	—
Hydrocodone	0.2	Oral	10	4–6 h	—	Combine with acetaminophen
Acetaminophen	15	Oral/rectal	1000	4 h	—	—
Ibuprofen	10	Oral	40	6–8 h	Asthma, anticoagulated	Cannot use before age 6 mo
Ketorolac	0.5–1	IV/IM	15–30	4–6 h	Same as ibuprofen	Not to exceed 48 h of tx

Abbreviations: IM, intramuscular; IN, intranasal; SQ, subcutaneous; tx, treatment.
Data from Tschudy M, Arcara K. The Harriet Lane handbook: a manual for pediatric house officers. 19th edition. Philadelphia: Mosby Elsevier; 2012.

Fentanyl citrate is 100 times more potent then morphine. It is a useful agent for PSA because it has a rapid onset within 2 to 3 minutes. However, fentanyl has a short duration of 30 to 60 minutes. Fentanyl lacks the histamine release side effect associated with morphine and is preferential for patients with hemodynamic instability. Fentanyl can be given intranasally and has a treatment profile that is comparable with IV morphine sulfate. Dosing of fentanyl is 1 to 2 μg/kg/dose (maximum 50–100 μg/dose).[30]

Remifentanil is a potent ultra–short-acting synthetic opioid analgesic drug. Because the medication is so short acting, an infusion is often needed to have continuous analgesia. Thus the goal of analgesia for a given procedure must be considered. Typical dosage is 1 μg/kg given over 30 to 60 seconds followed by an infusion of 0.01 to 2 μg/kg/min. Maximum effect begins within 30 to 90 seconds, and its context-sensitive half-life is less than 5 minutes because it is metabolized by plasma esterases rather than the liver.

Well-described Adverse Reactions to Opiates

Opiates have common well-described side effects. Adverse reactions seen in children using opioids include nausea, vomiting, hypotension, respiratory depression, and pruritus caused by histamine release. A well-known and serious side effect of fentanyl is chest wall rigidity. The treatment of rigid chest syndrome is aggressive respiratory support, which may require intubation and chemically induced paralysis, and use of an opioid reversal agent such as naloxone. The dosing for naloxone when needed for opiate reversal is 0.1 mg/kg, which can be repeated every 2 to 3 minutes.[30]

DISSOCIATIVE AGENTS
Ketamine

Ketamine is a dissociative anesthetic related to phencyclidine. The mechanism of action is disconnection between the thalamocortical and limbic systems. The end result is that the patient is moderately sedated and in a state in which amnesia and analgesia are also accomplished. This dissociative agent is the most commonly used sedative in the United States. Having both anesthetic and analgesic properties have made the drug an attractive choice for the emergency physician.[11] Therefore, ketamine can be used for painful procedures while maintaining airway patency and cardiac function.

Prior guidelines strongly urged against the use of ketamine in children between the ages of 3 and 12 months. A recent meta-analysis showed that the previous concerns for higher risks of airway compromise are anecdotal.[31] The latest absolute contraindications for the use of ketamine include infants less than 3 months old because of a higher risk of airway compromise. Several studies show an increase in airway obstruction, apnea, and laryngospasm in this age group.[31]

There is potential for excess secretions with ketamine use, which use to prompt the prophylactic use of antisialagogues. Atropine and glycopyrrolate as pretreatment adjuncts to ketamine sedation seem to be unnecessary. The rationale was that these measures would help reduce accumulated secretions in the posterior pharynx and potentially reduce the incidence of aspiration or other adverse airway events.[32] A large case series of patients showed the safety profile of ketamine when coadministered anticholinergics were omitted and excessive salivation was uncommon.[33] With ketamine use there has been concern for laryngospasm, which is uncommon. Laryngospasm is typically easily corrected with bag-valve mask ventilation. In a large meta-analysis, 0.3% of children were reported to have this complication. In the same meta-analysis, for 8282 pediatric ketamine sedations, the overall incidence of airway and respiratory adverse events was minimal at 3.9%. This study identified the following independent predictors of airway and respiratory events: younger than 2 years, aged 13 years or older, high IV dosing (ie, ≥2.5 mg/kg or total dose ≥5 mg/kg), coadministered anticholinergic, and coadministered benzodiazepine.[34]

Green and colleagues'[31] clinical practice guideline for emergency department ketamine use suggests that a minimum dissociative dose is achieved with 1.5 mg/kg IV and 4 to 5 mg/kg IM. Once the dissociative state is achieved, further dosing does not deepen sedation and the only need for titration is to maintain the dissociative state over time.[31] The IM route seems to cause more vomiting and causes a prolonged recovery time compared with the IV route.[31] The IV route is preferred for longer procedures and especially with the need for repeat dosing. Repeated IV doses can be achieved with 0.5 to 1.0 mg/kg if needed for prolonged sedation, whereas IM doses can be achieved with half of a dose or full dose.[31] IV ketamine should be given over 30 to 60 seconds to avoid transient respiratory depression.

Well-described Adverse Reactions to Ketamine

Ketamine is commonly used in pediatric emergency medicine. It is useful as a sedative-analgesic for painful procedures of short duration. Examples of procedures for which this agent is commonly used include incision and drainage of an abscess, closed fracture reduction, and wound repair. Negative effects of ketamine include emetogenesis, increased intracranial pressure, increased ocular pressure, increased secretions, apnea, and emergence phenomena.[35]

Ketamine is thought to be emetogenic and lead to feared emergence reactions. Some studies suggest that ondansetron administered before sedation may significantly reduce the associated nausea and vomiting. An 8% decrease in the rate of emesis has been achieved by some study groups.[31,36] Children receiving ketamine have low rates of emergence phenomena. They may dream and hallucinate during recovery, but these dreams are rarely frightening.[37] No variable predicts ketamine-associated airway complications, which are the most concerning to the emergency physician and there is no dose relationship for emesis or recovery agitation.[38]

The contraindication for patients with increased intracranial pressure is a topic of debate. New evidence suggests that the effect is likely minimal.[39] Some argue that the agent can be used safely in patients with acute traumatic brain injury, but more research is needed for this proposal and alternative agents should be the first choice in patients who have traumatic injury, and should definitively be the drug of choice in hydrocephalus or central nervous system abnormalities.

Laryngospasm is also a known adverse reaction. Should this occur, the practitioner may use bag-mask ventilation, and apply digital pressure at the superior jaw notch between the ear and the mandible. Other adverse effects from ketamine include tachycardia, hypertension, nystagmus, and muscle rigidity. Its use is contraindicated in patients with psychosis. Because of ketamine's sympathomimetic effects on the cardiovascular system, its use is contraindicated in patients with certain cardiovascular diseases.

SEDATIVE/HYPNOTIC AGENTS

Sedative/hypnotics are useful for the patient who requires sedation, and in some cases amnesia, for a stressful or painful procedure. The benzodiazepines are the most common agents used in this class. Most agents act by modulating gamma-aminobutyric acid receptors. One should keep in mind that several of these agents have no analgesic properties, and they should provide analgesia in the form of an opiate or other suitable class of medication to treat pain adequately. Each agent is discussed later with both pros and cons (**Table 4** shows details of sedative/hypnotics and dissociative agents).

Midazolam

Midazolam is a short-acting benzodiazepine with rapid onset of action. The benzodiazepine class is used for its sedative-hypnotic, anxiolytic, and amnestic effects; they do not have analgesic properties. Several studies assessing the effectiveness of midazolam have concluded the agent to be safe and effective in children.[40] They can be given with opioids for analgesia. Midazolam has also been used with ketamine to decrease emergence dysphoria. Titrated benzodiazepines seem to decrease such reactions effectively but not prophylactically.[41] An additional advantage of midazolam is that it can be given via multiple routes (ie, IM, intranasal, rectal, and oral).

Midazolam's time to peak effect is 2 to 3 minutes. The duration of action may be up to 45 minutes to 1 hour by the IV route. The IV and IM dose of midazolam is 0.1 mg/kg. Oral midazolam can also be used as an anxiolytic for nonpainful procedures. It is best when administered to a child with an empty stomach. When a child has recently eaten, its absorption can be erratic. The usual dose is 0.5 mg/kg.[30]

Well-described Adverse Reactions to Midazolam

Midazolam can be used as a premedication to reduce anxiety surrounding laceration repair and local anesthetic administration, and before obtaining IV access. Midazolam has several well-described adverse reactions of which the clinician should be aware. Major complications with benzodiazepines include respiratory depression and hypotension. Paradoxic reactions that can occur include combativeness, disorientation, inconsolable crying, agitation, and restlessness. Other side effects noted with midazolam, in decreasing order of frequency, include oxygen desaturation, apnea, hypotension, and hiccups.[42,43] With coadministration with opioids there is risk of hypoxia and apnea that is greater than with either agent used alone. Flumazenil is a benzodiazepine antagonist that can be used when iatrogenic overdose has occurred or when undesired effects occur. The pediatric dose of flumazenil is 0.01 mg/kg up to a maximum of 1 mg. The onset of action is 1 to 3 minutes.[30]

Propofol

Propofol is a sedative-hypnotic often used as a general anesthetic. Propofol is useful in children because of the short duration of action (shorter than that of ketamine) and the ability to achieve motionlessness for the patient. These advantages make it an ideal agent for obtaining diagnostic imaging and quick procedures such as lumbar puncture, reduction of dislocations, and laceration repair. When given intravenously there is an immediate effect, and when ceased there is immediate recovery for the patient, which is helpful when attempting quick procedures at the bedside. Another advantage is that propofol has antiemetic properties. However, compared with ketamine, propofol provides no analgesia, prompting the use of parenteral, local, or regional analgesics to be coadministered.

Propofol is dosed 1 mg/kg with repeat dosing at 0.5 mg/kg.[30] Propofol reduces intracranial pressure, making it a potential choice in hemodynamically stable patients with head trauma.[44] Propofol is contraindicated in any patient with a known allergy to eggs, soy products, or propofol itself.

Table 4
Commonly used sedative agents

Class	Drug	Route	Dose	Onset	Duration	Disadvantages
Anxiolytic	Midazolam	PO, PR, IV, IM, IN	PO/PR 0.5 mg/kg IV/IM 0.1 mg/kg IN 0.2 mg/kg	PO/PR 20–30 min, IV 1 min, IM 5–10 min, IN 5 min	1–4 h	No analgesia, paradoxic reaction, respiratory depression and hypotension
	Ativan	PO, IV	0.05	PO 60 min, IV 15–30 min	8–12 h	Prolonged duration of action
Hypnotic/ sedative	Propofol	IV	1–2 mg/kg Maximum unit dose (100 mg) Repeat 0.05 mg/kg	Seconds	Minutes (~6–10 min)	No analgesia, respiratory and CV depression
	Etomidate	IV	0.1–0.3 mg/kg Maximum unit dose (300 mg)	Seconds	Minutes (15–20 min)	No analgesia, myoclonus, respiratory depression
	Methohexital	IV	1 mg/kg Maximum unit dose (100 mg)	Seconds	10–90 min	No analgesia, respiratory and CV depressant
	Pentobarbital	IV	2–5 mg/kg Maximum unit dose (200 mg)	<1 min	30–90 min	No analgesia, respiratory and CV depressant
Dissociative	Ketamine[a]	IV, IM, PO	IV 1–2 mg/kg IM 3–4 mg/kg PO 6–10 mg/kg	IV 1–2 min, IM 3–5 min, PO 30 min	IV 0.5–1 h, IM 1–2 h, PO 2–3 h	Increased ICP, intraocular pressure, emetogenesis, hypersalivation, emergence
Combinations[b]	Fentanyl + midazolam	IV	Fentanyl 1–2 µg/kg, midazolam 0.05–0.1 mg/kg	IV 1–2 min	1–3 h	Respiratory depressant increased with combination
	Ketofol (ketamine + propofol)	IV	Propofol 1 mg/kg, ketamine 0.5 mg/kg	1 min	Propofol (minutes); ketamine 15–45 min	Dose regimens vary. Modest advantage profile

Abbreviations: CV, cardiovascular; ICP, intracranial pressure; PO, by mouth; PR, per rectum.

[a] Dosing of atropine (0.01 mg/kg, minimum 0.15 mg, maximum 0.5 mg) or glycopyrrolate 0.005 mg/kg maximum 0.25 mg for increased secretions. Unnecessary as prophylaxis.

[b] Decrease dose of each agent. Begin with narcotic and titrate in sedative. Apnea risk proportional to each agent used.[11,30,31,46]

Data from Tschudy M, Arcara K. The Harriet Lane handbook: a manual for pediatric house officers. 19th edition. Philadelphia: Mosby Elsevier; 2012.

Barbiturates

Barbiturates including pentobarbital are beneficial for their short-acting duration, which makes them ideal for sedation for imaging procedures that may be time consuming. They are also a more attractive agent used in the setting of intracranial injury, in which ketamine is contraindicated or its use is in question. When used alone in the proper dose, adverse reactions are rare. When sedation doses are used, no analgesia is accomplished when using barbiturates.

Methohexital

Methohexital is an ultra–short-acting barbiturate with an onset of 30 to 60 seconds. The duration of effect is only 5 to 10 minutes. A study from a 2009 *Pediatric Emergency Care* article showed that methohexital was superior to pentobarbital for the purpose of sedating emergency department patients for head computed tomography (CT).[45] The IV dose is 1 mg/kg.[46] For diagnostic imaging (eg, magnetic resonance imaging [MRI] and CT), rectal administration can be performed. Per rectum dosing is 25 mg/kg, with a maximum dose of 1 g.

Thiopental

Like methohexital, thiopental is a short-acting drug. The dose is 2.5 to 5 mg/kg given by the IV route. The maximum unit dose that can be given is 300 mg. Thiopental has a duration of action of 20 to 60 minutes. Like other barbiturates, a concerning side effect is respiratory depression. Thiopental can decrease intracranial pressure, making it a viable option if there is baseline concern for increased intracranial pressure (eg, patients with head injuries). Thiopental also can be given rectally for procedural sedation in children.

Pentobarbital

Pentobarbital also is commonly used as a sedative during radiologic procedures. The drug has an onset of action at approximately 3 to 5 minutes with a duration of action of 30 to 45 minutes. Pentobarbital can also be given via the IV, oral, or rectal route. The rectal route may lead to a delayed onset of sedation up to 45 minutes. The oral, IV, and rectal dosing recommendation is 2 to 5 mg/kg.

Well-described Adverse Reactions to Propofol and Barbiturates

Propofol side effects include respiratory depression, apnea, and hypotension.[44] Negative effects of barbiturates include hypotension, respiratory depression, and longer recovery times. When proper dosing of barbiturates is achieved, adverse reactions are rare. For methohexital, adverse reactions include oxygen desaturation, hypoventilation, cough, hypersalivation, and hiccups.

Etomidate

Etomidate works at the gamma-aminobutyric acid receptor to produce hypnosis without analgesia. With etomidate, protective airway reflexes may be significantly reduced or briefly lost. The hypnotic is typically associated with rapid sequence intubation but also can be used for PSA. Procedures in which immobility is desired, such as diagnostic imaging, are ideal. The Pediatric Sedation Research Consortium conducted a study to compare the efficacy, sedation duration, and adverse events after administration of etomidate or pentobarbital for diagnostic CT scans. Etomidate as given by emergency physicians was more effective and efficient than pentobarbital, with rare adverse events.[47] Another randomized study in the emergency department compared patients administered either 0.2 mg/kg of etomidate or 0.1 mg/kg of midazolam, and induction and recovery times were shorter with etomidate compared with midazolam.[48]

For children 10 years and older the recommended dosing is in the range of 0.1 to 0.3 mg/kg.[11] Repeat dosing is accomplished at 0.05 mg/kg every 5 minutes to a maximum total dose of 0.6 mg/kg to achieve the desired effect. The advantage of etomidate is the relative lack of hemodynamic effects compared with other sedating agents. Etomidate has also shown a useful effect on the CNS by lowering cerebral metabolism, cerebral blood flow, and intracranial pressure. Etomidate has no analgesic properties. It is best to treat the patient's pain with an analgesic such as morphine or fentanyl before formal sedation.

Well-described Adverse Reactions to Etomidate

Undesired effects with the use of etomidate include respiratory depression or apnea. It is recommended that it be given with a slow IV push to prevent this unwanted effect. There has been a concern regarding adrenal suppression, and this is a topic of much debate. Etomidate may directly inhibit 11β-hydroxylase, which blocks the conversion of 11-deoxycortisol to cortisol. Adrenal suppression has occurred with repeated dosing; therefore, etomidate is not ideal for prolonged procedures and for now should be avoided in patients at risk for sepsis or serious bacterial illness. Other adverse reactions include emesis (during and after the procedure) and myoclonus. Some report myoclonus with etomidate use. This reaction must be considered when planning for a painless diagnostic procedure, but the studies reviewed suggest that its frequency is minimal.

Nitrous Oxide

Given availability, an inhaled nitrous oxide–oxygen combination is useful.[49] The advantages of nitrous oxide are a quick onset of action, low incidence of complications, and the rapid return to the patient's baseline level of consciousness. In pediatrics, the use of nitrous oxide is favored even more because it can be administered without inflicting pain. Disadvantages are that the effects can be unpredictable and depend on a cooperative patient inhaling the agent. Nitrous oxide can provide the effects of amnesia, sedation, anxiolysis, and mild analgesia, making it an attractive choice for mild procedures.

Nitrous oxide can be delivered by a single tank system that has a fixed ratio of 50% nitrous oxide and 50% oxygen delivery, or varying concentrations with a multiple tank system. Concentrations of 33% to 70% nitrous oxide delivered by mask have led to clinically significant alleviation of anxiety and pain in the pediatric population. The most cited complications include vomiting and respiratory depression, but these are infrequent and tend to easily resolve once administration is ceased. This method is ideal for children between the ages of 2 and 5 years, because younger patients tend to not tolerate the mask apparatus.

A study by Babl and colleagues[50] showed that high-concentration continuous-flow nitrous oxide (70%) was safe in patients aged 1 to 17 years and in children aged 1 to 3 years. Out of 762 patients, 63 patients sustained 70 mild and self-resolving events (vomiting [5.7%], agitation [1.3%], nausea [0.9%]), and less than 0.1% serious adverse events such as chest pain or oxygen desaturation. The concerns with nitrous oxide use have largely focused on the need for a scavenging system and the risk of diversion.

MEDICATION COMBINATIONS
Fentanyl/Midazolam

Fentanyl/midazolam can be less predictable for sedation and analgesia. This combination carries a similar risk of hypotension and respiratory depression to propofol.

Both ketamine and propofol, with or without adjunct medications, are superior in their effectiveness and safety profiles.

Ketamine/Propofol

The combination of ketamine and propofol either in separate syringes or in a single syringe mixed 1:1 (termed ketofol) was described by Andolfatto and colleagues,[51] who argued that the benefit was to use drug doses lower than are typically required for each agent alone. The nausea-inducing and psychic recovery effects of ketamine are counterbalanced by the sedative and antiemetic effects of propofol. A potential advantage of ketofol compared with ketamine alone includes shorter recovery time and a theoretic lower incidence of recovery agitation. It was similarly argued that the hypotension seen with propofol is counterbalanced by the mild sympathomimetic properties of ketamine. The combination has been shown to be chemically stable and physically compatible when mixed in a single syringe.[52,53] A potential advantage of ketofol compared with propofol alone is the allowance for deep sedation with lower doses of propofol.

A reduction of side effects when using the ketofol combination is arguable. Andolfatto and colleagues[51] failed to find superiority in patients who received ketofol for emergency department procedural sedation when assessing reduced incidence of adverse respiratory events compared with propofol alone. This study included 284 patients who were ASA class 1 to 3 status and 14 years or older. The median ages for both groups that received ketofol versus propofol alone were between 48 and 54 years, respectively.

Shah and colleagues[53] specifically studied patients aged 2 to 17 years. Some patients received an initial IV bolus dose of ketamine 0.5 mg/kg and propofol 0.5 mg/kg, and the other group received solely a dose of 1 mg/kg ketamine. The ketamine/propofol had modest differences in total sedation time, time to recovery, adverse events, and satisfaction scores. Median sedation time was 3 minutes less in the ketamine/propofol group, median recovery time was faster in the ketamine/propofol group by 2 minutes, and there was less vomiting in this group as well (12%). Satisfaction scores were higher in the ketamine/propofol group.[52] The ketamine/propofol group had patients that required greater than 4 doses, whereas the ketamine group did not need redosing after 3 doses. The clinical significance of the modest advantages shown in this study is unclear.

Andolfatto and colleagues[54] performed an earlier study in patients with a median age of 13 years. A single-syringe 1:1 mixture of ketamine and propofol (ketofol) with a median dose of 0.8 mg/kg was highly effective. Shorter recovery times were reported (14 minutes).[54] Sharieff and colleagues,[55] in a pilot study of 20 patients aged 3 to 17 years, showed a rapid recovery and 38 minutes to discharge suitability. In this study, 0.5 mg/kg of ketamine followed by 1 mg/kg of propofol were used.

Dexmedetomidine

Dexmedetomidine is a potent selective alpha-2 adrenergic agonist that provides sedation, anxiolysis, and some analgesia without depressing the respiratory drive.[56] Its use in pediatric procedural sedation is new and experience is limited. It may have a role in painless procedures such as diagnostic imaging. Several studies have suggested its superiority when used as a sedative for imaging studies.[57] The dose for adults per the packet insert is an initial IV load of 0.5 to 1 μg/kg over 10 minutes followed by an infusion of 0.5 to 1 μg/kg/h. It has been noted that higher doses are often needed to achieve sedation in the pediatric population, such as an IV load of 2 to 3 μg/kg followed by a continuous infusion of 1 to 2 μg/kg per hour. The data that are available in pediatrics use a wide range of doses and more studies are needed to confirm a dose for effect.

Dexmedetomidine can have biphasic effects with initial increase in blood pressure and a reflex decrease in heart rate. Because of this, it often has to be loaded for a minimum of 10 to 30 minutes, which should be considered in the emergency setting. Studies comparing propofol and dexmedetomidine found no difference for success of MRI imaging procedures in pediatric sedation. Propofol had the advantage of immediate induction, faster recovery times, and faster discharge times.[58]

Dexmedetomidine can be administered to children via the intranasal or buccal routes, although no studies exist regarding the use of these routes for pediatric procedural sedation. In dentistry literature, intranasal dosing at 1.5 µg/kg has been shown to be as effective as oral midazolam and is associated with lower postprocedural pain scores. Buccal administration of 3 to 4 µg/kg results in moderate sedation without reported respiratory complications.

DISCHARGE CRITERIA

Discharge criteria following procedural sedation are based on stable serial vital sign assessments. This assessment is typically performed by a nurse trained in pediatric advanced life support (PALS) or advanced pediatric life support (APLS) and includes blood pressure and pulse oximetry. The patient should return to presedation mental status and preferably tolerate clear liquids.[59] If the patient is asleep, the emergency department staff should easily be able to rouse patients to their presedation mental status. The patient should be able to sit unaided (except when this is not a baseline developmental skill).

SUMMARY

Pain and anxiety in the pediatric population have historically been undermanaged. There is no justification for this. In the emergency department, pain and procedures are addressed routinely. The emergency physician should be well versed in providing analgesia and performing procedural sedation. Emergency physicians performing these procedures need to be in control of the airway, because compromise is the most serious complication. A broad understanding of the available safe and effective agents is key. Emergency clinicians should be fully prepared for the sedation and analgesia route they choose to use.

REFERENCES

1. American Academy of Pediatrics. Committee on Psychosocial Aspects of Child and Family Health, Task Force on Pain in Infants, Children, and Adolescents. The assessment and management of acute pain in infants, children, and adolescents. Pediatrics 2001;108(3):793-7.
2. Fein JA, Zempsky WT, Cravero JP, The Committee on Pediatric Emergency Medicine and Section on Anesthesiology and Pain Medicine. Relief of pain and anxiety in pediatric patients in emergency medical systems. Pediatrics 2012;130(5):e1391-405.
3. Alexander J, Manno M. Underuse of analgesia in very young pediatric patients with isolated painful injuries. Ann Emerg Med 2003;41(5):617-22.
4. Koh JL, Palermo T. Conscious sedation: reality or myth? Pediatr Rev 2007;28(7): 243-8.

5. American Society of Anesthesiologists Task Force on Sedation and Analgesia by Non-Anesthesiologists. Practice guidelines for sedation and analgesia by non-anesthesiologists. Anesthesiology 2002;96(4):1004–17.
6. American Academy of Pediatrics Child Life Council and Committee on Hospital Care, Wilson JM. Child life services. Pediatrics 2006;118(4):1757–63.
7. Cohen M, Duncan P, Tate R. Does anesthesia contribute to operative mortality? JAMA 1988;260(19):2859–63.
8. American Society of Anesthesiologists Committee. Practice guidelines for preoperative fasting and the use of pharmacologic agents to reduce the risk of pulmonary aspiration: application to healthy patients undergoing elective procedures: an updated report by the American Society of Anesthesiologists Committee on Standards and Practice Parameters. Anesthesiology 2011; 114(3):495–511.
9. Cravero JP, Blike GT, Beach M, et al. Incidence and nature of adverse events during pediatric sedation/anesthesia for procedures outside the operating room: report from the Pediatric Sedation Research Consortium. Pediatrics 2006;118(3):1087–96.
10. Hogan K, Sacchetti A, Aman L, et al. The safety of single-physician procedural sedation in the emergency department. Emerg Med J 2006;23(12):922–3.
11. Krauss B, Green SM. Procedural sedation and analgesia in children. Lancet 2006;367(9512):766–80.
12. Nagler J, Krauss B. Capnography: a valuable tool for airway management. Emerg Med Clin North Am 2008;26(4):881–97, vii.
13. Krauss B, Hess DR. Capnography for procedural sedation and analgesia in the emergency department. Ann Emerg Med 2007;50(2):172–81.
14. Hummel P, Puchalski M, Creech SD, et al. Clinical reliability and validity of the N-PASS: neonatal pain, agitation and sedation scale with prolonged pain. J Perinatol 2008;28(1):55–60.
15. Beyer JE, Denyes MJ, Villarruel AM. The creation, validation, and continuing development of the oucher: a measure of pain intensity in children. J Pediatr Nurs 1992;7(5):335–46.
16. Wong DL, Baker CM. Pain in children: comparison of assessment scales. Pediatr Nurs 1988;14(1):9–17.
17. Cramton RE, Gruchala NE. Managing procedural pain in pediatric patients. Curr Opin Pediatr 2012;24(4):530–8.
18. Stevens B, Yamada J, Ohlsson A. Sucrose for analgesia in newborn infants undergoing painful procedures. Cochrane Database Syst Rev 2010;(1):CD001069.
19. Johnston CC, Stremler R, Horton L, et al. Effect of repeated doses of sucrose during heel stick procedure in preterm neonates. Biol Neonate 1999;75(3):160–6.
20. Kennedy RM, Luhmann JD. The "ouchless emergency department". Getting closer: advances in decreasing distress during painful procedures in the emergency department. Pediatr Clin North Am 1999;46(6):1215–47, vii–viii.
21. Resch K, Schilling C, Borchert BD, et al. Topical anesthesia for pediatric lacerations: a randomized trial of lidocaine-epinephrine-tetracaine solution versus gel. Ann Emerg Med 1998;32(6):693–7.
22. Berde CB. Toxicity of local anesthetics in infants and children. J Pediatr 1993; 122(5):14–20.
23. Ferayorni A, Yniguez R, Bryson M, et al. Needle-free jet injection of lidocaine for local anesthesia during lumbar puncture: a randomized controlled trial. Pediatr Emerg Care 2012;28(7):687–90.

24. Klein EJ, Brown JC, Kobayashi A, et al. A randomized clinical trial comparing oral, aerosolized intranasal, and aerosolized buccal midazolam. Ann Emerg Med 2011;58(4):323–9.
25. Harcke HT, Grissom LE, Meister MA. Sedation in pediatric imaging using intranasal midazolam. Pediatr Radiol 1995;25(5):341–3.
26. Lane RD, Schunk JE. Atomized intranasal midazolam use for minor procedures in the pediatric emergency department. Pediatr Emerg Care 2008;24(5):300–3.
27. Kusre SR. Towards evidence based emergency medicine: best BETs from the Manchester Royal Infirmary. Bet 4: is intranasal fentanyl better than parenteral morphine for managing acute severe pain in children? Emerg Med J 2011; 28(12):1077–8.
28. Warrington SE, Kuhn RJ. Use of intranasal medications in pediatric patients. Orthopedics 2011;34(6):456.
29. Miner JR, Kletti C, Herold M, et al. Randomized clinical trial of nebulized fentanyl citrate versus I.V. fentanyl citrate in children presenting to the emergency department with acute pain. Acad Emerg Med 2007;14(10):895–8.
30. Tschudy M, Arcara K. The Harriet Lane handbook: a manual for pediatric house officers. 19th edition. Philadelphia: Mosby Elsevier; 2012. Formulary.
31. Green SM, Roback MG, Kennedy RM, et al. Clinical practice guideline for emergency department ketamine dissociative sedation: 2011 update. Ann Emerg Med 2011;57(5):449–61.
32. Green SM, Roback MG, Krauss B, Emergency Department Ketamine Meta-analysis Study Group. Anticholinergics and ketamine sedation in children: a secondary analysis of atropine versus glycopyrrolate. Acad Emerg Med 2010; 17(2):157–62.
33. Brown L, Christian-Kopp S, Sherwin TS, et al. Adjunctive atropine is unnecessary during ketamine sedation in children. Acad Emerg Med 2008;15(4):314–8.
34. Green SM, Roback MG, Krauss B, et al. Predictors of airway and respiratory adverse events with ketamine sedation in the emergency department: an individual-patient data meta-analysis of 8,282 children. Ann Emerg Med 2009; 54(2):158–68.e1–4.
35. Melendez E, Bachur R. Serious adverse events during procedural sedation with ketamine. Pediatr Emerg Care 2009;25(5):325–8.
36. Langston WT, Wathen JE, Roback MG, et al. Effect of ondansetron on the incidence of vomiting associated with ketamine sedation in children: a double-blind, randomized, placebo-controlled trial. Ann Emerg Med 2008;52(1):30–4.
37. Sherwin TS, Green SM, Khan A, et al. Does adjunctive midazolam reduce recovery agitation after ketamine sedation for pediatric procedures? A randomized, double-blind, placebo-controlled trial. Ann Emerg Med 2000;35(3):229–38.
38. Green SM, Kuppermann N, Rothrock SG, et al. Predictors of adverse events with intramuscular ketamine sedation in children. Ann Emerg Med 2000;35(1): 35–42.
39. Bourgoin A, Albanese J, Wereszczynski N, et al. Safety of sedation with ketamine in severe head injury patients: comparison with sufentanil. Crit Care Med 2003;31(3):711–7.
40. Sievers TD, Yee JD, Foley ME, et al. Midazolam for conscious sedation during pediatric oncology procedures: safety and recovery parameters. Pediatrics 1991;88(6):1172–9.
41. Wathen JE, Roback MG, Mackenzie T, et al. Does midazolam alter the clinical effects of intravenous ketamine sedation in children? A double-blind, randomized, controlled, emergency department trial. Ann Emerg Med 2000;36(6):579–88.

42. Golparvar M, Saghaei M, Sajedi P, et al. Paradoxical reaction following intrave-nous midazolam premedication in pediatric patients – a randomized placebo controlled trial of ketamine for rapid tranquilization. Paediatr Anaesth 2004; 14(11):924–30.

43. Singh R, Kumar N, Vajifdar H. Midazolam as a sole sedative for computed tomography imaging in pediatric patients. Paediatr Anaesth 2009;19:899–904.

44. Bassett KE, Anderson JL, Pribble CG, et al. Propofol for procedural sedation in children in the emergency department. Ann Emerg Med 2003;42(6):773–82.

45. Chun TH, Amanullah S, Karishma-Bahl D, et al. Comparison of methohexital and pentobarbital as sedative agents for pediatric emergency department patients for computed tomography. Pediatr Emerg Care 2009;25(10):648–50.

46. Bjorkman S, Gabrielsson J, Quaynor H, et al. Pharmacokinetics of I.V. and rectal methohexitone in children. Br J Anaesth 1987;59(12):1541–7.

47. Baxter AL, Mallory MD, Spandorfer PR, et al. Etomidate versus pentobarbital for computed tomography sedations: report from the pediatric sedation research consortium. Pediatr Emerg Care 2007;23(10):690–5.

48. Di Liddo L, D'Angelo A, Nguyen B, et al. Etomidate versus midazolam for procedural sedation in pediatric outpatients: a randomized controlled trial. Ann Emerg Med 2006;48(4):433–40, 440.e1.

49. Gamis AS, Knapp JF, Glenski JA. Nitrous oxide analgesia in a pediatric emer-gency department. Ann Emerg Med 1989;18(2):177–81.

50. Babl FE, Oakley E, Seaman C, et al. High-concentration nitrous oxide for proce-dural sedation in children: adverse events and depth of sedation. Pediatrics 2008;121(3):e528–32.

51. Andolfatto G, Abu-Laban RB, Zed PJ, et al. Ketamine-propofol combination (ketofol) versus propofol alone for emergency department procedural sedation and analgesia: a randomized double-blind trial. Ann Emerg Med 2012;59(6): 504–12.e1–2.

52. Andolfatto G, Willman E. A prospective case series of single-syringe ketamine-propofol (ketofol) for emergency department procedural sedation and analgesia in adults. Acad Emerg Med 2011;18(3):237–45.

53. Shah A, Mosdossy G, McLeod S, et al. A blinded, randomized controlled trial to evaluate ketamine/propofol versus ketamine alone for procedural sedation in children. Ann Emerg Med 2011;57(5):425–33.e2.

54. Andolfatto G, Willman E. A prospective case series of pediatric procedural sedation and analgesia in the emergency department using single-syringe ke-tamine-propofol combination (ketofol). Acad Emerg Med 2010;17(2):194–201.

55. Sharieff GQ, Trocinski DR, Kanegaye JT, et al. Ketamine-propofol combination sedation for fracture reduction in the pediatric emergency department. Pediatr Emerg Care 2007;23(12):881–4.

56. Carroll CL, Krieger D, Campbell M, et al. Use of dexmedetomidine for sedation of children hospitalized in the intensive care unit. J Hosp Med 2008;3(2):142–7.

57. McMorrow S, Abramo T. Dexmedetomidine sedation. Pediatr Emerg Care 2012; 28(3):292–6.

58. Koroglu A, Teksan H, Sagir O, et al. A comparison of the sedative, hemody-namic, and respiratory effects of dexmedetomidine and propofol in children undergoing magnetic resonance imaging. Anesth Analg 2006;103(1):63–7 [table of contents].

59. Sury M, Bullock I, Dermott K, Guideline Development Group. Sedation for diag-nostic and therapeutic procedures in children and young people: summary of NICE guidance. BMJ 2010;341:c6819.

Emergency Department Evaluation of Child Abuse

Aaron N. Leetch, MD[a,b,*], Dale Woolridge, MD, PhD[a,b]

KEYWORDS

- Nonaccidental trauma • Child abuse • Child maltreatment • Sexual abuse
- Emergency • Rib fractures • Shaken baby syndrome • Retinal hemorrhage

KEY POINTS

- The key to diagnosing child abuse early is to keep a high clinical suspicion.
- High-risk chief complaints for child abuse include the 6 Bs: bruises, breaks, bonks, burns, bites and baby blues.
- Medical evaluation and treatment should always supersede a forensic evaluation but should be as simultaneous as possible.
- All physical examination findings should be corroborated with a history and developmental level before they can be considered abusive.
- All emergency providers are mandatory reporters of a reasonable suspicion of abuse.

EMERGENCY DEPARTMENT EPIDEMIOLOGY

Child abuse or nonaccidental trauma (NAT) is a common occurrence in the United States. It is a diagnosis that many emergency providers (EPs) find both clinically and personally challenging to diagnose. However, it is imperative that these diagnoses be made to prevent further physical, mental, and emotional harm to the affected children.

The most recent reported incidence of NAT estimates that nearly 1.25 million cases or 1 in 58 children are abused annually in the United States.[1] An estimated 12% of these cases presented to hospitals initially. Recent data also show that, in 2010, an estimated 1560 children died of abuse and neglect. Survivors of child abuse have a high propensity for mood disorders, anxiety disorders, and substance abuse.

The emergency department (ED) is a common place for child abuse to present, whether overtly or latently. An estimated 2% to 10% of children visiting the ED are victims of either abuse or neglect. A study of 44 children who died of child abuse showed

[a] Department of Emergency Medicine, University of Arizona, Tucson, AZ 85724, USA;
[b] Department of Pediatrics, University of Arizona, 1501 North Campbell Avenue, Tucson, AZ 85724, USA
* Corresponding author. Department of Emergency Medicine, University of Arizona, Tucson, AZ 85724.
E-mail address: aleetch@aemrc.arizona.edu

Emerg Med Clin N Am 31 (2013) 853–873
http://dx.doi.org/10.1016/j.emc.2013.04.003
0733-8627/13/$ – see front matter © 2013 Elsevier Inc. All rights reserved.

that 19% of them had been evaluated by a physician within a month of their death. Nearly 71% of those evaluations were in an ED for complaints ranging from fussiness to vomiting to poor feeding.[2] A 2010 study showed that nearly one-fifth of abuse-related fractures had at least 1 previous physician visit in which the abuse was missed.[3] Without appropriate intervention, abuse may recur in nearly 35% of cases.[4] These children present to hospitals around the country, so the key to accurate diagnosis is a high level of clinical suspicion and a good understanding of the definitions.

DEFINITIONS IN CHILD ABUSE

There is no universally agreed definition for child abuse because it can range from blatant physical or sexual abuse to varying degrees of neglect or emotional abuse. However, a good understanding of the legal or research descriptions of child abuse is imperative for EPs making the diagnosis and appropriate referrals in the clinical setting. According the 2010 revised Child Abuse Prevention and Treatment Act, child abuse and neglect are defined as, "at a minimum, any recent act or failure to act on the part of a parent or caretaker, which results in death, serious physical or emotional harm, sexual abuse or exploitation, or an act or failure to act which presents an imminent risk of serious harm" (Public Law 104-235, Section 111; 42 USC 5106g).

The Department of Health and Human Services defines 4 main types of maltreatment in the Fourth National Incidence Study of Child Abuse and Neglect (NIS-4) Report to Congress as physical abuse, sexual abuse, neglect, and emotional abuse (**Table 1**).[1] Physical abuse is broadly defined as physical assault on a child. Sexual abuse is separated into intrusion, molestation, and other cases otherwise not described. Neglect entails failure to meet a child's basic needs of life, including physical, emotional, and educational neglect. Emotional abuse can include confinement, verbal abuse, or other unspecified forms.

For purposes of research, the Harm Standard and Endangerment Standard were devised to better qualify abuse.[1] The Harm Standard is stricter, necessitating that the victim experienced some type of harm or injury that is then qualified as fatal, serious injury/condition, moderate injury/condition, probable, or impairment. The Endangerment Standard allows for more inclusion of potential child abuse with these criteria as well as the category of endangered (**Box 1**).[1]

Special mention should be paid to Munchausen syndrome by proxy, because it is a specialized form of abuse that is often associated with a medical setting. It is a factious disorder in which caregivers derive an unknown (and hotly debated) benefit at the expense of the patient.[5,6] Allegations of abuse, whether physical or sexual, may be a type of Munchausen syndrome by proxy associated with repeated visits to EDs or primary care physicians claiming abuse. Although this should be considered, Munchausen is not a diagnosis easily made in the ED and is best determined using a multidisciplinary approach in an inpatient setting.[7]

Risk Factors in Patients

Patient characteristics most associated with increased rates of maltreatment include gender, age, race, disabilities, and school enrollment (**Table 2**). In the past and currently, there is no gender bias for physical abuse alone; however, girls are more often the victims of sexual abuse, which confers more overall abuse, compared with boys.[8] Children aged 6 to 8 years have the highest maltreatment rates, although there has been a recent increase in the youngest children, aged 0 to 2 years. The recent data show a significantly higher rate of maltreatment of African American children compared with white and Hispanic children, which is a new trend from the

Type of Abuse	Reports (%)	Examples
Table 1 **Types of abuse, percentage of reports, and cited examples from NIS-4**		
Physical abuse	58	Beating, burning, choking, biting Shaking, pushing, restraining, kicking Any other mechanism that may have been meant to hurt or punish the child
Sexual abuse	24	Intrusion: oral, anal, or genital penetration with any object Molestation: some form of genital contact without intrusion Other: cases of abuse without direct contact but includes exposure of a child or of a perpetrator to a child, lack of supervision of a child's sexual exposure, or touching areas other than the genitals with sexual intentions
Neglect	61	Abandonment or other refusal to maintain custody, such as desertion, expulsion from home, refusal to accept custody of a returned runaway Permitting or encouraging chronic maladaptive behavior, such as truancy, delinquency, prostitution, serious drug/alcohol abuse Refusal to allow needed treatment of a professionally diagnosed physical, educational, emotional, or behavioral problem; or failure to follow the advice of a competent professional's recommendation thereof Failure to seek, or unwarranted delay in seeking, competent medical care for a serious injury, illness, or impairment Consistent or extreme inattention to the child's physical or emotional needs, including needs for food, clothing, supervision, safety, affection, and reasonably hygienic living conditions Failure to register or enroll the child in school, as required by state law
Emotional abuse	27	Close confinement: binding a child to restrict movement or putting a child in a small space as a form of punishment Verbal abuse: threatening or demeaning words Other: allowing unspecified acts that have a profound effect on the child

Many different types of abuse are often inflicted on the same child, thus making the sum of percentages greater than 100%.

Adapted from Sedlak AJ, Mettenburg J, Basena M, et al. Fourth National Incidence Study of Child Abuse and Neglect (NIS-4). Washington, DC: US Department of Health and Human Services; 2010. Available at: http://www.acf.hhs.gov/programs/opre/research/project/national-incidence-study-of-child-abuse-and-neglect-nis-4-2004-2009. Accessed July 9, 2010.

previous data collection in 1996. Black children who are victims of NAT also carry a higher mortality than other races.[1]

Children with premature birth or children with disabilities/chronic medical illnesses traditionally were more often victims of abuse. However, the latest data show overall decreased rates of abuse, possibly owing to better recognition by medical providers and the widespread implementation of medical foster homes and respite care. However, when abused, these patients had higher morbidity and mortality.

Enrollment in school was evaluated for the first time in the most recent data collection. Children who were not enrolled in school were more likely to be sexually abused or neglected than those who were in school. In contrast, children who were enrolled

---

Box 1
Harm Standard and Endangerment Standard definitions for abuse according to NIS-4

- Fatal: the abuse or neglect is suspected to have led to the child's death.

- Serious injury/condition: injury or harm was significant enough to seriously impair the child's physical, mental, or emotional capacities long term or enough to require professional treatment to prevent such an outcome.

- Moderate injury/condition: injury or harm was significant enough to seriously impair the child's physical, mental, or emotional capacities for greater than 48 hours.

- Probable impairment: maltreatment that is so extreme or inherently traumatic that significant emotional injury or impairment may reasonably be assumed to have occurred, even though the child may show no obvious physical or behavioral signs of injury.

- Endangered: the child's health or safety was or is seriously endangered, but the child does not seem to have been harmed.

Adapted from Sedlak AJ, Mettenburg J, Basena M, et al. Fourth National Incidence Study of Child Abuse and Neglect (NIS-4). Washington, DC: US Department of Health and Human Services; 2010. Available at: http://www.acf.hhs.gov/programs/opre/research/project/national-incidence-study-of-child-abuse-and-neglect-nis-4-2004-2009. Accessed July 9, 2010.

---

in school had higher rates of physical abuse. The latter is not well explained, although there may be a component of selection bias caused by the presence of more caregivers (ie, teachers, coaches, principals), with those who attended school possibly being more apt to be identified. An important point for EPs is that the simple question of, "How is school going?" can elicit important social history pertaining to latent abuse.

Risk Factors in Caregivers/Families

Risk factors such as gender, relationship to the child, age of the perpetrator, unemployment, and a history of the perpetrator being abusive in the past are all associated with higher rates of abuse (see **Table 2**).[1,8] Biological parents were most often the perpetrators (81%) in physical abuse or neglect but were perpetrators in sexual abuse only a third of the time (36%). Female parents/caregivers are more likely to be perpetrators of physical abuse (75%), although NAT by men is more likely to result in the death of the child. Men are more often (87%) implicated in sexual abuse against children compared with women. Rates of child maltreatment by unemployed parents are 2 to 3 times higher than by employed parents. Studies are inconclusive on whether caregivers who were themselves abused are more likely to abuse others, although there seems to be a trend toward this being true.[8] Substance abuse and mental illness in abusers were also more common.[1]

Table 2
Risk factors for abuse

Victims	Perpetrators	Families
Women (sexual abuse)	Biological parents	Low socioeconomic status
Ages 0–1 and 6–8 y	(physical abuse, neglect)	Less than high-school education of
African American race	Women (physical abuse)	caregivers
Not in school	Men (sexual abuse)	Single parents with live-in partners
(sexual abuse, neglect)	Unemployed	
	Substance abuse	
	Mental health issues	

Low socioeconomic status, including income less than $15,000 annually, less than high-school education for caregivers, and participation in public assistance programs, contributed to increased maltreatment at 5 to 7 times the rates with higher socioeconomic status. Children living with their married biological parents had the lowest rate of maltreatment, whereas children living with a single parent and a live-in partner had the highest rates of abuse.[1]

THE APPROACH TO AN ABUSED CHILD

The forensic or legal evaluation is best performed by a trained team of law enforcement and child abuse specialists. However, EPs are best suited to medically evaluate a child first, with the data gathered during this evaluation often being used for further investigation. Medical examination and treatment should always supersede legal evaluation for the good of the child. The following initial evaluation of abuse has been adapted from the previous *Clinics of North America* review and the most recent American Academy of Pediatrics recommendations.[9,10]

History

An appropriate history should be taken from all involved, including the child, parents, caregivers, and any witnesses. In a critically ill patient, history should be focused to information that can guide lifesaving intervention.

If possible, the child should be interviewed alone. Sit down at or below eye level and, in a gentle manner, ask questions in terms that the child can understand. Ask open-ended questions and document the child's exact responses. Involvement of social work or a child life specialist can be useful to make the child comfortable and to help document pertinent information. If available, video or audio recording may be used.

Caregivers should also be interviewed alone when possible. It is important to remain objective and nonjudgmental because the EP's role is a medical evaluation, not a legal evaluation. Without assigning blame, EPs can ask plainly, "Are you concerned someone is abusing your child?" Documentation on the injury or abuse should include timing, mechanism, preceding events, and witnesses to the injury. Responses concerning for NAT include lack of explanation, dramatic changes in important details, wide variability of explanation between caregivers, and explanations inconsistent with the injury or the physical/developmental capacity of the child.

A complete medical history should be obtained from the primary caregiver. Past medical history should include birth history, chronic or congenital conditions, and history of prior trauma or hospitalizations. Familial history of bleeding, bone, genetic, or metabolic disorders should be elicited. Current progress in developmental milestones should be documented. Important social history includes identification of primary and other caregivers, history of similar trauma to other siblings, history of substance abuse in the household, and prior Child Protective Services (CPS) involvement.

Physical Examination

A complete physical examination should be performed with exact documentation of findings. Cardiovascular perfusion, work of breathing, and level of alertness can quickly identify a critically ill child. Lung auscultation can reveal a pneumothorax, and palpation of the chest and abdomen can uncover painful rib fractures or underlying solid organ injury. Symmetric and spontaneous movement of all extremities should be noted because failure to move one part can indicate a painful injury. The child should be completely undressed and the skin examined for patterned injuries such as bruising, burns, or bite marks. Examination of the head for hematomas or step-offs can uncover a skull fracture. A fundoscopic examination can disclose retinal hemorrhages, although this can be difficult without dilatation in an uncooperative child. Oral cavity injuries such as a torn frenulum are often associated with forced feeding or forced oral sex. A full neurologic examination should be documented in cases of traumatic brain injury. Anogenital examination should be performed in cases of sexual abuse but an external examination should also be performed in those with just physical abuse, and the two can be concurrent. General patterns of neglect can include cachexia, dental caries, severe diaper dermatitis, and poor wound care. Photography is useful to document injuries for legal purposes and is often done in conjunction with law enforcement. Further description of specific findings as well as the evaluation of sexual abuse is discussed later in this article.

HIGH-RISK CHIEF COMPLAINTS

Abused children often present to EDs with chief complaints unrelated or latently related to the abuse. They have a higher use of EDs compared with the general population.[11] Although it is unreasonable to treat every patient as if they are being abused, it is the role of EPs to keep a high index of suspicion. There have been numerous attempts at developing appropriate criteria for ED screening of abuse including reminder systems, scheduled education, and automatic screening based on risk factors.[12,13] Although observational studies suggest that these may be useful, none have been shown to be sufficiently accurate or reproducible.[14–16] A brief introspection of whether the child is being abused is often enough of a consideration, but there are several chief complaints that deserve further investigation. There are 6 B's that have high potentials for abuse and should heighten ED suspicion: bruises, breaks, bonks (head injury), burns, bites, and baby blues (**Box 2**).

THE 6 BS
Bruises

Bruising is one of the most common findings of abuse but is often overlooked on initial evaluation. Nearly 44% of fatal or near-fatal cases of child abuse had previous medical evaluations in which bruising was noted.[17] Patient age and motor developmental stage should be carefully considered when bruising is found on young children. Most children progress from crawling at about 6 months to cruising (walking with assistance) between 6 and 12 months to walking between 9 and 15 months, although some children show faster or slower gross motor development than others. The adage, "Those who don't cruise rarely bruise" was confirmed in a 1999 study by Sugar and colleagues.[18] In otherwise well children in whom abuse was not suspected,

---

Box 2
Six B's: high-risk chief complaints

- Bruises
- Breaks
- Bonks (head injuries)
- Burns
- Bites
- Baby blues (excessive crying, poor feeding)

bruising was found over the bony prominences (ie, shins, forehead, scalp, or upper leg) in 54% of walkers and nearly 21% of cruisers but in only 2% of precruisers.

Certain patterns of bruises also more strongly suggest abuse. A 2009 study by Pierce and colleagues[17] defined the TEN-4 (thorax, ears, neck) body region and age clinical decision rule, in which bruises on the torso (including genitals), ear, or neck on a child less than 4 years of age or any bruising on a child less than 4 months of age strongly suggested abuse, with a 97% sensitivity (**Box 3, Fig. 1**). However, specificity was only 84%, indicating that bruising in these areas or age groups is not necessarily diagnostic of abuse.

Any patterned bruising should also raise the suspicion for abuse (**Fig. 2**). Sharp demarcation, uniform shape, or clusters of bruising often can indicate that the child was assailed with an object.[19] Types of patterned bruises may include linear bruises from a rod, looped bruises from a cord, bandlike bruises from restraints around wrists or ankles, or mirror images of implements such as patterned belts or kitchen utensils.

In the past, dating bruises based on color was widely practiced to help distinguish accidental from nonaccidental trauma. However, recent literature suggests that dating of bruises by color has no scientific basis.[20,21] The accuracy of dating for fresh, intermediate, or old bruises was only 55% to 63% and interobserver reliability regarding color was poor whether the bruise was photographed or in vivo.[20–22] However, multiple bruises in various stages of healing should prompt concern.

Bruising around the abdomen should raise specific concern for intra-abdominal injury, but bruising is often absent even with severe blows.[23] Inflicted abdominal trauma related to abuse is associated with a delayed presentation, higher rate of solid and hollow viscous injury, and an overall higher morbidity and mortality.[24,25]

Pitfalls in evaluation of bruising

No bruise is diagnostic for abuse. It should prompt further investigation and should be correlated with a clinical history, development stage, and caregiver explanation. This information should ideally be confirmed by more than one source. Several normal childhood or medical conditions can cause or mimic bruising.

Hemophilia, leukemia, postinfectious vasculitides, and idiopathic thrombocytopenic purpura are well-described childhood illnesses that can cause easy bruising from poor clotting or platelet function. Minimal trauma can cause bruising similar that that described in abuse. A medical evaluation including a complete blood count with platelets, prothrombin time, and partial thromboplastin time may be indicated for evaluation.

Melanocytic nevus (previously called Mongolian spots) is a dark blue/green discoloration in the low back and buttocks that is well described and can initially be seen at

---

Box 3
TEN-4 rule for bruises suggesting abuse

- Bruises on the:
  - T: thorax (including genitals)
  - E: ears
  - N: neck
- Bruises on any child less than 4 months old

Data from Pierce MC, Kaczor K, Aldridge S, et al. Bruising characteristics discriminating physical child abuse from accidental trauma. Pediatrics 2010;125(1):67–74.

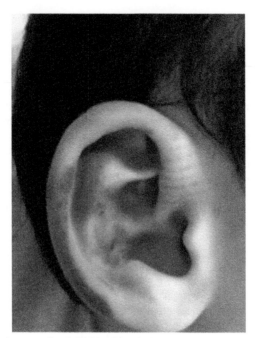

Fig. 1. Bruising on the ear of a child struck in the head.

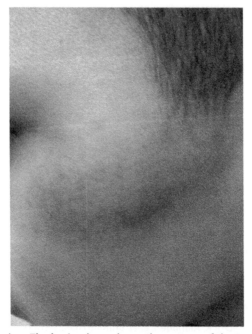

Fig. 2. Patterned bruises. The bruise shown bears the pattern of the tread on the bottom of the shoe the child was struck with.

birth. These marks can be large, sometimes covering the buttocks and extending up to the mid or upper back. They are most common in African American, Hispanic, Native American, and Asian ethnicities and the natural course is to self-resolve in 2 to 3 years.

Several cultural practices that are not abusive can cause patterned bruises that can initially alarm EPs. Cao giao, or coining, is a Vietnamese folk remedy in which a coin is vigorously rubbed against the skin to release sources of fever. The result is linear patterned bruises but no harm to the child. Cupping is similarly practiced by some Latin American cultures for relief of fever. Patterned circular bruises occur from a vacuum effect after a heated glass bowl is applied to the skin and allowed to cool.

When documenting bruises, color, size, and shape should still be documented, but always objectively (ie, U-shaped bruise rather than belt buckle–shaped bruise). Bruises may also prompt imaging studies because they may be the only visible clue to a deeper fracture or injury.

Breaks

Skeletal fractures are common in EDs. Childhood fractures occur most commonly in boys and usually affect the upper extremity. The mechanism is usually related to falls, sports, or motor vehicle collisions.[26] Fractures of abuse are less common but are also often found incidentally and without rational explanation.[27] Important risk factors of abusive fractures include age of the child, location of fracture, and number of fractures.

Toddlers and infants are most likely to have abusive fractures, with younger age being more suggestive.[28,29] Again, development plays a key role in diagnosis because infants do not become mobile enough even to roll until about 4 months of age. In this age group, the most commonly fractured bones are the clavicle and skull.[28]

The specific bone fractured must fit with the given history but some breaks more strongly suggest abuse than others. Rib fractures are frequently seen in abused children and are classically described as posteromedial, bilateral, and on contiguous ribs from a squeezing force as an infant is shaken (**Fig. 3**).[28] They can often be the only evidence of abuse. Rib fractures alone in children less than 3 years of age are associated with 95% positive predictive value (PPV) for NAT. This value increased to 100% when clinical scenario and history were considered.[29] Cardiopulmonary resuscitation rarely causes rib fractures, and when it does they are anterior and may be multiple.[30,31]

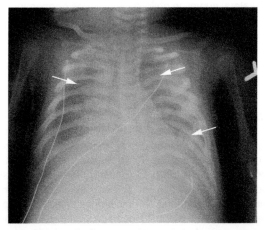

Fig. 3. Rib fractures. Multiple rib fractures (*arrows*) in various stages of healing in a 7-month-old abused child.

Long bone fractures highly associated with abuse include midshaft and metaphyseal fractures. Femoral fractures in the absence of a motor vehicle collision or other explained violent trauma conferred a significant probability that the inciting event was nonaccidental.[25] Humeral shaft fractures followed suit, especially when the child was less than 15 months of age.[32] Fractures are typically midshaft but neither spiral, transverse, nor oblique fractures correlated more with abuse.

In contrast with the direct force applied for midshaft fractures, metaphyseal fractures occur because of indirect forces. Shaking, pulling, or twisting mechanisms often cause rapid acceleration and deceleration that shear the immature spongiosa of the growing bone. Metaphyseal fractures are the classic fractures described by Caffey[33] that are often associated with other abusive injuries such as rib fractures, retinal hemorrhages, or head trauma. These bucket-handle or corner fractures are highly specific for abusive injury and are almost never seen in accidental trauma.[34]

ED-appropriate imaging in fractures

If the fracture is suspicious for abuse, current recommendations by the American Academy of Pediatrics (AAP) are for a complete skeletal survey to be performed in the ED, if the child is stable and less than 2 years old.[10] The usefulness of skeletal survey in children older than 5 years is poor, and variable in children between 2 and 5 years old.[35] Skeletal surveys should be separate, high-quality radiographs of every bone. A babygram with multiple areas on the same image is not acceptable and lowers the sensitivity of the survey. Skeletal survey alone does not identify all fractures and can be performed in conjunction with bone scintigraphy to increase the sensitivity. However, this is not an imaging modality that is readily available in the ED and should be considered as part of the inpatient evaluation. Neither skeletal survey nor bone scintigraphy is sensitive enough to identify all fractures and a repeat skeletal survey performed 2 weeks later will yield more findings. Repeat studies do not need to include the skull because it does not form calluses like cortical bones in the rest of the skeleton.[35]

The radiation exposure from a bone survey is estimated at 4 mSv and, although the concern of possible radiation effects is valid, the morbidity and mortality from missed abuse is well documented and high.

Skeletal survey is sensitive enough to be recommended for all suspected cases of abuse. A study of skeletal survey in children with burns concerning for abuse showed that 18% had concomitant fractures.[36] Finding these fractures not only helps identify further injuries in need of potential treatment but also helps build a case that the injuries sustained were nonaccidental. However, fractures cannot necessarily be correlated with exact injuries because dating of fractures is an inexact science reliant mostly on the radiologist's personal experience.[37]

Pitfalls in the evaluation of fractures

There are several medical conditions that confer bone fragility and a higher rate of fractures with minimal trauma. Osteogenesis imperfecta is an autosomal dominant defect in collagen that causes fragility. Children may also have bluish sclera, short stature, a large fontanelle, and tooth discoloration, although several types exist with variable penetrance. Nutritional deficiencies such as rickets (vitamin D deficiency) and scurvy (vitamin C deficiency), and chronic kidney disease with persistent electrolyte loss can cause osteopenia that can be seen on imaging. Pathologic fractures from childhood cancer can cause fractures that do not necessarily fit the mechanism of injury described.

Toddler fractures are important accidental fractures that initially appear suspicious. Fractures are associated with a twisting motion on a planted foot in children between 1 and 4 years old. At this age, the cartilage is stronger than the bones and resultant motion can cause a linear oblique fracture of the distal tibia (**Fig. 4**). Fractures of the midshaft tibia should be suspicious for abuse, as described earlier.[38]

Bonks

Head trauma is the most common cause of death caused by abuse.[39] Infants less than 1 year of age are specifically at risk and those who survive have significant morbidity related to neurologic sequelae. Children in this age group with intracranial injuries are frequently asymptomatic or have nonspecific symptoms so a high clinical suspicion must lead EPs to the diagnosis.[40] Symptoms can be as vague as poor feeding, excessive crying, lethargy, or seizures. Abusive head trauma should be considered in any young child presenting in extremis or cardiac arrest.

Skull fractures and intracranial hemorrhage (ICH) are commonly encountered in abusive head trauma, but are also seen in accidental trauma. Skull fractures associated with accidental trauma are usually linear and parietal.[27] Fractures that are bilateral, complex as opposed to linear, depressed, or crossing sutures lines should raise suspicion for abuse. History given by caregivers should always be evaluated in light of the patient's developmental level and the severity of trauma. The pediatric emergency care applied research network (PECARN) research group established an excellent decision rule to help identify those at low risk for clinically significant traumatic brain injury that can help in determining the plausibility of the caregiver's explanation.[41] Subdural hematomas are the most common type of ICH associated with abuse, whereas epidural hematomas are rarely associated with abuse (**Fig. 5**).[42] Of the subdural hematomas found, increasing number, location in the posterior fossa, and coincidence of cerebral edema were highly correlated with abuse.[43] A 2011 study showed 6 findings to be associated with abuse head trauma: rib fractures, retinal hemorrhages, long bone fractures, head/neck bruising, apnea, and seizures.[44] When 3 or more of these were present in children less than 3 years old, the PPV approached

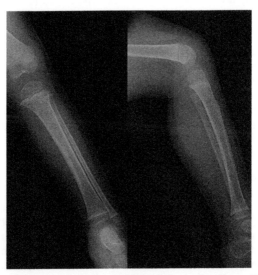

Fig. 4. Toddler fracture. Anteroposterior and lateral views of a tibia with a thin lucency.

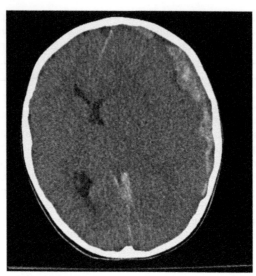

Fig. 5. Subdural hematoma. Subdural hematomas in an infant suspected of being shaken. Significant midline shift is evident.

100%. The combination of head injury and either retinal hemorrhages or rib fractures increased the PPV to nearly 100%.[44]

The triad of retinal hemorrhages, subdural hematomas, and posterior rib fractures is commonly known as shaken baby syndrome. The injury to the retina is similar in mechanism to that of the subdural hematomas and the rapid acceleration and deceleration causes a shearing injury to fragile vessels, resulting in hemorrhage. Although the term shaken baby syndrome has been argued in the legal realm, the presence of retinal hemorrhages has a high specificity for abuse, especially when the hemorrhages are bilateral, extensive, and multilayered.[45,46] Because these cases often go to trial, dilated evaluation by an ophthalmologist is recommended for all suspected cases of abuse less than 2 years of age.

ED-appropriate imaging in head injuries

The standard modality for diagnosing intracranial hemorrhage in the ED is computerized tomography (CT) of the head. However, with increasing concerns for radiation exposure of small children, there has been further investigation into the use of magnetic resonance imaging (MRI) as a primary alternative. However, the recommended sequence is CT head followed by MRI and diffusion-weighted imaging of the brain to further evaluate findings.[47]

Pitfalls in evaluation of head injuries

Abusive head trauma can be difficult to diagnose, especially when a patient is asymptomatic. Several conditions can predispose children to hemorrhage more readily. Glutaric aciduria type 1 is an inborn error of metabolism associated with macrocranium, subdural hematomas, and retinal hemorrhages. Hemorrhagic disease of the newborn can cause severe ICH in cases in which vitamin K prophylaxis is missed or refused. Simple birth trauma can cause ICH that is found incidentally and unrelated to the ED visit.

Burns

Burn injuries are most commonly sustained as scalds from hot liquids or direct contact with hot objects. Although not usually deadly, burns are a permanent physical reminder of abuse. Much like with bruising, patterned burns, uniform burns, and burns with sharp demarcation should be concerning for abuse outside a rational history. Accidental scald burns tend to be on the head and back because toddlers pull hot water onto themselves. Splashing also causes satellite burns. In contrast, forced immersion burns are sharply demarcated and have uniform depth, indicating that the child was held still while being burned.[48] Spared areas of skin where flexion or extension prevented infiltration of hot liquids strongly suggest inflicted burns. Diapers provide excellent burn protection so a history of a burn in the diaper area sustained while wearing a diaper should be suspicious for abuse. Contact burns often take the shape of the object used, such as cigarettes, irons, or heated kitchen utensils. Accidental contact burns often cause glancing injuries, as opposed to inflicted burns, which leave a more uniform mark.

Pitfalls in evaluating burns

Burns are common accidental injuries and must be explained by a rational history. Concerning history includes a supposedly unwitnessed burn, attribution of the burn to a sibling, and a delay in presentation.[49] Infectious or immunologic conditions such as staphylococcal scalded skin syndrome, Stevens-Johnson syndrome, or Kawasaki disease can cause sloughing of the skin and denuded areas similar to burns.

Bites

Bite marks on children are a disturbing sign of abuse. Often perpetrators lay blame on a sibling or animal, but careful history and measurement of the bite mark can help identify abuse. An intercanine distance of greater than 2.5 cm suggests an adult human bite rather than an animal or small child bite.[50] Photographs are helpful for documentation. Fresh bites are inoculated with the perpetrator's saliva and should be swabbed by forensic personnel for DNA evaluation.

Baby Blues

Pediatricians spend considerable time with new parents preparing them for the challenges of parenthood.[51] Screening for postpartum depression and education in ways to avoid succumbing to stressors are done at each newborn visit. However, this role can often extend into the ED during off-business hours. ED visits for complaints of excessive crying, poor feeding, or apparent life-threatening events (ALTE) can sometimes be clues to abuse. Infants with excessive crying are more likely to be slapped, smothered, or shaken than children who were not perceived to be excessive by caregivers.[52] The incidence curve of hospitalization for shaken baby syndrome mirrors the incidence curve for crying in both the starting point and shape of the curve.[53] Parents who seem to be excessively concerned or frustrated about their infant's crying should be cautioned on ways to avoid abuse, including leaving the child with a responsible caregiver for a brief time and avoidance of substance use. Nonspecific signs of poor feeding or lethargy are often the only symptom of abuse and children are often brought in by a caregiver other than the perpetrator. In cases of ALTE related to abuse, patients appeared well in the ED but were more likely to have focal findings and had the highest mortality of any other causes of ALTE.[54]

Sudden infant unexplained death syndrome (SUIDS) is clinically difficult to distinguish in an ED setting. SUIDS is differentiated from sudden infant death syndrome (SIDS) because the latter is a diagnosis that can only be made by exclusion after a full autopsy and forensic examination. Accidental causes, inborn causes, and non-accidental causes are best determined by a medical examiner. AAP clinical policy states that the rate of SUIDS is higher than infanticide and as such the family should be questioned in a nonjudgmental manner until a legal investigation can be completed.[55] Thorough objective documentation of history and physical examination findings as well as alerting law enforcement of a death is the appropriate role of the EP.

SEXUAL ASSAULT

Sexual assault of a child is a delicate scenario in the ED and deserves its own discussion. Victims should be prioritized in the ED. Prioritization is not always necessary for medical reasons but is necessitated for social and psychological reasons. These patients should be separated from the commotion of the waiting room into a quiet, nonthreatening area of the ED. Assign an advocate to the patient. This person is ideally a social worker trained as a sexual assault advocate. If not available, a social worker, nurse, or nurse assistant can remain with the patient. Be conscious of gender issues. The victim may not respond well to being isolated in a room with a male staff member. The following initial evaluation of sexual abuse has been adapted from the most recent AAP recommendations and the US Department of Justice National Protocol.[56–58]

The Interview

Extensive training exists on how to appropriately conduct a forensic interview. This interview is ideally conducted before the medical evaluation. If the forensic interview has not been conducted, the goal is to interview the patient to gain the critical medical information needed while being cautious to avoid altering the disclosure. To minimize impact, allow patients to tell their stories using their own terms, at their own pace, and always ask open-ended questions as opposed to leading questions.

Understanding the detailed events of an assault has the added benefit of directing your forensic collection. Listen without interruption, although occasional prompting with open-ended questions to encourage the victim through the disclosure may be warranted. As the victim divulges information, be meticulous to document exact words used so these can be quoted in documentation. Exact phrases during the initial medical interview have been shown to be powerful in court proceedings. Key features of the event that should be documented include: the type of contact (genital-genital; oral-genital, and so forth), characteristics of the assailant (name if known, number of assailants, gender, ethnicity, identifying features, and so forth), presence of body fluids (wet areas that may imply saliva, sweat, ejaculate, and so forth), cleansing events since the assault (showering, bathing, urination, stooling). It is also necessary to know whether the victim had consensual intercourse before the assault (within the last week) and the date of the last menstrual period if the patient is postpubertal.

The Kit

The forensic collection kit (so-called rape kit) is regularly supplied by the law enforcement agency investigating the case. The contents of these kits are, for the most part, standardized but may vary slightly from region to region. Before use, inspect the kit to make sure it is sealed and intact. From this point forward, a clearly defined chain of custody must be maintained until it is completed and handed back to law enforcement personnel. The common elements of the forensic collection kit are summarized in **Box 4.**

Box 4
Inventory of a standard sexual assault forensics kit

- Paper bags to package clothing and underwear
- Folded paper mat to collect foreign materials such as dried blood, dried secretions, fibers, loose hairs, vegetation, and soil/debris
- Envelope for collection of debris from pubic hair combings
- Swabs along with swab boxes for packaging of vaginal/cervical swabs and smears, penile swabs and smears, anal/perianal swabs and smears, oral swabs and smears, body swabs
- Known victim's blood, saliva sample, or buccal swab for DNA analysis
- Bulb syringe and vial for vaginal washings
- Nail pick for fingernail scrapings
- Sealing tape and stickers

Additional equipment (if available) that can augment data collection

- Alternative light source (fluorescent light or Wood light)
- Colposcope or other photographic device
- Speculum and/or anoscope
- Toluidine blue
  - 18-F Foley catheter with Luer lock syringe

The Examination

Make sure the patient is comfortable and explain everything that is going to happen. Unless they are suspects, have the parents involved as much as possible to keep the child comfortable. If possible, have the victim assist and direct during the examination. This involvement not only empowers the victim but also directs the collections (particularly combings and swabs) to regions of the body most likely to result in collection of biological evidence. Patients need to be fully disrobed and in a loose-fitting hospital gown. All regions of the body need to be inspected, including crevices, scalp, and fingernails (to check whether they are broken or retaining material). Positioning of the patient for the genital examination is critical not only for adequate visualization but for the comfort of the patient. For young girls, the knee-to-chest position is often comfortable when the child is in the parent's lap. The frog-legged and prone position can also help identify different aspects of the female genital examination for trauma or hymenal injury.

Keys to Processing and Packaging the Kit

Wear gloves at all times once the forensic kit is opened. Be cautious of what is touched. Work areas should be wiped clean with a disinfecting solution. Do not sneeze or cough onto the kit. Change gloves before and after each swab acquisition. Expect to change gloves more than 20 times through the examination. All evidence must be dried before storage. DNA within biological specimens is stable once desiccated. If specimens remain wet, fungus and bacteria can further degrade DNA in the collections. For this reason, material should never be packaged in plastic. Wet clothing can be laid out during the examination to dry but, if wet on packaging, law enforcement should be notified to expedite processing in the forensic laboratory. Commercial swab driers have a 1-hour timer with a swab compartment that gently circulates cool air over the swabs. An alternative can be a polystyrene cup turned upside down on the counter. Holes in the cup serve to hold and separate swabs while drying. Be careful to label the swabs in the swab rack or polystyrene cup.

Once dry, swabs and slides are packaged. Labeling should include the patient name, your name, body region of origin, and collection date/time on each package. Packages are then placed in separate envelopes once dry and tape sealed (it is important not to lick the envelope). Each envelope should be signed, with the signature extending across the tape. Once packaged, the outside of the kit has a region for the documentation of custody. On handing the completed kit to law enforcement, always witness their receipt and signature in the chain of custody section, thus documenting their receipt of the evidence.

ED MANAGEMENT AND DISPOSITION OF CHILD ABUSE

When abused children present to the ED, identification and treatment of life-threatening injuries take precedence compared with everything else. A thorough history and complete examination, both visual and by palpation, are indicated in every child, much like in patients with trauma. Once the child has been appropriately stabilized, then the legal evaluation can begin. Informing caregivers about the subsequent steps and need for mandatory reporting is vital and should be handled delicately because some caregivers do not respond positively to being investigated. EPs can simply state, "I am concerned someone is abusing your child and I am legally obligated to report this."

EPs are required by law to report cases in which there is a reasonable suspicion of child abuse. However, in addition to there being no firm definition of child abuse, child abuse experts disagree on what constitutes reasonable suspicion as a threshold for mandatory reporting.[57] Specific laws have minor variations from state to state but all allow for immunity from criminal or civil prosecution for mandatory reporters who file reports in good faith (specific statues can be found at the Web site for Administration for Children and Families, US Department of Health and Human Services; at www.childwelfare.gov/systemwide/laws_policies/search/index.cfm). Despite this, many EPs choose not to report cases of abuse.[59] In an attempt to simplify a complex interaction, the role of EPs in child abuse is proposed to be 6-fold:

1. Identify abuse
2. Facilitate a thorough investigation
3. Treat medical needs
4. Protect the patient
5. Provide an unbiased medical consultation to law enforcement
6. Provide an ethical testimony if called to court

The medical disposition of the child is determined by the EP. Even if the child does not medically meet inpatient criteria, an admission may still be warranted for the safety of the child until CPS can find another safe environment. This process is widely practiced and accepted by pediatricians, hospitals, and insurance companies.[60]

The ED is not the place to investigate suspects, accuse caregivers, or assign blame. Instead, it is important to stay focused on the medical evaluation of the child and allow law enforcement and CPS to investigate. Keeping objectivity allows an easier time testifying should the case go to court and the medical records and EP's testimony be subpoenaed.

Documentation

Documentation of abuse is carefully scrutinized in subsequent legal matters so a meticulous record is critical. It is important to be objective and use quotes when possible. History should include where and when the injury occurred as well as witnesses to the injury and explanations given for any delay in care. Events leading up to the event may elicit a cause for an abusive response. Physical examination should document color, size, and shape of any visible injuries. Developmental level of the child should be documented as what is given by history and what is observed in the ED encounter. The medical decision-making portion should give a concise opinion on whether the history and physical examination corroborate each other and whether the mechanism for injury is plausible or not.

For cases of sexual abuse, each forensic collection kit has documentation forms included and exact processing is vital. These forms are self-explanatory for the most part, with prompted fill-in sections and text areas for the examiner to complete. There is typically a signature line for consent from the victim's guardian. All pages need to be signed by the examiner, numbered, and have the victim's name and age along with the case number. Most paperwork is in triplicate (pressure-sensitive copy paper) for copies to law enforcement, crime laboratory, and medical facility. Examination portions of the documentation paperwork have body diagrams that can be marked to indicate location, with an associated page for the written description of each injury and finding. In general, the more verbose the better, because many of these cases take years to prosecute and no examiner can remember the examination over such a long period.

Photographic Documentation

Photographic evidence has been beneficial in prosecution and in reminding examiners of their findings for testimony. An additional benefit is that images can be evaluated at a later date by outside medical specialists. Photography is best performed by a law enforcement agency with approved forensic cameras, which is typically facilitated by the law enforcement agent, and in small rural agencies can be as rudimentary as an officer (using an agency-approved camera) taking the photographs with the direction of the examiner. Smartphones or personal cameras should not be used.

Box 5
Findings highly suspicious of abuse

- Aloof or inconsistent caregivers
- Young age
- Multiple injuries
- Patterned or sharply demarcated bruises or burns
- Bruises on the torso, ear, or neck
- Bruises in children less than 4 months of age
- Rib fractures
- Midshaft or metaphyseal fractures
- Subdural hematomas
- Retinal hemorrhages
  - Bite marks less than 2.5 cm in diameter

Table 3 Medical conditions that can mimic abuse	
Bruises	Hemophilia Leukemia Postinfectious vasculitides Idiopathic thrombocytopenic purpura Melanocytic nevus Cupping Coining
Breaks	Osteogenesis imperfecta Vitamin D deficiency (rickets) Vitamin C deficiency (scurvy) Chronic kidney disease Toddler fractures
Bonks	Bleeding diatheses Glutamic aciduria Vitamin K deficiency Birth trauma
Burns	Stevens-Johnson syndrome Staphylococcal scalded skin syndrome Kawasaki disease

SUMMARY

Child abuse is emotionally challenging and a common problem in EDs globally. EPs are in a prime position to act on immediate threats to life and limb and to identify abuse before significant morbidity or mortality ensues. Early identification of abuse can also lead to early treatment of the psychological and emotional scars, which EPs cannot adequately treat in the emergency setting. Although no single finding is 100% specific for abuse, several findings are suspicious for abuse (**Box 5**) but can have medical reasons that require evaluation first (**Table 3**). Maintaining a high clinical suspicion for high-risk cases of abuse remains the most important skill an EP can have to help curb this serious social problem.

REFERENCES

1. Sedlak AJ, Mettenburg J, Basena M, et al. Fourth National Incidence Study of child abuse and neglect (NIS-4). Washington, DC: US Department of Health and Human Services; 2010. Available at: http://www.acf.hhs.gov/programs/opre/research/project/national-incidence-study-of-child-abuse-and-neglect-nis-4-2004-2009. Accessed July 9, 2010.
2. King WK, Kiesel EL, Simon HK. Child abuse fatalities: are we missing opportunities for intervention? Pediatr Emerg Care 2006;22(4):211.
3. Ravichandiran N, Schuh S, Bejuk M, et al. Delayed identification of pediatric abuse-related fractures. Pediatrics 2010;125(1):60–6.
4. Skellern CY, Wood DO, Murphy A, et al. Non-accidental fractures in infants: risk of further abuse. J Paediatr Child Health 2000;36(6):590–2.
5. Schreier H. Munchausen by proxy defined. Pediatrics 2002;110(5):985–8.
6. Stirling J. Beyond Munchausen syndrome by proxy: identification and treatment of child abuse in a medical setting. Pediatrics 2007;119(5):1026–30.
7. Barker LH, Howell RJ. Munchausen syndrome by proxy in false allegations of child sexual abuse: legal implications. J Am Acad Psychiatry Law 1994;22(4):499–510.

8. Mulpuri K, Tredwell SJ. The epidemiology of nonaccidental trauma in children. Clin Orthop Relat Res 2011;469:759–67.
9. Jain AM. Emergency department evaluation of child abuse. Emerg Med Clin North Am 1999;17(3):575–93.
10. Kellogg ND. Evaluation of suspected child physical abuse. Pediatrics 2007; 119(6):1232–41.
11. Guenther E, Knight S, Olson LM, et al. Prediction of child abuse risk from emergency department use. J Pediatr 2009;154(2):272–7.
12. Mikton C, Butchart A. Child maltreatment prevention: a systematic review of reviews. Bull World Health Organ 2009;87(5):353–61.
13. Teeuw AH, Derkx BH, Koster WA, et al. Detection of child abuse and neglect at the emergency room. Eur J Pediatr 2012;171(6):877–85.
14. Woodman J, Lecky F, Hodes D, et al. Screening injured children for physical abuse or neglect in emergency departments: a systematic review. Child Care Health Dev 2010;36(2):153–64.
15. Newton AS, Zou B, Hamm MP, et al. Improving child protection in the emergency department: a systematic review of professional interventions for health care providers. Acad Emerg Med 2010;17(2):117–25.
16. Louwers EC, Affourtit MJ, Moll HA, et al. Screening for child abuse at emergency departments: a systematic review. Arch Dis Child 2010;95(3):214–8.
17. Pierce MC, Kaczor K, Aldridge S, et al. Bruising characteristics discriminating physical child abuse from accidental trauma. Pediatrics 2010;125(1):67–74.
18. Sugar NF, Taylor JA, Feldman KW. Bruises in infants and toddlers: Those who don't cruise rarely bruise. Arch Pediatr Adolesc Med 1999;153(4):399.
19. Maguire S, Mann MK, Sibert J, et al. Are there patterns of bruising in childhood which are diagnostic or suggestive of abuse? A systematic review. Arch Dis Child 2005;90(2):182–6.
20. Maguire S, Mann MK, Sibert J, et al. Can you age bruises accurately in children? A systematic review. Arch Dis Child 2005;90(2):187–9.
21. Schwartz AJ, Ricci LR. How accurately can bruises be aged in abused children? Literature review and synthesis. Pediatrics 1996;97:254–7.
22. Munang LA, Leonard PA, Mok JY. Lack of agreement on colour description between clinicians examining childhood bruising. J Clin Forensic Med 2002; 9(4):171–4.
23. Thompson S. Accidental or inflicted? Evaluating cutaneous, skeletal, and abdominal trauma in children. Pediatr Ann 2005;34:372–81.
24. Canty TG Sr, Canty TG Jr, Brown C. Injuries of the gastrointestinal tract from blunt trauma in children: a 12-year experience at a designated pediatric trauma center. J Trauma 1999;46:234–40.
25. Wood J, Rubin DM, Nance ML, et al. Distinguishing inflicted versus accidental abdominal injuries in young children. J Trauma Acute Care Surg 2005;59(5): 1203–8.
26. Rennie L, Court-Brown CM, Mok JY, et al. The epidemiology of fractures in children. Injury 2007;38(8):913–22.
27. Kemp AM, Dunstan F, Harrison S, et al. Patterns of skeletal fractures in child abuse: systematic review. BMJ 2008;337:a1518.
28. Clarke NM, Shelton FR, Taylor C. The incidence of fractures in children under the age of 24 months – in relation to non-accidental injury. Injury 2012;43:762–5.
29. Leventhal JM, Thomas SA, Rosenfield NS, et al. Fractures in young children: distinguishing child abuse from unintentional injuries. Arch Pediatr Adolesc Med 1993;147(1):87.

30. Bulloch B, Schubert CJ, Brophy PD, et al. Cause and clinical characteristics of rib fractures in infants. Pediatrics 2000;105(4):e48.

31. Barsness KA, Cha ES, Bensard DD, et al. The positive predictive value of rib fractures as an indicator of nonaccidental trauma in children. J Trauma Acute Care Surg 2003;54(6):1107–10.

32. Williams R, Hardcastle N. Humeral fractures and non-accidental injury in children. Emerg Med J 2005;22(2):124–5.

33. Caffey J. Some traumatic lesions in growing bones other than fractures and dislocations: clinical and radiological features. Br J Radiol 1957;30:225–38.

34. Kleinman PK, Perez-Rossello JM, Newton AW, et al. Prevalence of the classic metaphyseal lesion in infants at low versus high risk for abuse. AJR Am J Roentgenol 2011;197(4):1005–8.

35. Kemp AM, Butler A, Morris S, et al. Which radiological investigations should be performed to identify fractures in suspected child abuse? Clin Radiol 2006; 61(9):723–36.

36. DeGraw M, Hicks RA, Lindberg D. Incidence of fractures among children with burns with concern regarding abuse. Pediatrics 2010;125(2):e295–9.

37. Prosser I, Maguire S, Harrison SK, et al. How old is this fracture? Radiologic dating of fractures in children: a systematic review. AJR Am J Roentgenol 2005;184(4):1282–6.

38. Tenenbein M, Reed MH, Black GB. The toddler's fracture revisited. Am J Emerg Med 1990;8(3):208–11.

39. Duhaime AC, Christian CW, Rorke LB, et al. Nonaccidental head injury in infants—the "shaken-baby syndrome". N Engl J Med 1998;338(25):1822–9.

40. Laskey AL, Holsti M, Runyan DK, et al. Occult head trauma in young suspected victims of physical abuse. J Pediatr 2004;144(6):719–22.

41. Kupperman N, Holmes JF, Dayan PS, et al. Identification of children at very low risk of clinically-important brain injures after head trauma: a prospective cohort study. Lancet 2009;374:1160–70, 20.

42. Piteau SJ, Ward MG, Barrowman NJ, et al. Clinical and radiographic characteristics associated with abusive and nonabusive head trauma: a systematic review. Pediatrics 2012;130(2):315–23.

43. Kemp AM, Jaspan T, Griffiths J, et al. Neuroimaging: what neuroradiological features distinguish abusive from non-abusive head trauma? A systematic review. Arch Dis Child 2011;96(12):1103–12.

44. Maguire SA, Kemp AM, Lumb RC, et al. Estimating the probability of abusive head trauma: a pooled analysis. Pediatrics 2011;128(3):e550–64.

45. Togioka BM, Arnold MA, Bathurst MA, et al. Retinal hemorrhages and shaken baby syndrome: an evidence-based review. J Emerg Med 2009;37(1):98–106.

46. Bhardwaj G, Chowdhury V, Jacobs MB, et al. A systematic review of the diagnostic accuracy of ocular signs in pediatric abusive head trauma. Ophthalmology 2010;117(5):983–92.

47. Kemp AM, Rajaram S, Mann M, et al. What neuroimaging should be performed in children in whom inflicted brain injury (iBI) is suspected? A systematic review. Clin Radiol 2009;64(5):473–83.

48. Greenbaum AR, Donne J, Wilson D, et al. Intentional burn injury: an evidence-based, clinical and forensic review. Burns 2004;30(7):628–42.

49. Stone NH, Rinaldo L, Humphrey CR, et al. Child abuse by burning. Surg Clin North Am 1970;50(6):1419.

50. Wagner GN. Bitemark identification in child abuse cases. Pediatr Dent 1986; 8(1):96–100.

51. Flaherty EG, Stirling J Jr. The pediatrician's role in child maltreatment prevention. Pediatrics 2010;126(4):833–41.
52. Reijneveld SA, van der Wal MF, Brugman E, et al. Infant crying and abuse. Lancet 2004;364(9442):1340–2.
53. Barr RG, Trent RB, Cross J. Age-related incidence curve of hospitalized shaken baby syndrome cases: convergent evidence for crying as a trigger to shaking. Child Abuse Negl 2006;30(1):7–16.
54. Parker K, Pitetti R. Mortality and child abuse in children presenting with apparent life-threatening events. Pediatr Emerg Care 2011;27(7):591–5.
55. Hymel KP. Distinguishing sudden infant death syndrome from child abuse fatalities. Pediatrics 2006;118(1):421–7.
56. Kellogg N. The evaluation of sexual abuse in children. Pediatrics 2005;116(2): 506–12.
57. A national protocol for sexual assault medical forensic examinations 2004. The United States Department of Justice Website: Office on Violence Against Women: selected publications. Available at: http://www.ovw.usdoj.gov/publications.html. Accessed December 18, 2012.
58. Levi BH, Crowell K. Child abuse experts disagree about the threshold for mandated reporting. Clin Pediatr 2011;50(4):321–9.
59. Van Haeringen AR, Dadds M, Armstrong KL. The child abuse lottery–will the doctor suspect and report? Physician attitudes towards and reporting of suspected child abuse and neglect. Child Abuse Negl 1998;22(3):159.
60. Medical necessity for the hospitalization of the abused and neglected child. American Academy of Pediatrics, Committee on Hospital Care and Committee on Child Abuse and Neglect. Pediatrics 1998;101:715–6.

Common Indications for Pediatric Antibiotic Prophylaxis

Matthew B. Laurens, MD, MPH

KEYWORDS

- Antibiotic prophylaxis • Traumatic wounds • Meningococcal exposure
- Pertussis exposure • Influenza exposure

KEY POINTS

- Antibiotic prophylaxis of traumatic wounds should be individualized after taking pertinent risk factors into account: exposure, wound complexity, underlying host factors.
- All close contacts of patients with invasive meningococcal disease are considered at high risk for nasopharyngeal colonization and subsequent disease.
- Pertussis can present with nonspecific signs and/or symptoms; prompt diagnosis and antibiotic treatment limits spread to contacts and the community.
- Persons at risk for severe influenza should be offered antiviral prophylaxis as it is effective in preventing influenza disease.

INTRODUCTION

Physicians treating acute pediatric emergencies tend to focus on issues that are urgent and apparent. Although this approach is appropriate for initial evaluation and treatment of an acutely ill child, illness prevention is an essential component of comprehensive medical care in the emergency room setting. Many activities of illness prevention are directed by the entire medical care team and focus on education of parents and caregivers about fall and injury prevention, bicycle safety, poisoning prevention, pedestrian safety, and other important public health topics.

A separate focus of illness prevention can be grouped under the category of antimicrobial prophylaxis. These activities are generally physician-directed, although often prompted by suggestions from other members of the patient care team. Antimicrobial prophylaxis prevents infection and/or complications of infection, and is a routine practice for defined procedures in the hospital, including the perioperative setting. In contrast to perioperative protocols that often dictate antimicrobial prophylaxis be

Pediatric Infectious Diseases and Tropical Pediatrics, Howard Hughes Medical Institute/Center for Vaccine Development, University of Maryland School of Medicine, 685 West Baltimore Street, Room 480, Baltimore, MD 21201, USA
E-mail address: mlaurens@medicine.umaryland.edu

Emerg Med Clin N Am 31 (2013) 875–894
http://dx.doi.org/10.1016/j.emc.2013.05.006
0733-8627/13/$ – see front matter © 2013 Elsevier Inc. All rights reserved.

systematically given to patients based on the planned procedure, emergency rooms and pediatric acute care facilities do not have automated procedures for antimicrobial prophylaxis in place. The responsibility thus falls on the physician caring for the child to appropriately prescribe antibiotics to prevent infection and complications of infection. Common indications for antimicrobial prophylaxis in the pediatric acute care setting include traumatic wounds, meningococcal exposures, pertussis exposures, and influenza exposures. This listing is not comprehensive and other indications exist, including needlestick injuries, sexual assault, and endocarditis prophylaxis, each of which merits a separate discussion.

TRAUMATIC WOUNDS

One of the most common reasons for emergency room visits is for treatment of traumatic wounds. With the exception of a contusion, most traumatic wounds include compromise of the skin barrier and provide a portal for entry of microorganisms from the skin flora, the environment, or the object that penetrated the skin. Traumatic wounds can be classified based on risk for infection as either low risk or high risk and requiring antibiotic prophylaxis. Sometimes, this classification is not altogether clear. Regardless, the decision regarding antibiotic prophylaxis should always be individualized after taking pertinent risk factors into account.

Pathophysiology

Traumatic wounds manifest with local tissue damage, the extent of which depends on the mechanism of and site of injury. An inflammatory phase follows where cytokine release leads to localized swelling and erythema. These cytokines signal neutrophils, macrophages, and fibroblasts to localize at the wound site to clear bacteria and begin tissue regeneration. Fibroblasts direct epithelialization of damaged skin, stimulating collagen deposition, and cross-linking. The success of neutrophils and macrophages in cleaning up any bacteria depends on the bacterial types and load at the wound site, which is generally related to the mechanism of injury (eg, puncture vs laceration), and the object inflicting the wound.

In cases in which the bacterial load at the wound site is difficult to clear, antibiotic therapy may be indicated to prevent wound infection. Reasons for bacterial persistence include immune compromise with reduced phagocytic response, difficulty irrigating deep puncture wounds, contamination with heavy bacterial loads, and reduced circulation to relatively avascular or hypoperfused areas.

Classification

Low-risk wounds include clean, minor wounds in an immunocompetent host. High-risk wounds are classified as having one or more of the following risk factors: immunocompromised host; open fractures; penetrating injuries with retained foreign body; puncture wounds; crush injuries; bite wounds; wounds that penetrate relatively avascular areas, including tendons, joints, and cartilage; heavily contaminated wounds that cannot be adequately debrided; and wounds that are delayed more than 18 hours before presentation.

Although difficult to assess the degree of immunosuppression in the emergency department (ED) setting, patients with known immunodeficiency, including those with daily systemic corticosteroid use and patients with neutropenia on chemotherapy, should receive antimicrobial prophylaxis for wound management. Patients with open fractures benefit from antimicrobial prophylaxis,[1] likely because they are at risk of bacterial contamination with skin flora and/or environmental bacteria depending on the mechanism of injury and the setting where it occurred. A penetrating injury may include a retained foreign body after evaluation of risks and benefits of removal. The remaining foreign matter may contain bacteria and provide a nidus for infection. Puncture wounds are difficult to cleanse and thus may harbor organisms found on the skin surface or on the object that penetrated the skin barrier. Crush injuries harbor injured and devitalized tissue where bacteria are more likely to thrive. Both human and animal bite wounds are likely to contain many bacterial species due to oral bacterial colonization. The limited vascular supply to tendons and cartilaginous structures may restrict local neutrophil and macrophage activity, making it difficult to clear bacteria. Wounds contaminated with soil, feces, and other foreign matter are composed of high bacterial loads that may be inadequately debrided in a timely fashion and overwhelm the ability of local tissue to clear bacterial organisms. Similarly, wounds that remain open for more than 18 hours, whether by primary or secondary intention, are more likely to harbor bacteria and progress to infection.

Fingertip injuries are frequently considered to be high-risk wounds by many practitioners, but routine antibiotic prophylaxis does not appear to influence the rate of infection after repair of distal fingertip injuries,[2] and thus antibiotic therapy is generally not indicated.

Assessment and Management

The ultimate goal of traumatic wound management is to achieve skin healing that is intact and structurally and functionally similar to the pretraumatic state. All wounds should be adequately irrigated at high pressure to decrease bacterial load.[3] Studies demonstrate equivalent wound infection rates for irrigation with tap water compared with sterile saline.[4,5] Proper closure technique is also important in preventing infection.

Simple wounds are considered low risk and do not benefit from antimicrobial prophylaxis. In high-risk wounds, oral antimicrobial prophylaxis is indicated, and is generally continued for 3 to 5 days. In contrast, established wound infections that are not complicated by osteomyelitis or retained foreign bodies are generally treated for 7 to 10 days, or for 1 to 2 days after clinical resolution of the infection. A summary of suggested antimicrobial regimens is included in **Table 1**. The role of topical antibiotic therapy use in soft tissue wound repair in the ED is understudied, with one study supporting the use of topical antimicrobial therapy used 3 times daily with wound cleansing and dressing changes to reduce the risk of infection.[6]

Management of wounds resulting from bite injuries lacks a clear evidence base, as most clinical trials did not include appropriate anaerobic antimicrobials,[7] and few used optimal techniques for isolation of pathogens.[8] In general, bite wounds should be closed only after careful wound cleansing in areas where blood supply is plentiful and where cosmetic results are desired, such as the head and face.[9] Bite injuries to the hand and deep puncture wounds should not be closed because of higher risk of infection. Delayed closure after irrigation and observation for 3 to 5 days is an option for wounds that are difficult to decontaminate at presentation. A recent Cochrane review supports the use of antibiotic prophylaxis after any bite injury to the hand.[10] There is weak evidence that human bites should be given prophylactic antibiotics. There is limited but conflicting evidence on routine use of prophylaxis to reduce infection for dog and cat bites.[10–12] The decision to give antimicrobial prophylaxis should be individualized to each patient, but should strongly be considered, especially in high-risk wounds, given the limited evidence base and the potential to prevent infectious complications of cellulitis, osteomyelitis, septic arthritis, sepsis, and other potential life-threatening complications.

Table 1
Recommended antimicrobial therapy for high-risk traumatic wounds

Human bites; dog or cat bites (where indicated)	First-line therapy	Amoxicillin/clavulanate 40 mg/kg/d PO divided BID (maximum dose 875 mg PO BID)
	Penicillin-allergic patients	Clindamycin 30 mg/kg/d PO divided q6 or q8 h plus trimethoprim/ sulfamethoxazole 5 mg/kg PO BID
Open fractures	First-line therapy	1st generation cephalosporin ± MRSA therapy[a]
	Additional therapy for Type III open fractures	Gentamicin or amikacin
Plantar foot wounds distal to metatarsophalangeal joint and through shoe sole	First-line therapy	Ciprofloxacin, ceftazidime, or cefepime
All other high-risk wounds	First-line therapy	1st generation cephalosporin or dicloxacillin ± MRSA therapy[a]

Abbreviations: BID, twice a day; MRSA, Methicillin-resistant *Staphylococcus aureus*; PO, by mouth; q, every.
[a] MRSA therapy can be achieved with either oral clindamycin 30 mg/kg/d PO divided q6 or q8 hours or trimethoprim-sulfamethoxazole 5 mg/kg PO BID, or intravenous clindamycin, vancomycin, or linezolid depending on local resistance patterns. Alternatives for MRSA coverage in children ≥8 years include doxycycline and tetracycline. Anti-MRSA therapy should be individualized based on previous history of MRSA infections, colonization, and/or household contacts with MRSA.

For open fractures, the Eastern Association for the Surgery of Trauma established guidelines[13] that call for immediate initiation of gram-positive antimicrobial coverage with a first-generation cephalosporin in all open fractures. This group recommends additional gram-negative coverage with an aminoglycoside for Type III open fractures that involve a wound larger than 10 cm with extensive soft tissue injury, those requiring vascular repair, are open for 8 hours or more before treatment, or are traumatic amputations. This broad coverage should continue for 72 hours after the injury in Type III fractures. For open fractures with extensive fecal or potential clostridial contamination (especially farm-related injuries), high-dose penicillin should be added to the prophylactic regimen.

The case of penetrating plantar foot wounds requires special mention. The penetration of a nail or other object through a shoe sole is more likely to introduce bacteria harbored in the shoe, such as *Pseudomonas*, but most plantar foot wounds caused by penetration into skin are caused by *Staphylococcus* and *Streptococcus*.[14] Although controversial, penetrating plantar foot wounds generally do not warrant prophylactic antibiotics, except for those distal to the metatarsophalangeal joints[15] or in those at greater risk of infection (eg, immunocompromised or diabetic patients, or wounds with a retained foreign body). For these cases, recommendations for high-risk wound antimicrobials can be followed. For injuries in which objects penetrate through a shoe sole, anti-*Pseudomonas* coverage should be given. Two to 3 days after the injury, all penetrating foot injuries should be reassessed for evidence of cellulitis and/or osteomyelitis even if prophylactic antibiotics are given, because of the possibility of resistant organisms and/or a retained foreign body.

Those who are incompletely immunized against tetanus should be given tetanus toxoid with or without tetanus immune globulin therapy according to guidelines established by the American Academy of Pediatrics (AAP).[16] Tetanus prophylaxis should be given if more than 10 years have elapsed since the last tetanus booster in the setting of low-risk wounds and, if more than 5 years have elapsed, for high-risk wounds. DTaP is the recommended vaccine for children aged 6 weeks to 6 years, and Td for children aged 7 to 18 years. For children aged 7 to 10 years who are incompletely immunized against pertussis and for children aged 11 to 18 years who have not previously received Tdap, a single dose of Tdap should be used. Persons bitten by animals that are potentially rabid and who cannot be tested or observed for 10 days should be given rabies immune globulin (RIG) and a rabies vaccination series according to AAP guidelines.[16] In healthy individuals, the previously recommended 5-dose human rabies vaccine regimen has been reduced to 4 doses of 1 mL each, administered intramuscularly in the deltoid or anterolateral thigh as soon as possible after exposure on days 0, 3, 7, and 14. Immunocompromised patients, however, should still receive the fifth dose on day 28, as well as RIG on day 0. If a patient has been vaccinated with 3 doses of human rabies vaccine before rabies exposure, RIG is not indicated, but 2 additional 1-mL doses of human rabies vaccine should be given on days 0 and 3. In summary, care for the traumatic wound should include the following:

- Cleaning the skin around the bite
- Copious irrigation
- Inspection for foreign bodies
- Radiographs as needed to evaluate for fractures or foreign bodies
- Evaluation for wound closure if appropriate
- Consideration of antimicrobial prophylaxis for high-risk wounds
- Evaluation of tetanus status
- Time-specific discharge instructions for wound checks within 48 hours

Complications

Potential infectious complications of traumatic wounds include localized skin and soft tissue infections, osteomyelitis, and gangrene requiring amputation. Systemic complications that may develop include sepsis, tetanus, and rabies. Noninfectious complications that may result include reduced circulation with death and necrosis of damaged tissue requiring debridement, loss of sensation to areas supplied by severed or damaged nerve tissue, and hypertrophy of replacement tissue resulting in keloid scar formation.

Disposition and Follow-up

Patients should be discharged with instructions to return to their primary care physician in 24 to 48 hours for evaluation of wound healing. At the follow-up visit, signs of skin and soft tissue infection should prompt initiation or reevaluation of the antibiotic regimen and screening for osteomyelitis in areas overlying bone. Open wounds should be assessed for suitability for wound closure including revision of wound margins when devitalized tissue is present.

MENINGOCOCCAL EXPOSURES
Background

Neisseria meningitidis is a gram-negative diplococcus that inhabits the mucosal surfaces of the nasopharynx in approximately 10% of healthy persons.[17] The organism survives a short time in the environment, and humans are the only reservoir. Meningococcal disease manifestations include meningitis and meningococcemia and case fatality rates are 10% to 14%.[18] Survivors may experience significant morbidity, including neurologic disability, limb loss, and hearing loss. Twelve serogroups have been identified, 6 of which (A, B, C, W135, X, and Y) are associated with epidemics. Rates of meningococcal disease are highest among children younger than 2 years,[18] yet the overall rate of meningococcal disease has declined in the United States since 2000, reaching a historic low of 0.21 cases per 100,000 population in 2011.[19] At the same time, outbreaks of meningococcal disease continue to occur in the United States, with serogroups B, C, and Y each being responsible for approximately a third of outbreaks.[18,20] Serogroups A and W135 are mostly responsible for transmission in the "meningitis belt" that stretches through sub-Saharan Africa.

Transmission

The organism is spread via droplets from the upper respiratory tract of colonized individuals who are generally asymptomatic to their close contacts. Nasopharyngeal carriage increases with age, peaking in young adulthood. Increased carriage rates have been documented in household contacts of those with disease, as well as in military recruits and university students living in closed quarters where efficient transmission is facilitated.[21] Although incompletely understood, nasopharyngeal membranes may become compromised through drying or other mechanisms that allow the bacterium to invade and cause disease.[22] Studies of transmission from pilgrims to the Hajj to their household contacts found that among household members who acquired nasopharyngeal carriage, approximately 1 in 70 developed invasive disease.[23] Recently, occupational transmission from an unconscious adult to a police officer and a respiratory therapist was documented in California.[24] As the organism is typically highly susceptible to antimicrobials, droplet precautions can be stopped 24 hours after initiation of appropriate antimicrobial therapy when patients are no longer considered infectious.

Diagnosis

For patients with suspected invasive disease, culture and Gram stain of blood, cerebrospinal fluid (CSF), purpuric lesion scrapings, synovial fluid, and other normally sterile sites may be diagnostic. Nasopharyngeal culture positivity denotes colonization, but may not necessarily correlate with invasive disease. Antigen testing of CSF is used to support a probable diagnosis. In some settings, polymerase chain reaction (PCR) testing may be used, but availability is limited in the US clinical setting. Confirmed cases include individuals with compatible symptoms and isolation of the organism from a normally sterile site. Probable cases include those with clinically compatible symptoms and either positive antigen testing of CSF, positive immunohistochemistry testing, or a positive PCR test of blood or CSF. Cases are considered suspect if clinical symptoms are accompanied by gram-negative diplococci isolated from a normally sterile site, or when clinical purpura fulminans is present.

Management of Exposures

All close contacts of patients with invasive meningococcal disease are considered at high risk for nasopharyngeal colonization and subsequent disease, and should be given postexposure prophylaxis regardless of vaccination status. Reasons for this practice include the prevalence of serogroup B disease that is not prevented by vaccines currently available in the United States and incomplete protection conferred by vaccines against other circulating strains. Chemoprophylaxis should be initiated within 1 day after an index case is diagnosed, as household contacts are at highest risk of disease in the first week after case detection. Initiation of prophylaxis more than 14 days after exposure is not considered beneficial.

To determine the need for prophylactic measures, the intensity of contact with a case of meningococcal disease should be considered. **Table 2** lists the AAP-defined[16] risk categories and the corresponding recommendation for prophylactic antibiotics to eliminate the potential of nasopharyngeal carriage. Culture of the nasopharynx in exposed persons is not considered useful in determining the need for prophylaxis.

First-Line Treatment

Treatment for elimination of nasopharyngeal carriage is indicated both in those with invasive disease who are not treated with ceftriaxone and in close contacts. First-line therapies in children include rifampin and ceftriaxone. Ciprofloxacin is an alternate therapy in adults. The AAP recommends rifampin as first-line therapy in most clinical scenarios for eradication of nasopharyngeal carriage. A recent Cochrane review of 24 randomized clinical trials, mostly in adults, to evaluate chemoprophylactic regimens for meningococcal carriage eradication, found that rifampin, ciprofloxacin, ceftriaxone, and penicillin were effective, but cited concerns of rifampin resistance in isolates that persisted after treatment.[25] Despite this finding, persistent isolates were rare in the studies in which it was documented and is not likely of clinical importance. Although the simplest regimen may be azithromycin, this therapy has been evaluated in only one adult study,[26] and is not generally recommended because of a lack of confirmatory studies and data from Africa showing resistance of *N meningitidis* isolates to macrolide antibiotics.[27] Neither rifampin nor ciprofloxacin should be given

---

Table 2
Risk categories for meningococcal disease and recommendations for antimicrobial therapy

High risk: chemoprophylaxis recommended (close contacts)	1. Household contact, especially children younger than 2 y 2. Child care or preschool contact at any time during 7 d before onset of illness 3. Direct exposure to index patient's secretions through kissing or through sharing toothbrushes or eating utensils, markers of close social contact, at any time during 7 d before onset of illness 4. Mouth-to-mouth resuscitation, unprotected contact during endotracheal intubation at any time 7 d before onset of illness 5. Frequently slept in same dwelling as index patient during 7 d before onset of illness 6. Passengers seated directly next to the index case during airline flights lasting more than 8 h
Low risk: chemoprophylaxis not recommended	1. Casual contact: no history of direct exposure to index patient's oral secretions (eg, school or work) 2. Indirect contact: only contact is with a high-risk contact, no direct contact with the index patient 3. Health care personnel without direct exposure to patient's oral secretions
In outbreak or cluster	1. Chemoprophylaxis for people other than people at high risk should be administered only after consultation with local public health authorities

Adapted from American Academy of Pediatrics. 2012 Red Book: report of the Committee on Infectious Diseases. 29th edition. Elk Grove Village (IL): American Academy of Pediatrics; 2012.

to pregnant women. Some regions have documented resistance of *N meningitidis* to ciprofloxacin,[28] and its use in these areas should be avoided. A summary of suggested chemoprophylactic regimens for meningococcal exposures and those with invasive meningococcal disease is listed in **Table 3**.

In an outbreak setting where a circulating strain is preventable by a meningococcal vaccine (strains A, C, W135, and Y), a meningococcal conjugate vaccine can be administered as part of a disease control program.[18] Careful evaluation of the epidemiology of cases by public health authorities, including genotyping of isolates and calculation of a community attack rate, should be undertaken before mass vaccination campaigns are implemented because of the high cost, potential for heightened public anxiety, and the questionable benefit to the community.[29] There is currently no indication for routine meningococcal vaccination outside of the vaccine schedule for those exposed to an index case with invasive disease. See www.cdc.gov/vaccines for complete information on vaccine schedules, including special indications for meningococcal conjugate vaccination in those with a persistent complement component deficiency, anatomic or functional asplenia, and travelers to hyperendemic or epidemic areas.

Complications

Invasive meningococcal disease carries a relatively high mortality rate of 10% to 14%, and 11% to 19% of survivors have permanent effects, including neurologic disability, limb loss, or hearing loss.[18]

Chemoprophylaxis is effective in reducing carriage and avoiding invasive disease and associated complications, but is not completely without risk. Rifampin use is associated with hepatotoxicity, and gastrointestinal effects of nausea and dyspepsia. Rifampin is a potent inducer of the CYP450 3A4 metabolic pathway and may reduce serum levels of drugs, including antiseizure medications and protease inhibitors. Rifampin use is associated with the emergence of resistance to meningococcal isolates and should be used as a single agent only for short periods, including chemoprophylaxis, not for treatment of disease. In cases in which compliance is questionable, a single dose of ceftriaxone given intramuscularly is a good option for those without a hypersensitivity contraindication.

Disposition

Chemoprophylaxis of close contacts exposed to invasive *N meningitidis* infections relies on timely reporting to the health department of any confirmed, presumptive, or probable case of meningococcal disease. Health care practitioners should educate close contacts and their caregivers about the seriousness of meningococcal disease in an effort to increase acceptance of and compliance with the chemoprophylactic regimen. Those who refuse prophylaxis should be instructed to return for care without delay should fever, malaise, or petechiae develop.

PERTUSSIS EXPOSURES

Pertussis is one of the most highly communicable diseases, with attack rates of 100% recorded in susceptible individuals. It is also known as "whooping cough," because of the pronounced inhalational whoop that is classically heard after a series of coughs. Infants and young children have the highest rates of acquisition, and young infants experience the most serious manifestations of illness. In North America, pertussis disease usually occurs in summer and fall. In spite of widespread vaccination in the United States, a resurgence of pertussis has been documented

Table 3
Chemoprophylaxis regimens for close contacts and persons with meningococcal disease

Antimicrobial	Age of Infants, Children, and Adults	Dose	Duration	Efficacy %	Precautions
Rifampin[a]	<1 mo	5 mg/kg PO q 12 h	2 d		
	≥1 mo	10 mg/kg PO q 12 h (maximum 600 mg)	2 d	90–95	Can interfere with efficacy of oral contraceptives and some seizure and anticoagulant medications; can stain contact lenses
Ceftriaxone	<15 y	125 mg IM	Single dose	90–95	To decrease pain at injection site, dilute with 1% lidocaine
	≥15 y	250 mg IM	Single dose	90–95	To decrease pain at injection site, dilute with 1% lidocaine
Ciprofloxacin[a,b]	≥1 mo	20 mg/kg PO (maximum 500 mg)	Single dose	90–95	Not recommended routinely for people younger than 18 y of age; use may be justified after assessment of risks and benefits for the individual patient.

Abbreviations: IM, intramuscular; PO, by mouth; q, every.

[a] Not recommended for use in pregnant women.

[b] Use only if fluoroquinolone-resistant strains of *N meningitidis* have not been identified in the community.

Adapted from American Academy of Pediatrics. 2012 Red Book: report of the Committee on Infectious Diseases. 29th edition. Elk Grove Village (IL): American Academy of Pediatrics; 2012.

since 2005, and is thought to be because of increased awareness, better testing using PCR assays, and because the acellular pertussis vaccines used are less potent than the whole-cell vaccine in widespread use before the 1990s.[30] Other reasons include antigenic differences in circulating strains and increased production of pertussis toxin.[31] Although better vaccines and vaccine strategies are being pursued, physicians should remain vigilant to recognize, diagnose, and treat pertussis cases and their contacts.

Pertussis was isolated in 1906, and vaccination became available in the 1940s, made from killed whole *Bordetella pertussis* bacteria commonly referred to as whole-cell vaccines. There is wide variation in immune response to whole-cell vaccines,[32] likely in part because of differences in manufacturing and the bacterial strain used. Because of concerns of reactogenicity to whole-cell vaccines, recombinant acellular pertussis vaccines were developed and are currently used for routine vaccination in developed countries, whereas whole-cell vaccines continue to be used in developing countries because of lower cost. For the primary vaccination series, the 2013 Advisory Committee on Immunization Practices (ACIP) recommends 3 doses of acellular pertussis vaccine at 2, 4, and 6 months of age, with a booster at 15 to 18 months, and a second booster at 4 to 6 years. An additional booster is recommended at 11 to 12 years. For adults, a 1-time booster of acellular pertussis is recommended, but some experts argue that this should be repeated every 10 years, as protection is not lifelong.[33] In October 2012, the ACIP recommended that all pregnant women receive 1 booster dose of tetanus/diphtheria/acellular pertussis (Tdap) for every pregnancy at 27 to 36 weeks' gestation regardless of previous Tdap history to maximize maternal antibody response and passive antibody transfer to the infant.

Pathophysiology

Pertussis disease is caused by *B pertussis* (95%) and less commonly by *Bordetella parapertussis*. A related organism, *Bordetella bronchiseptica* is normally enzootic in animals and has been isolated from humans with coughlike illnesses. *Bordetella* are fimbriated gram-negative rods that express virulence factors, including filamentous hemagglutinin, periactin, and pertussis toxin, which causes a lymphocytic leukocytosis in unimmunized individuals.

Transmission is presumably via droplets from a coughing patient that reach the upper respiratory tract of susceptible individuals. One primary case can cause as many as 15 to 17 secondary cases among those who are susceptible, and even more contacts may have subclinical illness.[34]

Pertussis disease is most serious in young, unprotected infants. Deaths occur mostly in unimmunized infants younger than 6 months old. Complications of pertussis include pneumonia, apnea, seizures, encephalopathy, and cardiorespiratory failure. The death rate in young children who acquire disease is 1% to 2%.

Pertussis can present with nonspecific signs of rhinitis and mild cough that fail to improve after 7 to 14 days. Other clinical signs include cough with or without paroxysms, whoop, and vomiting. Diagnosis relies on clinical suspicion, but disease manifestations can be elusive.[35] Prompt diagnosis and antibiotic treatment limits spread to contacts and to the community. Transmission can be blocked if vaccine coverage rates are high and booster vaccines are given, but new vaccines with higher efficacy and additional control strategies are warranted.[36]

Acquisition of pertussis disease confers immunity, but similar to vaccine-induced immunity, this wanes over time and persons with a history of pertussis illness should still be considered susceptible.

Diagnosis

Laboratory testing to confirm pertussis disease includes culture on appropriate media, direct fluorescent antibody testing (DFA), or PCR. Nasopharyngeal specimens (swab, washing, or aspiration) are best for testing and are more likely to isolate the organism within the first 3 weeks of cough. Samples obtained by aspiration yield the highest rate of positive cultures. Nasopharyngeal testing using calcium alginate or Dacron swabs may also be used, and should ideally be left in the posterior pharynx for 10 seconds before withdrawing. Specimen swabs should then be placed in Regan-Lowe transport media to prevent drying en route to the laboratory and to increase culture yield.

Compared with culture, PCR testing of nasopharyngeal specimens increases sensitivity of detection fourfold. However, there is currently no standard PCR method for detection and false-positive PCR results have been reported; thus, culture specimens also should be obtained for confirmatory testing. DFA testing of secretions may be helpful in patients with symptoms for more than 3 weeks who may have negative culture or PCR testing, but these tests may cross-react with other antibodies to yield false-positive results or false-negative results in infants with pertussis disease due to limited antibody production.

Classification

Cases of pertussis fall into 2 categories: classic illness and mild illness. Pertussis that occurs as a primary infection in a previously unimmunized child is referred to as classic illness, whereas mild illness can occur in a previously vaccinated or unvaccinated host.[37] Classic illness presents in 3 stages: an initial stage with rhinorrhea, tearing, and mild cough; a paroxysmal stage where cough increases in frequency and number and when paroxysms of cough are interspersed with a significant inspiratory whoop that may be associated with posttussive vomiting; and a convalescent stage when coughing decreases in frequency and severity. Mild illness typically manifests as an indolent infection, and usually comes to medical attention because of chronic cough lasting 2 or more weeks in duration. Persons with mild illness may experience the characteristic paroxysmal cough and/or whoop, but not as commonly as those with classic illness.[38] Other manifestations of mild illness in older children and adults include serial coughing, air hunger, and headache, and should prompt clinicians to consider testing.

Infants with pertussis present with varying degrees of symptoms dependent on age, immunization status, and acquired maternal antibody. Infant death rates from pertussis approach 1% to 3%. Cough and whoop are not seen in infants, but common manifestations include apnea and seizures. Infants younger than 6 months presenting with apnea or seizures of unknown etiology should be tested for pertussis. Testing and presumptive treatment should be considered in infants with evidence of severe pertussis (eg, white blood cell count >30,000/μL, tachycardia, and hyperventilation) and in those with a history of recent exposure to an index case.

In adults, most have either been previously vaccinated and/or exposed to pertussis illness and thus may have some degree of immunity that can alter the initial clinical presentation to include only serial coughing, air hunger, and headaches.

First-Line Treatments

Treatment of those exposed to cases of pertussis includes a 2-pronged approach of vaccination and chemoprophylaxis.

Pertussis exposures should be evaluated for pertussis immunization status. Those not immunized or underimmunized should be vaccinated according to the recommended schedule at www.cdc.gov/vaccines. Completion of the primary 5-vaccination series for infants and children younger than 7 years should be documented. The fifth dose is not required if the fourth dose was given on or after the fourth birthday. Tdap should be given to children aged 7 to 10 years who did not complete the primary series, and to adolescents older than 10 years and adults who have no history of booster Tdap vaccination.

Chemoprophylaxis using the same regimen for treatment of pertussis should be given to several groups of those exposed to the index case regardless of immunization status, including all household contacts and children in child care. Special efforts should be made to give chemoprophylaxis to those at high risk for severe pertussis, including infants, pregnant women, and those in regular contact with these groups. First-line medications used for chemoprophylaxis include macrolide antibiotics: azithromycin, clarithromycin, and erythromycin. In a pediatric clinical trial, azithromycin was equally effective as erythromycin estolate in treating pertussis, had fewer gastrointestinal effects, was less likely to adversely affect therapy compliance,[39] had a shorter treatment course, and did not interfere with cytochrome p450 metabolism. Azithromycin should be given to infants younger than 6 months because of increased risk of hypertrophic pyloric stenosis associated with erythromycin use in this age group.[40] Alternative treatment can be given with trimethoprim-sulfamethoxazole in case of drug allergy or resistance to macrolides. A summary of chemoprophylactic regimens is outlined in **Table 4**.

Relapsing pertussis has been described posttreatment in a very low birth weight neonate and should be considered if symptoms recur after treatment is completed.[41]

In a recent study of 86 health care workers vaccinated with Tdap and subsequently exposed to pertussis, daily symptom monitoring for 21 days after exposure was found to be noninferior to antibiotic prophylaxis.[42] As a result, the ACIP recommends antibiotic prophylaxis for exposed health care workers in regular contact with high-risk patients (neonates and pregnant women), whereas other health care workers should either receive postexposure prophylaxis or monitor symptoms for 21 days in the absence of prophylaxis. Hospital-specific infection-control procedures for health care workers should be followed where available.

For persons who were exposed to pertussis more than 21 days prior, vaccination status should still be verified and pertussis vaccine updated as needed. Chemoprophylaxis is unlikely to benefit exposures after 21 days, but these individuals should be evaluated for pertussis disease if they are symptomatic.

Contraindications

Pertussis vaccination should not be administered to any patient who has a history of allergy or anaphylaxis to pertussis-containing vaccines, or who developed encephalopathy within 7 days of receiving vaccine. Those with a progressive neurologic disorder should also not receive DTaP vaccination.

Complications

Pertussis vaccination and chemoprophylaxis each carry a risk of side effects. Although these adverse effects are outweighed by the reduction in risk of pertussis disease and transmission, patients and their parents should be educated regarding common signs and symptoms that may follow pertussis vaccination and chemoprophylaxis.

Common side effects of DTaP and Tdap vaccination include erythema (26%–39%) and swelling (15%–30%) at the injection site, drowsiness (40%–47%), anorexia (19%–25%), fussiness (14%–19%), and vomiting (7%–13%).[43]

Table 4
Recommended antimicrobial therapy and postexposure prophylaxis for pertussis in infants, children, adolescents, and adults

Age	Recommended Drugs			Alternative
	Azithromycin	Erythromycin	Clarithromycin	TMP-SMX
≤1 mo	10 mg/kg/d as a single dose for 5 d	Only give if azithromycin not available because of risk of pyloric stenosis: 40 mg/kg/d divided q6 h for 14 d	Not recommended	Contraindicated <2 mo of age
1 mo–5 mo	See above	40 mg/kg/d divided q6 h for 14 d	15 mg/kg/d divided BID for 7 d	≥2 mo of age: TMP, 8 mg/kg/d; SMX, 40 mg/kg/d divided BID for 14 d
≥6 mo and children	10 mg/kg as a single dose on day 1 (maximum 500 mg), then 5 mg/kg as a single dose on days 2 through 5 (maximum 250 mg/d)	40 mg/kg/d divided q6 h for 7–14 d (maximum 1–2 g/d)	15 mg/kg/d divided BID for 7 d (maximum 1 g/d)	See above
Adolescents and adults	500 mg as a single dose on day 1, then 250 mg as a single dose on days 2 through 5	2 g/d divided q6 h for 7–14 d	1 g/d divided BID for 7 d	TMP, 320 mg/d; SMX, 1600 mg/d divided BID for 14 d

Abbreviations: BID, twice a day; q, every; SMX, sulfamethoxazole; TMP, trimethoprim.
Adapted from Centers for Disease Control and Prevention. Recommended antimicrobial agents for the treatment and postexposure prophylaxis of pertussis: 2005 CDC guidelines. MMWR Recomm Rep 2005;54(RR-14):1–16.

Side effects of macrolide antibiotics are typically related to the gastrointestinal system, including diarrhea, nausea, abdominal pain, and loose stool.

Disposition

All persons exposed to pertussis should be observed for 21 days after exposure to ensure they do not display signs or symptoms of pertussis. Those with symptoms or with confirmed pertussis should be excluded from day care, school, work, and other public settings until they have completed at least 5 days of antimicrobial therapy. Parents of exposed children should be notified so that appropriate treatment can be given. Patients who are not treated with antimicrobials after exposure should be excluded from day care and school for 21 days after the last exposure. In the school setting, public health authorities should be notified so they can assist with control efforts. As health care workers are more likely to transmit pertussis to high-risk groups, such as newborns, exposed persons in this group should be evaluated by infection-control staff to maximize preventive efforts.

INFLUENZA EXPOSURES

Influenza viruses are RNA viruses and classified into 3 types: A, B, and C. Type A is the most common and is further subdivided based on surface antigens hemagglutinin and neuraminidase. Type B displays less genetic diversity compared with type A, and type C causes only mild disease in children. Current seasonal influenza vaccines for the 2012–2013 season in the United States are trivalent and protect against 2 type A strains (H1N1 and H3N2) and 1 B strain. The Food and Drug Administration (FDA) recently approved a quadrivalent live attenuated influenza vaccine for children older than 3 years for the 2013–2014 season that will include 2 type A strains and 2 type B strains.[44]

Influenza is spread by the respiratory route when large, virus-laden droplets are coughed or sneezed into the environment, or other contact with respiratory secretions. Transmission requires close contact, as large droplets can travel approximately 1 m and rapidly fall from the air after being expelled. The incubation period is from 1 to 4 days, with most cases occurring on day 2 postexposure. Although adults are deemed infectious from the day before symptom onset for the next 6 to 11 days, children transmit virus from several days before symptoms develop until up to 10 days after onset. Host immunity depends on underlying immune status and previous exposure to either naturally circulating virus or vaccine strains. As a result of limited host immunity, influenza disproportionately affects children younger than 2 years, with the highest rates of hospitalization in children younger than 6 months.

Influenza attack rates are understudied. In a relatively unvaccinated population in Nicaragua, where influenza vaccination of children aged 6 to 23 months was introduced in 2007,[45] annual attack rates from 2007 to 2009 for seasonal influenza in a cohort of children aged 2 to 14 years ranged from 12% to 24%.[46] In the United States, influenza transmission occurs from late fall to winter, sometimes extending to early spring.

Diagnosis

Influenza is diagnosed using viral culture, PCR, or immunofluorescent or rapid diagnostic testing and is easiest to detect during the first 3 days of clinical symptoms when viral shedding is highest. Nasopharyngeal testing using a swab, aspirate, or washing is preferred. Influenza virus can be grown in culture within 2 to 6 days, a period after which antiviral medications may not provide maximal benefit.

Reverse-transcriptase PCR (RT-PCR) testing is available in some settings, with more rapid results than culture while maintaining high sensitivity and specificity. Direct fluorescent and immunofluorescent testing can yield results in 3 to 6 hours, and can be used as a basis for treatment and prophylaxis of high-risk contacts. A common influenza test used in the United States is rapid influenza diagnostic testing (RIDT). RIDTs are based on immunochromatographic lateral flow and membrane-based assays that are advantageous in their quick turnaround time and ease of use. Disadvantages include high false-negative rates during high influenza activity, high false-positive rates during low influenza activity, and some tests do not distinguish between influenza A and B or pandemic strains. Both viral culture and RT-PCR methods are considered the gold standard for influenza testing. In a community setting where circulating influenza virus is documented, diagnostic testing is not required. In this situation, children with suspected influenza and their high-risk contacts may be treated and given prophylaxis on the basis of symptoms alone.

Indications for Postexposure Prophylaxis

Persons at increased risk of severe influenza should be offered antiviral prophylaxis, as it is 70% to 90% effective in preventing influenza disease. Exposures that occurred more than 48 hours prior generally do not merit prophylaxis, as the incubation period has likely passed. Children considered high risk include those with the following conditions: underlying pulmonary disease such as asthma, cardiac disorders, pregnancy, chronic metabolic disease such as diabetes mellitus, renal dysfunction, hemoglobinopathies, or long-term immunosuppressive therapy. According to AAP guidelines, chemoprophylaxis following influenza exposures should be considered in the following scenarios involving high-risk children[16]:

- Protection of unimmunized high-risk children or children who were immunized less than 2 weeks before influenza circulation, because adequate immune response develops 2 weeks after immunization
- Protection of children at increased risk of severe infection or complications, such as high-risk children for whom the vaccine is contraindicated
- Protection of unimmunized close contacts of high-risk children
- Protection of immunocompromised children who may not respond to vaccine
- Control of influenza outbreaks in a closed setting, such as an institution with unimmunized high-risk children
- Protection of immunized high-risk children if the vaccine strain poorly matches circulating influenza strains

First-Line Treatment

Drugs available in the United States for treatment or chemoprophylaxis of influenza exposures include the neuraminidase inhibitors oseltamivir and zanamivir, and the adamantanes amantadine and rimantadine. Neuraminidase inhibitors are active against both A and B strains, as well as the 2009 pandemic H1N1 strain, whereas the adamantanes are active only against A strains. Because of resistance of circulating A strains against the adamantanes, including pandemic H1N1 influenza, use of this class of drugs has not been recommended for use since 2005. Antivirals indicated for chemoprophylaxis and treatment depend on circulating influenza strains and resistance patterns to available drugs that is tracked by the Centers for Disease Control and Prevention. Updated information regarding preferred antivirals can be found at www.cdc.gov/flu/professionals/antivirals/index.htm. Dosing of the neuraminidase inhibitors varies by age and weight and is summarized in **Table 5**. Recommendations

Table 5
Recommended antiviral prophylaxis and therapy for influenza in infants, children, adolescents, and adults

Antiviral Agent	Indication	Premature Neonate	Infants ≤8 mo	Infants 9–11 mo	Age Group ≥12 mo	Adults
Oseltamivir	Prophylaxis	Suggested dose: 1 mg/kg/dose once daily; currently not FDA approved for prophylaxis in infants <12 mo	Suggested dose: 3 mg/kg/dose once daily; currently not FDA approved for prophylaxis in infants <12 mo	Suggested dose: 3.5 mg/kg/dose once daily; currently not FDA approved for prophylaxis in infants <12 mo	≤15 kg: 30 mg once daily; 15–23 kg: 45 mg once daily; 23–40 kg: 60 mg once daily; >40 kg: 75 mg once daily	75 mg once daily
	Treatment	1 mg/kg/dose BID[47]; not FDA approved	3 mg/kg/dose BID for 5 d; not FDA approved for infants <2 wk	3.5 mg/kg/dose BID for 5 d[48]	≤15 kg: 30 mg BID; 15–23 kg: 45 mg BID; 23–40 kg: 60 mg BID; >40 kg: 75 mg BID	75 mg BID
Zanamivir	Prophylaxis				Not indicated for <5 y; ≥5 y: 10 mg (2 inhalations) once daily	10 mg (2 inhalations) once daily
	Treatment				Not indicated for <7 y; ≥7 y: 10 mg (2 inhalations) BID	10 mg (2 inhalations) BID

Abbreviations: BID, twice a day; FDA, Food and Drug Administration.

for oseltamivir prophylaxis is based on data extrapolated from the 2009 FDA emergency use of oseltamivir for infants older than 3 months for pandemic H1N1 influenza and another clinical study.[47] This population is particularly at risk for serious complications and death from influenza, and the benefits of prophylaxis should be weighed against the risk of potential side effects of antiviral medication. The duration of antiviral prophylaxis is for 7 days after exposure. For outbreaks in long-term care facilities, such as nursing homes and hospitals, prophylaxis should be given for a minimum of 2 weeks or up to 1 week after the last known case was identified. Treatment dosing is continued for 5 days and extended in those who remain severely ill.

Optimal timing of initiation of antiviral therapy is as soon as possible after exposure has occurred for prophylaxis and within 48 hours of symptom onset for treatment. When used against H5N1, oseltamivir was highly effective in reducing mortality, even when given 6 to 8 days after symptom onset.[49] For this reason, initiation of treatment dosing more than 48 hours after symptom onset should be considered, especially in high-risk groups.

For those with compromised renal function, oseltamivir, amantadine, and rimantadine dosing should be adjusted. Only zanamivir does not require adjustment in renal insufficiency.

Complications

Potential complications of influenza illness include respiratory failure requiring mechanical ventilation and bacterial superinfection. Rare complications include encephalopathy, myocarditis, myositis, pericarditis, Reye syndrome, and transverse myelitis.

Potential complications of antiviral medications used for treatment and prophylaxis include nausea and vomiting associated with oseltamivir and bronchospasm associated with zanamivir. Because of potential exacerbation of underlying conditions, such as asthma, zanamivir is contraindicated in people with underlying respiratory disease.

Disposition

Education of patients and their caregivers regarding the need for prophylaxis and compliance with the prophylactic regimen is essential. For those who are not at increased risk or who refuse prophylaxis, physicians should offer anticipatory guidance to return for care and treatment should symptoms develop.

SUMMARY

Opportunities to prevent illness in the ED using antimicrobial prophylaxis are frequent and are based on clinical evidence. The challenge for physicians is to recognize patients at risk for infection or complications of infection, educate patients and their caregivers about the risks and benefits of prophylaxis to ensure compliance, prescribe an appropriate antibiotic regimen, and provide complete instructions at discharge, including circumstances in which a return for further care is indicated.

Emergency room physicians are commonly on the front lines of medical care when patients with traumatic wounds present for treatment, when close contacts with exposure to meningococcal disease or pertussis seek treatment, and when influenza is diagnosed in a household. In each circumstance, there exists an opportunity to prevent morbidity and mortality that is not often tangible, but impacting disease prevention using appropriate antimicrobial prophylaxis can be highly rewarding.

REFERENCES

1. Gosselin RA, Roberts I, Gillespie WJ. Antibiotics for preventing infection in open limb fractures. Cochrane Database Syst Rev 2004;(1):CD003764.
2. Altergott C, Garcia FJ, Nager AL. Pediatric fingertip injuries: do prophylactic antibiotics alter infection rates? Pediatr Emerg Care 2008;24(3):148–52.
3. Hollander JE, Singer AJ. Laceration management. Ann Emerg Med 1999;34(3): 356–67.
4. Moscati RM, Mayrose J, Reardon RF, et al. A multicenter comparison of tap water versus sterile saline for wound irrigation. Acad Emerg Med 2007;14(5):404–9.
5. Valente JH, Forti RJ, Freundlich LF, et al. Wound irrigation in children: saline solution or tap water? Ann Emerg Med 2003;41(5):609–16.
6. Dire DJ, Coppola M, Dwyer DA, et al. Prospective evaluation of topical antibiotics for preventing infections in uncomplicated soft-tissue wounds repaired in the ED. Acad Emerg Med 1995;2(1):4–10.
7. Talan DA, Citron DM, Abrahamian FM, et al. Bacteriologic analysis of infected dog and cat bites. Emergency Medicine Animal Bite Infection Study Group. N Engl J Med 1999;340(2):85–92.
8. Abrahamian FM, Goldstein EJ. Microbiology of animal bite wound infections. Clin Microbiol Rev 2011;24(2):231–46.
9. Wu PS, Beres A, Tashjian DB, et al. Primary repair of facial dog bite injuries in children. Pediatr Emerg Care 2011;27(9):801–3.
10. Medeiros I, Saconato H. Antibiotic prophylaxis for mammalian bites. Cochrane Database Syst Rev 2001;(2):CD001738.
11. Cummings P. Antibiotics to prevent infection in patients with dog bite wounds: a meta-analysis of randomized trials. Ann Emerg Med 1994;23(3):535–40.
12. Quinn JV, McDermott D, Rossi J, et al. Randomized controlled trial of prophylactic antibiotics for dog bites with refined cost model. West J Emerg Med 2010;11(5): 435–41.
13. Hoff WS, Bonadies JA, Cachecho R, et al. East Practice Management Guidelines Work Group: update to practice management guidelines for prophylactic antibiotic use in open fractures. J Trauma 2011;70(3):751–4.
14. Eidelman M, Bialik V, Miller Y, et al. Plantar puncture wounds in children: analysis of 80 hospitalized patients and late sequelae. Isr Med Assoc J 2003;5(4): 268–71.
15. Wedmore IS, Charette J. Emergency department evaluation and treatment of ankle and foot injuries. Emerg Med Clin North Am 2000;18(1):85–113, vi.
16. American Academy of Pediatrics. 2012 Red Book: report of the Committee on infectious diseases. 29th edition. Elk Grove Village (IL): American Academy of Pediatrics; 2012.
17. Claus H, Maiden MC, Wilson DJ, et al. Genetic analysis of meningococci carried by children and young adults. J Infect Dis 2005;191(8):1263–71.
18. Bilukha OO, Rosenstein N. Prevention and control of meningococcal disease. Recommendations of the Advisory Committee on Immunization Practices (ACIP). MMWR Recomm Rep 2005;54(RR-7):1–21.
19. Centers for Disease Control and Prevention (CDC). Infant meningococcal vaccination: Advisory Committee on Immunization Practices (ACIP) recommendations and rationale. MMWR Morb Mortal Wkly Rep 2013;62(3):52–4.
20. Centers for Disease Control and Prevention (CDC). Outbreak of meningococcal disease associated with an elementary school—Oklahoma, March 2010. MMWR Morb Mortal Wkly Rep 2012;61(13):217–21.

21. Caugant DA. Genetics and evolution of *Neisseria meningitidis*: importance for the epidemiology of meningococcal disease. Infect Genet Evol 2008;8(5):558–65.
22. Mueller JE, Gessner BD. A hypothetical explanatory model for meningococcal meningitis in the African meningitis belt. Int J Infect Dis 2010;14(7):e553–9.
23. Wilder-Smith A, Goh KT, Barkham T, et al. Hajj-associated outbreak strain of *Neisseria meningitidis* serogroup W135: estimates of the attack rate in a defined population and the risk of invasive disease developing in carriers. Clin Infect Dis 2003;36(6):679–83.
24. Centers for Disease Control and Prevention (CDC). Occupational transmission of *Neisseria meningitidis*—California, 2009. MMWR Morb Mortal Wkly Rep 2010; 59(45):1480–3.
25. Zalmanovici TA, Fraser A, Gafter-Gvili A, et al. Antibiotics for preventing meningococcal infections. Cochrane Database Syst Rev 2011;(8):CD004785.
26. Girgis N, Sultan Y, Frenck RW Jr, et al. Azithromycin compared with rifampin for eradication of nasopharyngeal colonization by *Neisseria meningitidis*. Pediatr Infect Dis J 1998;17(9):816–9.
27. Lubell Y, Turner P, Ashley EA, et al. Susceptibility of bacterial isolates from community-acquired infections in sub-Saharan Africa and Asia to macrolide antibiotics. Trop Med Int Health 2011;16(10):1192–205.
28. Centers for Disease Control and Prevention (CDC). Emergence of fluoroquinolone-resistant *Neisseria meningitidis*—Minnesota and North Dakota, 2007-2008. MMWR Morb Mortal Wkly Rep 2008;57(7):173–5.
29. Iser BP, Lima HC, de Moraes C, et al. Outbreak of *Neisseria meningitidis* C in workers at a large food-processing plant in Brazil: challenges of controlling disease spread to the larger community. Epidemiol Infect 2012;140(5):906–15.
30. Shapiro ED. Acellular vaccines and resurgence of pertussis. JAMA 2012;308(20): 2149–50.
31. Mooi FR, van der Maas NA, De Melker HE. Pertussis resurgence: waning immunity and pathogen adaptation—two sides of the same coin. Epidemiol Infect 2013 [Epub ahead of print]. Available at: http://www.ncbi.nlm.nih.gov/pubmed/23406868.
32. Cherry JD. Epidemiology of pertussis. Pediatr Infect Dis J 2006;25(4):361–2.
33. Rodriguez-Cobo I, Chen YF, Olowokure B, et al. Clinical and economic assessment of different general population strategies of pertussis vaccine booster regarding number of doses and age of application for reducing whooping cough disease burden: a systematic review. Vaccine 2008;26(52):6768–76.
34. Cherry JD. The epidemiology of pertussis and pertussis immunization in the United Kingdom and the United States: a comparative study. Curr Probl Pediatr 1984;14(2):1–78.
35. Mink CM, Cherry JD, Christenson P, et al. A search for *Bordetella pertussis* infection in university students. Clin Infect Dis 1992;14(2):464–71.
36. Libster R, Edwards KM. Re-emergence of pertussis: what are the solutions? Expert Rev Vaccines 2012;11(11):1331–46.
37. Gordon JE, Hood RI. Whooping cough and its epidemiological anomalies. Am J Med Sci 1951;222(3):333–61.
38. Schlapfer G, Cherry JD, Heininger U, et al. Polymerase chain reaction identification of *Bordetella pertussis* infections in vaccinees and family members in a pertussis vaccine efficacy trial in Germany. Pediatr Infect Dis J 1995;14(3):209–14.
39. Langley JM, Halperin SA, Boucher FD, et al. Azithromycin is as effective as and better tolerated than erythromycin estolate for the treatment of pertussis. Pediatrics 2004;114(1):e96–101.

40. Maheshwai N. Are young infants treated with erythromycin at risk for developing hypertrophic pyloric stenosis? Arch Dis Child 2007;92(3):271–3.

41. Bonacorsi S, Farnoux C, Bidet P, et al. Treatment failure of nosocomial pertussis infection in a very-low-birth-weight neonate. J Clin Microbiol 2006;44(10): 3830–2.

42. Goins WP, Edwards KM, Vnencak-Jones CL, et al. A comparison of 2 strategies to prevent infection following pertussis exposure in vaccinated healthcare personnel. Clin Infect Dis 2012;54(7):938–45.

43. Arcara K, Tschudy M. Harriet Lane handbook: a manual for pediatric house officers. 19th edition. Philadelphia: Mosby Elsevier; 2012.

44. Domachowske JB, Pankow-Culot H, Bautista M, et al. A randomized trial of candidate inactivated quadrivalent influenza vaccine versus trivalent influenza vaccines in children aged 3-17 years. J Infect Dis 2013;207(12):1878–87.

45. Ropero-Alvarez AM, Kurtis HJ, Danovaro-Holliday MC, et al. Expansion of seasonal influenza vaccination in the Americas. BMC Public Health 2009;9:361.

46. Gordon A, Saborio S, Videa E, et al. Clinical attack rate and presentation of pandemic H1N1 influenza versus seasonal influenza A and B in a pediatric cohort in Nicaragua. Clin Infect Dis 2010;50(11):1462–7.

47. Acosta EP, Jester P, Gal P, et al. Oseltamivir dosing for influenza infection in premature neonates. J Infect Dis 2010;202(4):563–6.

48. Kimberlin DW, Acosta EP, Prichard MN, et al. Oseltamivir pharmacokinetics, dosing, and resistance among children aged <2 years with influenza. J Infect Dis 2013;207(5):709–20.

49. Adisasmito W, Chan PK, Lee N, et al. Effectiveness of antiviral treatment in human influenza A (H5N1) infections: analysis of a Global Patient Registry. J Infect Dis 2010;202(8):1154–60.

Erratum

An error was made in the February 2013 issue of *Emergency Medicine Clinics*. On page 117 in the article "Ultrasound-Guided Procedures in the Emergency Department— Diagnostic and Therapeutic Asset" Dr Stephanie G. Cohen's name was omitted from the title page. Dr Cohen contributed to this article and her affiliations are as follows:

Stephanie G. Cohen, MD
Assistant Professor of Pediatrics and Emergency Medicine
Emory University School of Medicine
Atlanta, GA

Emerg Med Clin N Am 31 (2013) 895
http://dx.doi.org/10.1016/j.emc.2013.05.008   emed.theclinics.com
0733-8627/13/$ – see front matter © 2013 Elsevier Inc. All rights reserved.

Erratum

Index

Note: Page numbers of article titles are in **boldface** type.

Emerg Med Clin N Am 31 (2013) 897–905
http://dx.doi.org/10.1016/S0733-8627(13)00063-1
0733-8627/13/$ – see front matter © 2013 Elsevier Inc. All rights reserved.

emed.theclinics.com

EmergencyMed **Advance**

All the latest emergency medicine news and research you need, all in one place

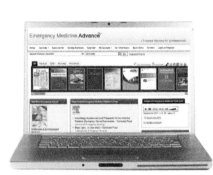

EmergencyMedAdvance.com is a new essential online resource offering valued high-quality content and news for the global community of Emergency Medicine professionals to save time and stay current—from physicians and nurses to EMTs.

Stay current
• Emergency Medicine news   • Upcoming meetings and events

Save time
• Access relevant articles in press   • Search across 500+ health sciences journals
  from 16 participating journals   • Learn how to submit a manuscript

And more...
• Journals' profiles   • Sign up for free e-Alerts
• Personalized search results   • Emergency Medicine jobs
• Emergency Medicine bookstore

**Bookmark us today at
EmergencyMedAdvance.com**

ELSEVIER

Printed and bound by CPI Group (UK) Ltd, Croydon, CR0 4YY

03/10/2024

01040489-0010